825

BXB

£15 50

D1556208

Clinical
Cardiac Radiology

To our wives
Denys and Jacquy

Clinical Cardiac Radiology

Keith Jefferson, M.A., F.R.C.P., F.F.R.

Consultant Radiologist, National Heart Hospital and St. George's Hospital, London; Lecturer, Cardiothoracic Institute, University of London

and

Simon Rees, M.A., M.R.C.P., F.F.R.

Consultant Radiologist, National Heart Hospital and St. Bartholomew's Hospital, London; Lecturer, Cardiothoracic Institute, University of London

BUTTERWORTHS

ENGLAND: BUTTERWORTH & CO. (PUBLISHERS) LTD.
               LONDON: 88 Kingsway, WC2B 6AB

AUSTRALIA: BUTTERWORTHS PTY. LTD.
               SYDNEY: 586 Pacific Highway, 2067
               MELBOURNE: 343 Little Collins Street, 3000
               BRISBANE: 240 Queen Street, 4000

CANADA: BUTTERWORTH & CO. (CANADA) LTD.
               TORONTO: 14 Curity Avenue, 374

NEW ZEALAND: BUTTERWORTHS OF NEW ZEALAND LTD.
               WELLINGTON: 26–28 Waring Taylor Street, 1

SOUTH AFRICA: BUTTERWORTH & CO. (SOUTH AFRICA) (PTY) LTD.
               DURBAN: 152–154 Gale Street

Suggested U.D.C. Number 616·12–073·7

ISBN 0 407 13575 8

Made and printed in Great Britain by
William Clowes & Sons, Limited, London, Beccles and Colchester

Contents

CONTENTS

SECTION VI: Obstruction and Regurgitation

SECTION VII: Myocardial and Pericardial Disease

Appendices

Introduction

This book is about the chest x-ray in heart disease. It is intended to be a practical book for radiologists and for physicians and surgeons who use the chest x-ray as part of their clinical examination of the patient. X-ray examination of the heart is not new, but until recently the true significance of many of the appearances could be verified only by the occasional autopsy. Cardiac catheterization, angiocardiography and open heart surgery have changed this. The book is based on a study of films in over 1,500 patients in whom the anatomy of the heart and the physiology of the circulation were known. The significance of the numerous radiological signs has been evaluated and, in many cases, re-evaluated in relation to anatomy and physiology. Computer techniques have been employed when appropriate. Standard postero-anterior, penetrated postero-anterior and lateral views only have been used. There is very little reference to oblique views, as the authors feel that no more useful information is obtained provided a penetrated frontal view is available: also, technically satisfactory oblique films can often be obtained only after screening, which as a routine involves an unacceptably high radiation dose. Fluoroscopy of the heart, however, may be clinically indicated and the findings are described. Barium swallow is also not used as a routine, but only when additional information might be obtained. Angiocardiographic appearances are described and related to plain film findings.

The first half deals with changes in the size, shape and position of the heart, its chambers and the great arteries and veins, followed by the appearances of the lungs resulting from alterations in pressure and flow. There is also a section on skeletal and other extracardiac changes in heart disease, much of the material being based on the St. Cyres lecture for 1971 delivered by one of us (K.J.). In the second half, lesions are considered individually in clinical groups, stressing where the chest x-ray is of help in differential diagnosis and in deciding the severity or relative importance of a lesion.

The approach throughout is a clinical one, because the authors feel that the x-ray should be interpreted in the light of the clinical findings and form an integral part of the clinical examination of the patient.

How to Use the Book

PART ONE

Part One of this book is devoted to the general radiology of the heart, the lungs and the other systems in heart disease.

The radiology of the heart (Section I, Chapters 1–6) provides information more about anatomy than about physiology. The two most important exercises are to determine whether the heart is enlarged and which chamber is enlarged. Large right and left ventricles have characteristic shapes, but they are often misleading, particularly in biventricular enlargement in rheumatic heart disease. Right atrial size is difficult to assess unless the chamber is obviously dilated. The left atrium can be quite accurately assessed on the penetrated anterior and lateral views. This is of much importance in left-sided lesions; when the left atrium is normal, lesions affecting the left ventricle are suggested, but if it is more than slightly enlarged, mitral valve disease of some variety is likely. Other features one should particularly look for are the size and position of the pulmonary trunk and aorta, and the presence of cardiac calcification.

The lungs in heart disease (Section II, Chapters 7–12) provide much information about haemodynamics and often show on which side of the heart the lesion lies; the Table below relates lung changes to haemodynamics and outlines their basic anatomical significance.

Lungs	*Haemodynamic significance*	*Anatomical significance*
Normal (Chapter 7)	Normal pulmonary flow and pressures	Lesion in either side of the heart not affecting haemodynamics
Plethora (Chapter 8)	Left-to-right shunt	Chamber enlargement depends on site of shunt
Oligaemia (Chapter 8)	Reduced pulmonary flow	Lesion in right heart
Proximal vessel dilatation (Chapter 9)	Pulmonary arterial hypertension	Right heart affected by pulmonary vascular disease from many causes
Proximal vessel dilatation and plethora (Chapters 8 and 9)	Pulmonary arterial hypertension with left-to-right shunt	Chamber enlargement depends on site of shunt and degree of pulmonary hypertension
Upper zone vessel dilatation; oedema (Chapter 10)	Pulmonary venous hypertension	Lesion in left heart or pulmonary veins
Upper zone vessel dilatation: lower lobe vessel narrowing (Chapter 10)	Pulmonary venous and arterial hypertension: elevated pulmonary vascular resistance	Lesion in left heart or pulmonary veins
Upper zone vessel dilatation and plethora (Chapters 8 and 10)	Left-to-right shunt and pulmonary venous hypertension	Chamber enlargement depends on site of shunt and left heart lesion

The thoracic cage and general disease associated with the heart are discussed in Section III, Chapters 13, 14 and 15. This section is set out in some detail particularly for clinicians who may not be familiar with extracardiac radiology.

PART TWO

Whereas Part One is a general narrative description of cardiac radiology, Part Two is designed to help the radiologist or clinician make a diagnosis as precisely as possible from the chest x-ray. Lesions with common clinical and radiological features are grouped into sections. Sections IV and V deal with defects of cardiac septation in which there are shunts with or without cyanosis. Section V forms a classification of lesions causing central cyanosis in congenital heart disease. Section VI is concerned with lesions primarily involving endocardial structures, producing obstruction or regurgitation. Section VII deals with diseases primarily involving the myocardium or pericardium. The Table below is a précis of Part Two, and is a simplified guide showing the salient clinical and radiological features common to each section.

SECTION IV—SHUNTS WITHOUT CYANOSIS

	Lungs	*Heart*	*Clinical features*
Atrial shunts (Chapter 16)	Plethora Anomalous veins	Right ventricle + Heart displaced to left Pulmonary trunk + Aorta small	Right ventricle+ Fixed split of second sound Ejection systolic murmur
Ventricular shunts (Chapter 17)	Plethora	Pulmonary trunk normal or slightly + Aorta normal Left atrium +	Left ventricle + Right ventricle + Pan-systolic murmur
Aorto-pulmonary shunts (Chapter 18)	Plethora	Left ventricle + Left atrium + Pulmonary trunk variable Aortic knuckle + in ductus	Left ventricle + Continuous murmur

SECTION V—SHUNTS WITH CYANOSIS

Right-to-left shunts due to obstruction in right heart

	Lungs	*Heart*	*Clinical features*
Fallot's tetralogy (Chapter 19) and its differential diagnosis (Chapter 20)	Oligaemia	Right ventricle + Bay in left border (rarely post-stenotic dilatation of pulmonary trunk) Aorta +	Right ventricle + Single second sound

Right-to-left shunts due to obstruction in the lungs

	Lungs	*Heart*	*Clinical features*
Eisenmenger syndrome (Chapter 21)	Proximal vessel dilatation	Heart normal or slightly + Right ventricle + Pulmonary trunk +	Right ventricle + Pulmonary second sound + Ejection sound

Right-to-left shunts without obstruction in right heart

	Lungs	*Heart*	*Clinical features*
Veno-arterial mixing lesions (Chapter 22)			
(a) Proximal to lungs Complete transposition Total anomalous pulmonary venous drainage Single atrium Single ventricle Double outflow right ventricle Truncus arteriosus	Proximal vessel dilatation Plethora	Variable chamber enlargement	Pulmonary arterial hypertension Other features variable

(b) In lungs

	Lungs	*Heart*	*Clinical features*
Arteriovenous fistula	Solid opacity with large vessels	Normal	Silent or continuous murmurs

(c) Distal to lungs

Superior or inferior vena cava draining to left atrium	Normal if isolated lesion	Normal if isolated lesion	No murmurs unless associated with other lesions

SECTION VI—OBSTRUCTION AND REGURGITATION

	Lungs	*Heart*	*Clinical features*
Diseases of tricuspid valve and right atrium (Chapter 23)	Normal or oligaemia	Right heart + Left ventricle and left atrium + in tricuspid atresia	Right ventricle + Left ventricle + in tricuspid atresia Inspiratory murmurs left sternal edge
Diseases of pulmonary valve and right ventricular outflow (Chapter 24)	Normal or oligaemia	Normal heart size Pulmonary trunk +	Right ventricle + Pulmonary second sound late and diminished Inspiratory murmurs in pulmonary area
Diseases of mitral valve, left atrium and pulmonary veins (Chapter 25)	Upper zone vessel dilatation Lower zone vessel narrowing Oedema	Left atrium + Calcification mitral valve	Mitral murmurs Expiratory apical murmurs
Diseases of aortic valve, left ventricular outflow and aorta (Chapter 26)	Normal or upper zone vessel dilatation	Left ventricle + Ascending aorta + Calcification aortic valve	Left ventricle + Expiratory basal murmurs

SECTION VII—MYOCARDIAL AND PERICARDIAL DISEASE

	Lungs	*Heart*	*Clinical features*
Ischaemic heart disease (Chapter 27)	Normal or upper zone vessel dilatation	Normal or left ventricle + Left ventricular aneurysm Calcification in coronary arteries or aneurysm	Ischaemic pain ECG changes
Cardiomyopathy (Chapter 28)	Normal or upper zone vessel dilatation	Left ventricle + Right ventricle + less often	Left ventricle + Right ventricle + Dysrhythmia Failure
Cardiac aneurysm, tumour and cyst (Chapter 29)	Normal or upper zone vessel dilatation	Localized bulge Bizarre shape Calcification	Mimics valve disease Failure Dysrhythmia
Pericardial effusion (Chapter 30)	Normal Upper zone vessel dilatation only with large heart	Enlarged heart difficult to tell from chamber dilatation	Chest pain Pericardial rub ECG changes
Constrictive pericarditis (Chapter 30)	Normal or upper zone vessel dilatation	Heart usually enlarged but may be normal Pericardial calcification	High venous pressure Small pulse Pulsus paradoxus Quiet heart Diastolic sound

Acknowledgements

We owe much to our clinical colleagues at the National Heart Hospital, whose material we have used and whose clinical skills have been a stimulus to the writing of this book. We acknowledge with gratitude the expertise of our radiographers under Miss Daphne Beauchamp, and the cheerful service of Mrs. Jill Leggatt and Miss Margaret Hill who retrieved from the files endless numbers of films for us. We thank the Board of Governors of the National Heart Hospital for their generous grants for the computer analysis. P.M.A. Consultants Ltd. of Victoria Road, Horley, Surrey carried out the computer work and we are especially grateful to Mr. A.M. Evans for his help. The Department of Medical Illustration at the National Heart Hospital under Mr. Barry Richards with Mr. Geoffrey Lambert, Miss Tina Raynham and Miss Roberta Young made nearly all the illustrations and we particularly thank them for their skill and patience. We are grateful to Mrs. Tricia Tyrall, Mrs. Margerie Chandler, Miss Elizabeth Bruzaud and Mrs. Denys Jefferson for typing the many drafts of the manuscript. We thank our publishers for their guidance. We owe a special debt of gratitude to Mrs. Denys Jefferson who devoted a great deal of her time to recording the computer results, an invaluable service without which our book could not have been completed in a reasonable time.

Finally we are indebted to the following for permission to reproduce illustrations:

Dr. George Simon—*Figures 6, 37* and *155*.

The Editor of *Proceedings of the Royal Society of Medicine*—*Figure 106a–c* (Figs. 2, 7 and 9 from Jefferson, 1965, *Proc. R. Soc. Med.* **58**, 677).

The Editor of *Radiology*—*Figure 152* (Fig. 1 from Currarino and Silverman, 1958, *Radiology* **70**, 532).

E. & S. Livingstone Ltd.—*Figure 158* (Fig. 42 from *A Textbook of Radiology*, ed. by David Sutton, 1971).

Dr. E.H. Allen—*Figure 174*.

Professor E.G.L. Bywaters—*Figure 175*.

Dr. Ronald Murray—*Figures 176, 178, 181–184* and *187*.

Dr. A.C. Young—*Figure 180*.

The Editor of *British Heart Journal*—*Figure 246* (Fig. 1b from Miller *et al.*, 1973, *Br. Heart J.* **35**, 9); *Figure 266a* and *b* (Fig. 1 from Elliott, Anderson and Edwards, 1964, *Br. Heart J.* **26**, 289); and *Figure 288a* and *b* (Fig. 1 from Neufeld *et al.*, 1962, *Br. Heart J.* **24**, 393).

The Editor of *Surgical Clinics of North America*—*Figure 289* (after Collett and Edwards, 1949, *Surg. Clins N. Am.* **29**, 1245).

The Scientific Council on Paediatric Cardiology of the International Society of Cardiology—*Figure 320* (from *Classification of Heart Disease in Childhood*, ed. by Hamish Watson, 1970).

Dr. Otto Hernandez and Dr. Eduardo Morales—*Figures 360–362*.

Dr. Cecil Symons—*Figures 363a, b* and *364a, b*.

PART ONE
General Radiology

SECTION I
The Heart

CHAPTER I

Radiological Anatomy and Assessment of Heart Size

RADIOLOGICAL ANATOMY

As changes in heart size and shape are so often accompanied by important alterations in the arteries and veins of the mediastinum, all cardiovascular structures within the mediastinum are considered together and regarded as forming the cardiovascular shadow on the anterior and lateral views of the chest. They can be identified on plain radiography if they are bordered by radiolucent lung or if, by enlargement or acquisition of calcium, they produce a shadow of greater radio-density than the surrounding structures.

On the anterior view the normal border-forming cardiovascular structures are as follows (*Figure 1*).

Right upper border
Innominate vein and superior vena cava or innominate artery and ascending aorta.

Right lower border
Right atrial appendix and right atrium.
Inferior vena cava.

Left upper border
Left subclavian artery.
Aortic arch (aortic knuckle).

Left middle border
Pulmonary trunk (main pulmonary artery).
Left atrial appendix.

Left lower border
Left ventricle.

In children under the age of two years the thymus often obscures the upper cardiovascular borders. Thymic enlargement may occasionally persist in normal children until the age of about six years and is occasionally unilateral (*Figure 2*).

On the lateral view of the chest, the following are the normal border-forming cardiovascular structures (*Figure 3*).

Anterior upper border
Superior vena cava.
Ascending aorta.
Pulmonary trunk.

Anterior lower border
Right ventricle.

Posterior upper border
Left atrium and pulmonary veins.

Posterior lower border
Left ventricle (sometimes right atrium).
Inferior vena cava.

3

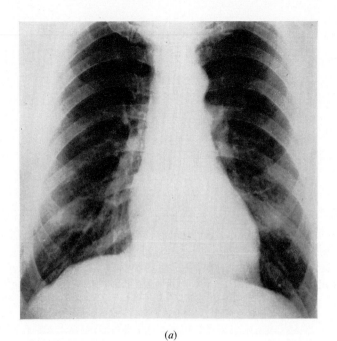

(a)

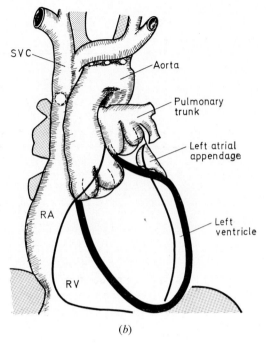

(b)

Figure 1 (above). (a) Normal chest radiograph—anterior view. (b) Diagram of border-forming structures—anterior view. SVC=superior vena cava; RA=right atrium; RV=right ventricle

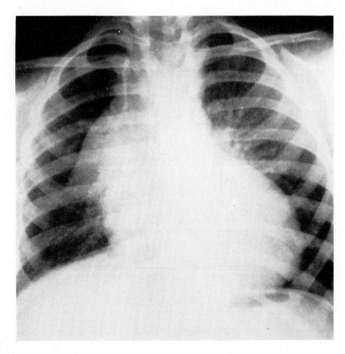

Figure 2 (left). Enlarged thymus in child

Superiorly the anterior border-forming structures limit the posterior extent of the retrosternal air space, and inferiorly a variable amount of right ventricle is in contact with the posterior surface of the sternum. The pulmonary veins prevent a clear-cut view of the posterior contour of the left atrium, but the posterior borders of the left ventricle and inferior vena cava are well seen.

Important cardiovascular structures which may be rendered visible because of their increased density are as follows.

(1) The left atrium (*Figure 4*), the proximal ascending aorta, the descending aorta and the azygos vein (*see Figure 14*) on the anterior view.

(2) The aortic arch and descending aorta on the lateral view.

(3) Any calcified structures, particularly the aortic and mitral valves, the pericardium, the coronary arteries and the left atrium (*see page* 52).

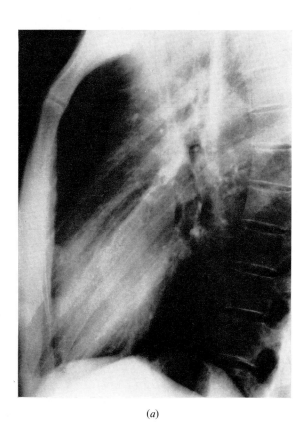

(a)

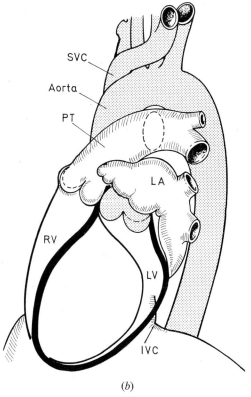

(b)

Figure 3 (above). (a) Normal chest radiograph—lateral view. (b) Diagram of border-forming structures—lateral view. SVC = superior vena cava; PT = pulmonary trunk; LA = left atrium; RV = right ventricle; LV = left ventricle; IVC = inferior vena cava

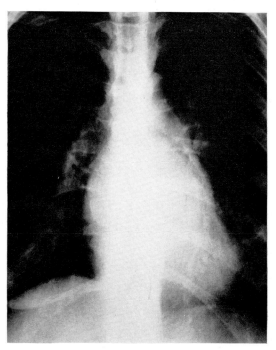

Figure 4 (right). Penetrated anterior view. Enlarged left atrium showing increased density

HEART SIZE

Heart size may be recorded by:
  (1) Grading it subjectively.
  (2) Measuring the cardio-thoracic ratio.
  (3) Calculating the heart volume.

Subjective grading

The subjective method consists of assessing the heart in terms of normal size and grades 1, 2 and 3 enlargement. Expressed in descriptive terms, grade 1 is slight but definite, grade 2 obvious, and grade 3 gross. For the experienced observer this method has the great advantage of speed, but the inexperienced would be well advised to check his assessment with one of the other methods as explained below. A lateral view is essential for subjective assessment as the heart may be unduly deep or shallow, thus influencing the grading.

Cardio-thoracic ratio

The cardio-thoracic ratio, expressed as a percentage, is the ratio between the maximum transverse diameter of the heart and the maximum width of the thorax. Methods for determining the latter vary, but the generally accepted way is to take the maximum width above the costo-phrenic angles measured from the inner edges of the ribs.

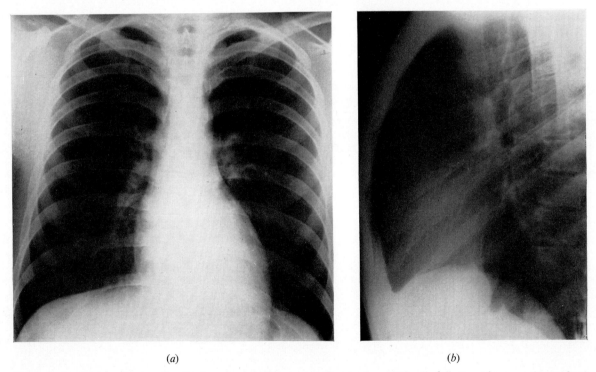

(a)   (b)

Figure 5. Aortic regurgitation. Cardio-thoracic ratio 44 per cent. Heart volume 650 ml/m² body surface area (upper limit of normal 550 ml/m²)

The upper limit of normal is traditionally 50 per cent, but rigid acceptance of such a figure may result in false positive and negative diagnoses of cardiac enlargement. For example, in aortic regurgitation, enlargement of the left ventricle may occur downwards more than laterally, thus hardly increasing the ratio, which may be under 50 per cent in the presence of obvious cardiac enlargement (*Figure 5*). Conversely, it may exceed 50 per cent with no enlargement if the heart is compressed as a result of sternal depression (*see Figure 151*) or a flat chest or if the diaphragm is high because of obesity or exposure of the radiograph in expiration. In children the upper limit of normal is above 50 per cent and varies inversely with age, so that some account must be taken of this when interpreting serial readings during growth. Measurement of the transverse cardiac diameter rather than the ratio may be of some help (*Figure 6*).

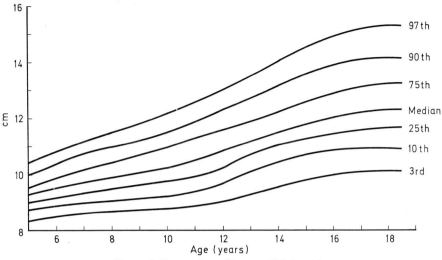

Figure 6. Percentiles of heart width in males

Heart volume

The calculation of heart volume is based on the assumption that the heart is an ellipsoid. Anterior and lateral views are required, and measurements are taken in centimetres as follows (*Figures 7 and 8*).

Figure 7. See text for explanation. RA–SVC = right atrium–superior vena cava junction; PT–LAA = pulmonary trunk–left atrial appendix junction; RCPA = right cardio-phrenic angle

Figure 8. See text for explanation

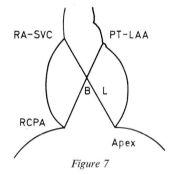

Figure 7

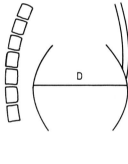

Figure 8

Long diameter (L)
   From the superior vena caval/right atrial junction to the cardiac apex.

Broad diameter (B)
   From diaphragm/right atrial junction to pulmonary trunk/left atrial appendix junction.

Depth diameter (D)
   The greatest horizontal depth of the heart.

The volume of the heart (*V*), expressed in millilitres per square metre of body surface area, is calculated by the formula

$$V = \frac{L \times B \times D \times K \times M}{A}$$

where *K* is the ellipsoid constant (0·63), *M* is the magnification factor, and *A* is the body surface area in square metres derived from height and weight tables (Du Bois standards—*Figures 9 and 10*). The magnification factor (*M*) depends on the radiographic technique used. At the National Heart Hospital, the

7

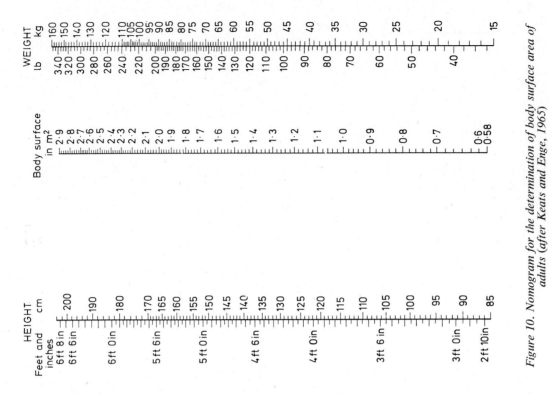

Figure 10. Nomogram for the determination of body surface area of adults (after Keats and Enge, 1965)

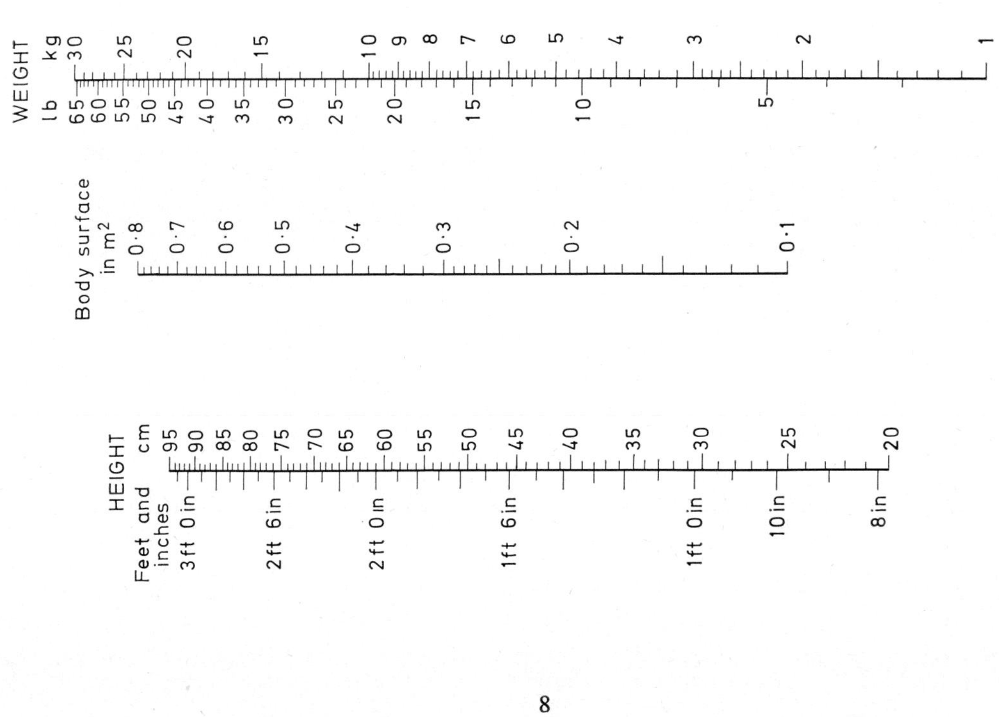

Figure 9. Nomogram for the determination of body surface area of children (after Keats and Enge, 1965)

anterior view is taken at a focus/film distance of 5 feet (1·5 metres) and the lateral at 4 feet (1·2 metres); in these circumstances $M = 0·68$ and $M \times K = 0·43$. The upper limits of normal for adults (Keats and Enge, 1965) are 550 ml/m² body surface area for males and 500 ml/m² for females. Those for children (after Mannheimer, 1949) are given in Table 1.

TABLE 1

Upper Limit of Normal Heart Volumes in Children
(After Mannheimer, 1949)

Age	Heart volume (ml/m² body surface)
0–30 days	120
30–90 days	250
90–360 days	320
1–2 years	325
2–9 years	350
9–12 years	380
12–14 years	425
14–16 years	460
Adult women	500
Adult men	550

Calculation of heart volume is time-consuming and is not practical in a busy department except for special purposes. Its main uses are:

(1) As an adjunct to subject assessment in a patient with doubtful cardiac enlargement.

(2) In providing an accurate measurement for future reference, such as the effect of medical and surgical treatment on heart size.

TABLE 2

Cardio-thoracic Ratio in 678 Adult Patients

Subjective	Normal	+1	+2	+3
Count	125	214	235	104
Mean	45·74	51·37	57·31	65·84
Standard deviation	3·18	3·50	4·32	6·47
Mean + 1 S.D.	48·92	54·87	61·63	

TABLE 3

Heart Volume Measurements in 470 Adult Patients

Subjective	Normal	+1	+2	+3
Count	84	139	162	85
Mean	459·25	590·73	779·10	1,240·00
Standard deviation	78·82	91·14	133·04	344·55
Mean + 1 S.D.	538·07	681·87	912·14	

Subjective assessment of heart size is the most practical method and is the one recommended for general use, except for the beginner. In the authors' experience there is a statistically significant correlation between subjective assessment, cardio-thoracic ratio and volume measurements, as is shown in Tables 2 and 3. Mean and standard deviations have been calculated for cardio-thoracic ratios and volumes in a large group of adult patients, subdivided by subjective assessment of heart size into normal and three grades of enlargement. By taking the mean plus one standard deviation as the arbitrary upper limit of a group it will be seen that the dividing points between normal, +1, +2 and +3 subjective enlargement roughly correspond to cardio-thoracic ratios of 50, 55 and 60 per cent and to volumes of 550, 700 and 900 ml/m². For the inexperienced, such guidelines are put forward as a means of checking the accuracy of a subjective assessment.

CHAPTER 2

The Systemic Veins and Atria

RIGHT SUPERIOR VENA CAVA

The superior vena cava borders the right upper mediastinum on the anterior view until about the age of 40 years, at which time the aorta begins to elongate and bulge to the right beyond the margin of the superior vena cava. The normal superior vena cava is not often identified as such because it usually overlies the ascending aorta within the mediastinum. It may, however, be projected outside the aorta, and then appears less dense than the rest of the cardiovascular shadow as it possesses little antero-posterior depth. The superior vena cava is occasionally displaced laterally by an elongated or dilated aorta.

Superior vena caval dilatation may be due to increased pressure or flow (*Figure 11*). The causes are as follows.

Increased venous or right atrial pressure
   (1) Congestive cardiac failure.
   (2) Tricuspid obstruction and regurgitation (*see* Chapter 23).
   (3) Constrictive pericarditis, pericardial tamponade (*see* Chapter 30).
   (4) Restrictive cardiomyopathy (*see* Chapter 28).
   (5) Right atrial tumour (*see* Chapter 29).
   (6) Mediastinal tumour, mediastinitis.

Increased venous flow
   Partial or total anomalous pulmonary venous drainage to:
   (1) Left superior vena cava or left innominate vein.

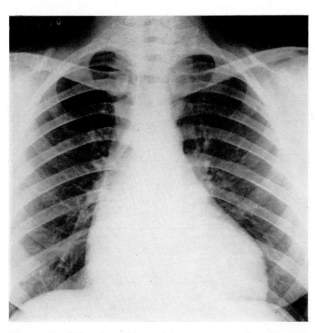

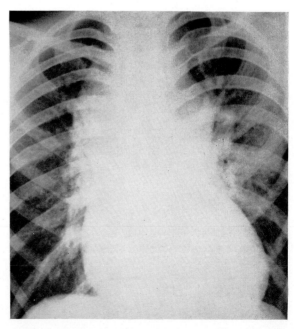

Figure 11. Dilatation of superior vena cava and azygos vein in tricuspid stenosis

Figure 12. Dilatation of both superior venae cavae in total anomalous pulmonary venous drainage

(2) Right superior vena cava.

(3) Azygos vein.

A dilated superior vena cava as a result of high right atrial pressure is frequently invisible because of overlap by the aorta. The greatest dilatation is seen as a result of increased flow in total anomalous pulmonary venous drainage to the left superior vena cava; both venae cavae are dilated, but the right superior vena cava is usually larger than the left because it receives systemic venous return as well as the anomalous pulmonary venous return (*Figure 12*). The superior vena cava may appear very large in normal children under the age of two years due to venous distension if the chest x-ray is exposed after a deep inspiration: it may resemble an enlarged thymus. A dilated superior vena cava can sometimes be distinguished from a prominent aorta as superiorly it always fades away into the neck, whereas the aorta may have a partly visible upper border which curves medially across the mediastinum.

LEFT SUPERIOR VENA CAVA

The presence of a left superior vena cava may be detected on the anterior view as a straight vertical border in the left upper mediastinum merging inferiorly with the heart (*Figure 13*). Its edge may be just outside or may cross the aortic knuckle and pulmonary trunk. However, in approximately half the cases it lies entirely within the borders of the cardiovascular shadow and is then invisible as a separate shadow. The left superior vena cava drains into the coronary sinus except in anomalous pulmonary venous drainage, when it usually joins the left innominate vein. Rarely it drains into the left atrium and may cause cyanosis in the absence of cardiac murmurs (*see* page 212). A left superior vena cava draining into the coronary sinus may be associated with most types of congenital heart disease, particularly the following defects of the atrial septum (Somerville, 1972):

Single atrium 60–70 per cent.
Complete canal 50 per cent.
Sinus venosus defect 18 per cent.
Ostium primum defect 17 per cent.
Fossa ovalis defect 10 per cent.

The right superior vena cava is usually but not invariably present (Harris *et al.*, 1972), and the two are connected via the left innominate vein. Bilateral superior vena cava is a feature of supracardiac total anomalous pulmonary venous drainage and other complex anomalies associated with absence of the spleen or polysplenia (*see* Chapter 5).

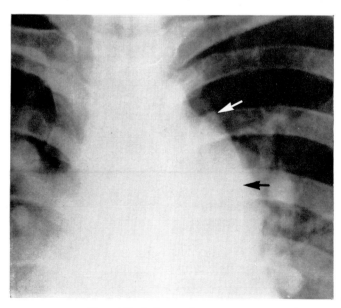

Figure 13. Left superior vena cava

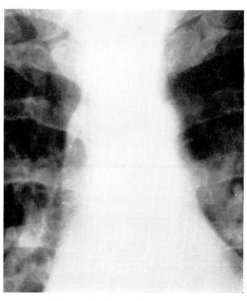

Figure 14. Normal azygos vein

AZYGOS VEIN

The azygos vein ascends in the right paravertebral gutter and arches forward over the right main bronchus to enter the back of the right superior vena cava. It is joined by the hemiazygos vein, which lies in the left paravertebral gutter, by connection across the midline. Both veins receive intercostal veins and are an important collateral pathway between the superior and inferior vena caval systems in mediastinal and portal venous obstruction. The horizontal portion of the normal azygos vein may sometimes be identified as an oval or ribbon-like opacity in the right tracheo-bronchial angle. When dilated, it appears more rounded or oval and may be mistaken for an enlarged tracheo-bronchial lymph node (*Figure 14*). The causes of azygos vein dilatation are as follows.

Increased venous or right atrial pressure
    Similar to superior vena caval dilatation (*see* page 10).

Increased flow
    Pulmonary venous drainage into azygos vein.
    Portal venous obstruction.
    Superior vena caval obstruction.
    Absence of hepatic portion of inferior vena cava.

Congenital aneurysm

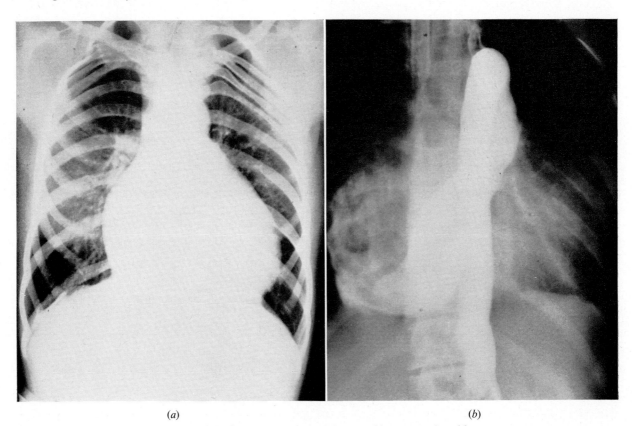

(a)   (b)

Figure 15. Enlarged hemiazygos vein resembling aortic knuckle

In portal venous obstruction the azygos vein forms part of the collateral circulation from portal to systemic venous systems. If superior vena caval obstruction lies above the azygos vein, it acts as a by-pass collateral to the right atrium. When the hepatic segment of the inferior vena cava is absent, the pre-hepatic segment is continued as the azygos vein, which is dilated and joins the right superior vena cava. Similarly, a left-sided inferior vena cava may continue as the hemiazygos vein which joins the left superior vena cava and coronary sinus, or connection may occur across the midline to the azygos vein and the right superior vena cava. In the former situation the dilated hemiazygos vein may be mistaken for the aortic knuckle (*Figure 15*), and in the latter there may be the rare situation of viscero-atrial discordance (right atrium and larger lobe of the liver on opposite sides of the body) (*Figure 16—also see* page 43).

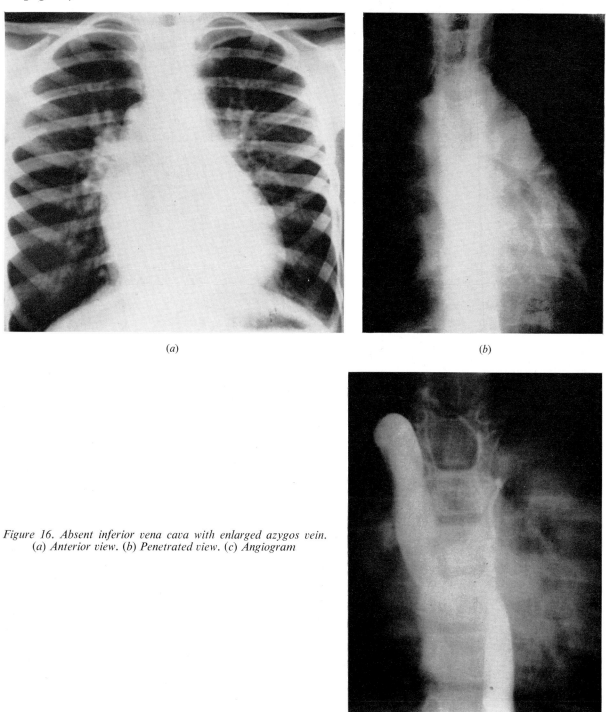

(a)

(b)

*Figure 16. Absent inferior vena cava with enlarged azygos vein.
(a) Anterior view. (b) Penetrated view. (c) Angiogram*

(c)

Accessory azygos vein

The azygos vein may be displaced laterally into the lung and lie in the inferior recess of an accessory fissure. This vein may become dilated in the same way as the normal azygos vein, for example in congestive failure (*Figure 17*).

13

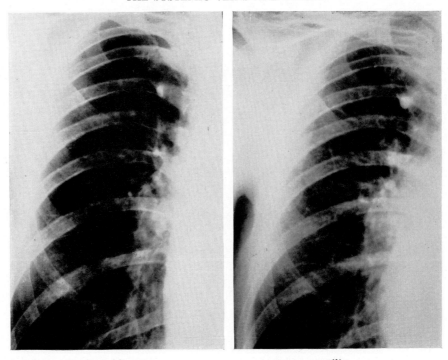

(a)   (b)

Figure 17. Azygos vein in azygos fissure. (a) Normal size. (b) Enlarged in right-sided heart failure

INFERIOR VENA CAVA

The post-hepatic segment of the inferior vena cava has a short intrathoracic segment, which is occasionally visible in the right cardio-phrenic angle on the anterior view of the chest but is nearly always seen on the lateral view. It may rarely enlarge in right heart failure. Anomalous right pulmonary veins may connect with it by a long curved vein descending close to the right border of the heart (scimitar syndrome, *Figure 18—also see* page 141). The part played by the inferior vena cava in the diagnosis of ventricular enlargement on the lateral view is discussed on page 26.

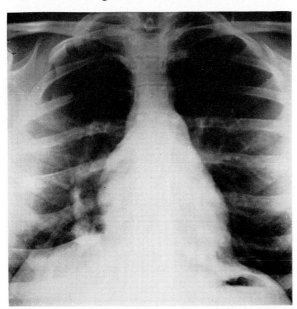

Figure 18. Anomalous venous drainage of right lung into inferior vena cava (scimitar syndrome)

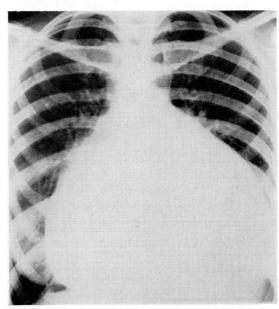

Figure 19. Enormous right atrium in tricuspid regurgitation: lung changes of severe additional mitral valve disease unimpressive

RIGHT ATRIUM

On the anterior view the right atrium forms less than the lower half of the right mediastinal border in adults, but in children it may represent about half this contour. It is not always uniformly convex, but may show a secondary bulge towards its upper part caused by the base of the appendix. Its lower contour may be somewhat flat, particularly when the heart is rotated slightly into the left anterior oblique. The right atrium and inferior vena cava may form part of the lower posterior cardiac border on the lateral view, particularly if the right side of the patient is rotated slightly backwards.

The causes of right atrial dilatation are as follows.

(1) Shunts into right atrium (*see* Chapters 16, 17 and 18):
  (*a*) Atrial septal defect, single atrium.
  (*b*) Anomalous pulmonary venous drainage.
  (*c*) Left ventricular/right atrial shunt.
  (*d*) Ruptured aortic sinus into right atrium.
  (*e*) Coronary artery fistula to right atrium or coronary sinus.
(2) Tricuspid obstruction and regurgitation (*see* Chapter 23).
(3) Pulmonary obstruction and regurgitation (*see* Chapter 24).
(4) Pulmonary arterial hypertension (*see* Chapter 9).
(5) Right-sided cardiomyopathy (*see* Chapter 28).
(6) Right atrial tumours (*see* Chapter 29).

The differential diagnosis is:

(1) Pericardial effusion.
(2) Pericardial cyst.
(3) Cardiac tumour.
(4) Mediastinal tumour (particularly ectopic thymus).

Estimation of right atrial size on plain radiography is fraught with difficulties. To establish with certainty that the right atrium is dilated, its convex border should project abnormally far into the right lower lung field, and it should be at least half as long as the total height of the right border of the

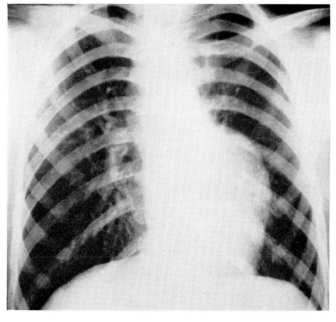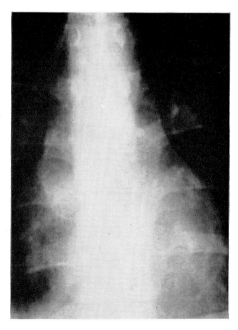

Figure 20 (left). Left juxtaposition of atrial appendices. Bulge of left upper cardiac border from appendices. Flat right atrial border. (Tricuspid atresia)

Figure 21 (right). Normal-sized left atrium visible on penetrated view

mediastinum (*Figure 19*). A large right atrium, however, may not produce these signs, as dilatation may occur mainly anteriorly and medially and the atrial convexity may be hidden by the spine if the heart is displaced to the left (as is so often the case in atrial septal defect). The border of a right atrium, thought to be normal in size before closure of an atrial septal defect, not infrequently appears less convex and shorter after operation due to reduction in chamber size. Right atrial dilatation may be mistakenly diagnosed when an abnormally convex border results from right atrial displacement caused by enlargement of the right ventricle, left ventricle or left atrium. A greatly enlarged left atrium may itself form most or all of the right lower cardiac border and be mistaken for a big right atrium. In a large heart it is often impossible to tell whether the abnormal right lower contour is produced by the right or the left atrium: it is not infrequently produced by both. A grossly enlarged right atrium may form both the anterior and the posterior margin of the heart on the lateral view.

The convex bulge of the right atrium may be unimpressive in some cases of tricuspid atresia. This may be due to the smallness of the right atrium in conjunction with a large atrial septal defect or to medial displacement of the right atrium as a result of right ventricular hypoplasia, but is most often due to left juxtaposition of the atrial appendices. In juxtaposition the upper part of the right atrial border is flattened because the right atrial appendix is displaced to the left behind the aorta and lies beside the left atrial appendix (*Figure 20*). It is important to be familiar with this appearance, as tricuspid atresia is common and transposition invariable (*see* page 221). Flattening of the right atrial border is also seen in constrictive pericarditis (*see* page 286).

LEFT ATRIUM

The left atrium is placed centrally in the posterior and upper part of the heart. Occasionally the normal left atrium can be seen on the anterior view as an increased density well within the right cardiac border (*Figure 21*). The appendix forms a short straight segment on the left heart border below the pulmonary trunk. On the lateral view the left atrium forms the upper posterior border of the heart, but its outline is indistinct as it is overlapped by the four pulmonary veins. Sometimes the right lower pulmonary veins, just before entering the left atrium, form a confluence or small chamber visible on the anterior view as a dense shadow which may be mistaken for a tumour mass (*see Figure 109*).

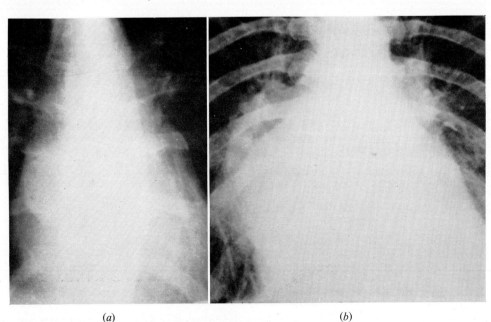

Figure 22. Enlarged left atrium. (a) Increased density within heart border. Descending aorta displaced to left. (b) Left atrial border outside heart border

(a)　　　　　　　　　　(b)

The causes of left atrial enlargement are:
  (1) Mitral obstruction and regurgitation (*see* Chapter 25).
  (2) Aortic obstruction and regurgitation (*see* Chapter 26).
  (3) Systemic hypertension.

(4) Ischaemic heart disease (*see* Chapter 27).
(5) Cardiomyopathy (*see* Chapter 28).
(6) Shunts at ventricular or aorto-pulmonary levels (*see* Chapters 17 and 18).
(7) Left atrial tumour (*see* Chapter 29).

The left atrium attains a large size only in severe congenital anomalies of the mitral valve, particularly severe mitral regurgitation, and in rheumatic heart disease. With enlargement from any other cause, its wall remains relatively incompliant and dilatation is modest. In rheumatic heart disease its size depends on the degree of rheumatic involvement of its wall, the duration and severity of the left atrial hypertension, and the presence or absence of atrial fibrillation. Severe mitral regurgitation into the healthy left atrium, as may occur with chordal rupture or papillary muscle dysfunction, is frequently accompanied by signs of pulmonary hypertension and oedema as the large systolic wave is reflected directly back into the pulmonary venous and arterial bed. Conversely, a copious left atrium in rheumatic mitral valve disease will absorb the high pressure, and signs of pulmonary venous and arterial hypertension tend to occur late in the course of the disease. This is typically seen in mitral regurgitation with an aneurysmal left atrium, when important pulmonary hypertension occurs only when the left ventricle fails.

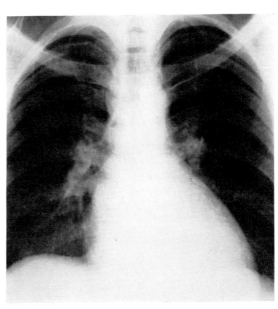

Figure 23 (right). Aortic root aneurysm simulating enlarged left atrium

Figure 24 (below). Large left atrial appendix contained within heart border. (a) Anterior view. (b) Angiogram

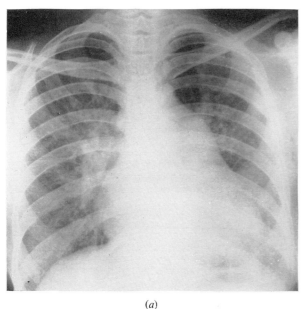

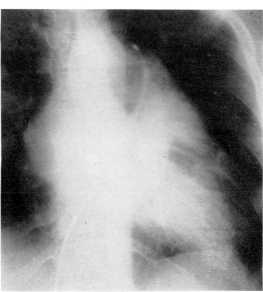

(*a*)

(*b*)

Enlargement of the left atrium may occur to the right, to the left, posteriorly or inferiorly, or in any combination of the four directions. Enlargement to the right is seen as an increased density with a convex outer margin which may be within, coincident with or outside the right heart border (*Figure 22*). When within the heart shadow, this increased density may be confused with a dilated aortic root (*Figure 23*).

Enlargement to the left is manifested by convex bulging of the appendix on the left heart border. However, occasionally the appendix may be large but contained with a straight left heart border and produce no localized convexity (*Figure 24*). Although a normal-sized appendix may sometimes produce

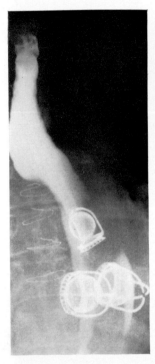
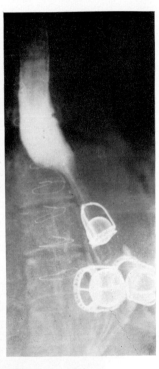

Figure 25 (left). Large left atrium displacing oesophagus to left and causing holding of barium. Triple Starr valve replacement

Figure 26 (below). Large left atrium. (a) Wide carinal angle. (b) Normal carinal angle but with elevation of left lower lobe bronchus

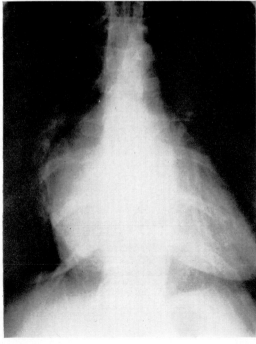

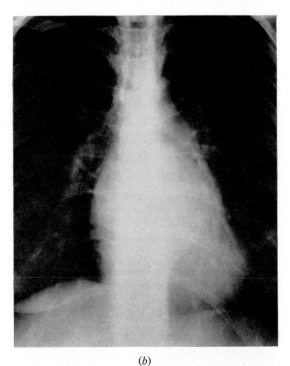

(a)

(b)

a slight bulge, any convexity usually indicates enlargement of the appendix. Bulging of the appendix without any dilatation of the body of the left atrium is seen in partial left pericardial defect (*see* page 288). A prominent appendix bulge as a part of left atrial enlargement is rarely seen except in rheumatic heart disease. This rule is useful in distinguishing rheumatic mitral valve disease from functional and other causes of mitral regurgitation.

Posterior enlargement is detected by an increased density within the heart shadow on the penetrated anterior view and by posterior displacement of the back of the left atrium and pulmonary veins on the lateral view. In minor degrees of left atrial enlargement, increased density on the anterior view is an earlier sign than displacement of the barium-filled oesophagus. Posterior enlargement may deviate the middle of the descending aorta to the left (Bedford's sign—*see Figures 22a* and *26a*). Although this sign is of most value in young patients in whom the aorta is normally straight, distinction from an elongated aorta can usually be made, because in aortic unfolding the point of maximum deviation is rarely at the level of the mid-atrium. Aortic displacement is most likely to occur in patients with a narrow antero-posterior diameter to the chest, and in such patients left atrial enlargement does not have to be marked to push the aorta away from the spine. Posterior enlargement of the atrium may compress the oesophagus and produce dysphagia: this is probably more liable to occur if the oesophagus is deviated to the left, as in this position it is squashed between the atrium, the spine and the descending aorta (*Figure 25*) (usually the oesophagus is displaced to the right and posteriorly).

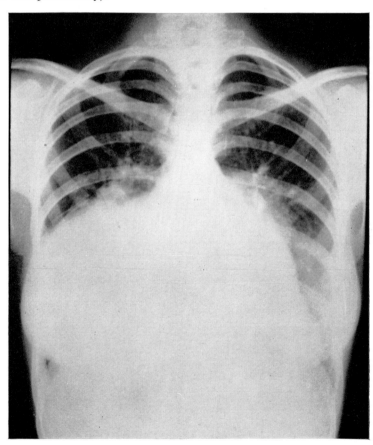

Figure 27. Aneurysmal left atrium. The atrium touches the right lateral chest wall. The appendix bulges to the left

Upward displacement of the roof of the left atrium with widening of the carinal angle is a late sign of left atrial enlargement (*Figure 26a*). The carinal angle is widest in short thickset people with a high diaphragm, but normally does not exceed 90 degrees. The upward displacement of the distal half of the left bronchus without widening of the carina is the earliest sign of superior enlargement; it is associated with outward and upward bowing of the left lower lobe bronchus (*Figure 26b*). Inferior extension to the diaphragm on the right side does occur, but is seen only when the atrium is very large. It may then be difficult to differentiate left atrial from right atrial dilatation, but the left atrium usually forms a more acute angle with the diaphragm than the right atrium.

The term aneurysmal left atrium is used when the right border approaches the right chest wall and the appendix is very large (*Figure 27*). Usually the atrium also forms the whole of the posterior heart border; it touches the diaphragm, and the carinal angle approaches 180 degrees. The right descending pulmonary artery is displaced outwards and may be mistaken for a hilar mass. The middle lobe and either lower lobe, particularly the left, may be collapsed as a result of pulmonary or bronchial compression. The oesophagus may be compressed with the production of dysphagia (*see Figure 25*) (Chesshyre and Braimbridge, 1971; Whitney and Croxon, 1971), and rare cases of vertebral erosion have been reported (Ashworth and Morgan-Jones, 1946). Calcification of the left atrium is discussed on page 53.

CHAPTER 3

The Ventricles

INTRODUCTION

The normal ventricles

The right ventricle is roughly triangular in shape, with its apex at the pulmonary valve and its base resting on the diaphragm. The left ventricle is ellipsoid in shape and related to the left postero-lateral aspect of the triangular right ventricle (*Figure 28*). The left ventricle forms the whole of the left lower cardiac border, the ventricular border, on the anterior view. It is responsible for the normal smooth convex contour of this border. The base/apex axis of the right ventricle is nearly vertical, whereas the long axis of the left ventricle is roughly 45 degrees to the vertical. The most convex point on the ventricular border is the apex of the heart, which normally lies just above the left leaf of the diaphragm.

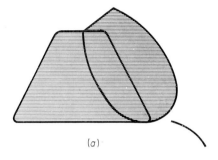

(a)

Figure 28. (a) Diagram of normal right and left ventricles. (b) Angiogram of right ventricle. (c) Angiogram of left ventricle

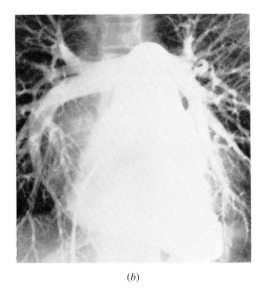

(b)

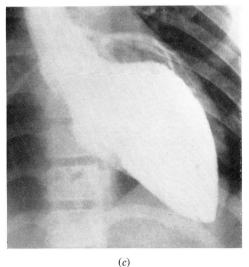

(c)

Ventricular enlargement

Radiological enlargement of the ventricles usually results from dilatation, although the dilatation is normally accompanied by some hypertrophy. Ventricular cavity enlargement is seen in conditions of diastolic overload (increased diastolic filling) such as valve regurgitation and left-to-right shunts. It also occurs when the ventricle begins to fail as a pump—in ischaemic heart disease, congestive cardiomyopathy, or failure of either ventricle from any cause. As well as resulting in cardiac enlargement, ventricular dilatation often causes an alteration of heart shape characteristic of the right or left ventricle.

Hypertrophy is a response to systolic overload or contraction against an abnormally high resistance. It has to be massive in order to produce cardiac enlargement; an enlarged heart from pure hypertrophy is most often seen in hypertrophic cardiomyopathy and in severe obstructive lesions in children such as pulmonary stenosis. Hypertrophy, however, frequently results in an abnormal heart shape which is similar to that seen in dilatation and usually enables right and left ventricular hypertrophy to be distinguished. Because dilatation may not be distinguishable from hypertrophy, the term enlargement is preferred when applied to the heart or either ventricle. Thus ventricular enlargement produces an alteration in cardiac shape which in most cases is characteristic of one or other ventricle, in some is non-specific, and in a few is positively misleading. The following account refers to the characteristic changes of ventricular enlargement.

RIGHT VENTRICULAR ENLARGEMENT

When the right ventricle enlarges, it does so mainly by a broadening of its triangular shape (*Figure 29*). In moderate enlargement, the left ventricle along its left lateral border is displaced upwards and outwards, resulting in prominence of the upper part of the ventricular border. The apex is elevated but still formed by the left ventricle. The border below the apex is related to the left inferior angle of the right ventricle and usually turns abruptly medially. Thus two distinct contours of the ventricular border are usually distinguished: a long prominent upper contour above the apex, and a second shorter contour turning medially below the apex (*Figure 30*). With increasing right ventricular enlargement, the left ventricle is rotated further upwards and outwards but also backwards. The right ventricle may ultimately form the whole of the ventricular border in front of the left ventricle; sometimes the right ventricle is border-forming only in diastole, while in systole the upper part of the border is formed by the left ventricle and the lower part by the right ventricle. The shape of the ventricular border in right ventricular enlargement is similar whether it is formed by a displaced left ventricle or by a very large right ventricle (*Figure 31*); a common exception is Ebstein's anomaly (*Figure 32*).

A large right ventricle also dilates anteriorly and may be demonstrated on a lateral film of the chest as an increased heart contact with the sternum. This sign must be interpreted with extreme caution, as a narrow flat chest or a depressed sternum may result in similar appearances. Cardiac contact with more than the lower half of the body of the sternum in a chest of normal shape, however, is a good but rather late sign of right ventricular dilatation. Normal or even absent contact of the heart with the sternum may be seen with important right ventricular enlargement when the heart is rotated backwards as in a barrel-shaped chest. The best sign of right ventricular enlargement on the lateral view is an increase in bulk of the anterior portion of the heart, however it lies in the chest (*Figure 33*). The posterior border of the heart on the lateral chest x-ray is rarely altered by right ventricular enlargement, but posterior and superior displacement of the left ventricle may result in a postero-inferior border which slopes steeply downwards and forwards. This type of contour is not easily distinguished from normal, but denies important left ventricular dilatation (*Figure 34*).

Prominence of the right atrium and dilatation of the pulmonary trunk are seen in diseases in which the right ventricle is enlarged and supply important supporting evidence. Signs of pulmonary arterial hypertension may also be used as secondary evidence of right ventricular enlargement provided that changes of pulmonary venous hypertension are absent. If the latter are present, the left ventricle may be enlarged as well as the right, for example in mitral regurgitation and pulmonary hypertension. If the left atrium is enlarged, its dilated appendix may obscure the upper part of the ventricular border and render differentiation between an enlarged right and left ventricle impossible.

In right ventricular hypertrophy, outward and upward displacement of the left ventricle may produce a similar cardiac contour to that seen with dilatation, but in a heart which is normal in size or slightly enlarged (*Figure 35*). A convex lower anterior border may be seen on the lateral view. It must be emphasized, however, that ventricular contours in right ventricular hypertrophy may be normal in both views.

Right ventricular hypertrophy in conjunction with right ventricular outflow hypoplasia, as occurs in Fallot's tetralogy and pulmonary atresia, deserves special mention. On the anterior view, a concavity is seen below the aortic knuckle due to smallness of the pulmonary trunk and right ventricular outflow. The lower part of the ventricular border is convex. The convexity may be high, producing a *cœur en sabot*

22

heart (*Figure 36*). It may be maximal in the middle of the ventricular contour, which will then appear round (*Figure 37*), or it may be lower in position as in classical right ventricular enlargement (*Figure 38*). Quite frequently the contour is normal, while occasionally it may resemble left ventricular hypertrophy

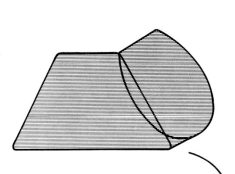

Figure 29. Right ventricle enlarged: normal left ventricle

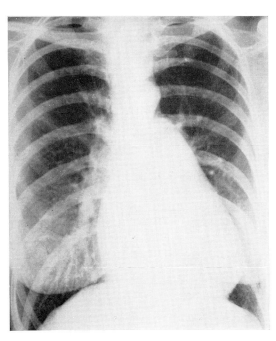

Figure 30. Typical right ventricular enlargement (atrial septal defect)

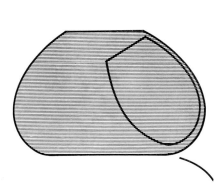

Figure 31. Right ventricle grossly enlarged: normal left ventricle

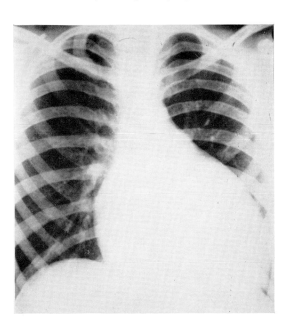

Figure 32. Gross right ventricular enlargement simulating left ventricular enlargement (Ebstein's anomaly)

(*see* page 175). The left ventricle may still form the ventricular border, but if the right ventricle is large and the left ventricle is small, the right ventricle is often border-forming. The right ventricle may be rotated on its antero-posterior axis in such a way that the outflow tract points abnormally to the right and the left inferior angle of the ventricle is displaced upwards, exaggerating the high apex and *cœur en sabot* shape of the heart.

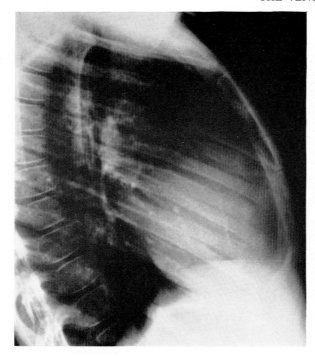

Figure 33. Lateral view of right ventricular enlargement—increased bulk of anterior portion of the heart

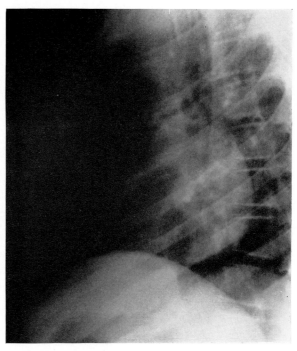

Figure 34. Lateral view of right ventricular enlargement—postero-superior displacement of left ventricle

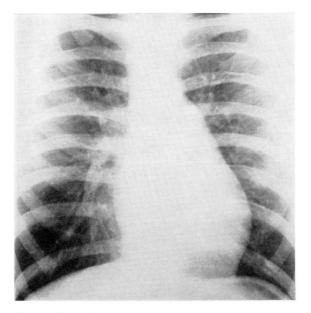

Figure 35. Right ventricular hypertrophy in pulmonary stenosis—similar shape to right ventricular dilatation

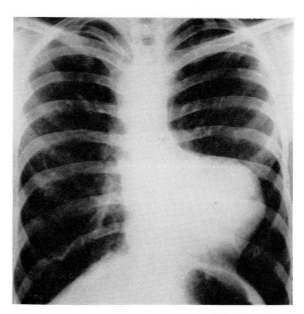

Figure 36. Cœur en sabot in pulmonary atresia

The causes of right ventricular enlargement are:
    (1) Tricuspid regurgitation (*see* Chapter 23).
    (2) Pulmonary obstruction and regurgitation (*see* Chapter 24).
    (3) Fallot and its differential diagnosis (*see* Chapters 19 and 20).
    (4) Atrial shunts (*see* Chapter 16).
    (5) Right-sided cardiomyopathy (*see* Chapter 28).
    (6) Pulmonary arterial hypertension (*see* Chapter 9).
    (7) Secondary to pulmonary venous hypertension (*see* Chapter 10).

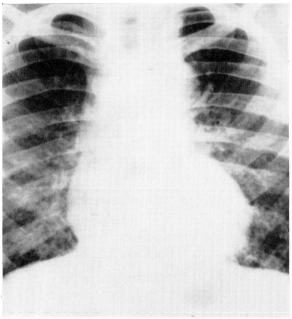

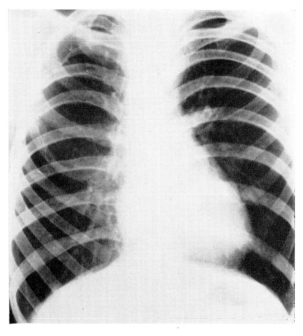

Figure 37. Right ventricular hypertrophy in Fallot's tetralogy—rounded ventricular contour

Figure 38. Right ventricular hypertrophy in Fallot's tetralogy—apex of typical right ventricular enlargement

SUMMARY OF RIGHT VENTRICULAR ENLARGEMENT

Dilatation of the right ventricle causes cardiac enlargement, often with a characteristic alteration in the shape of the heart. Hypertrophy of the right ventricle may not be associated with abnormality of cardiac size or shape: if severe, however, it may cause cardiac enlargement and the characteristic alteration in shape.

The signs of right ventricular enlargement are as follows.

Direct signs

Abnormal ventricular contour on anterior view
(1) Upward and outward displacement of the ventricular border.
(2) Elevation of the apex.
(3) An upper longer arc above the apex and a lower short arc turning medially below the apex.

Abnormal anterior border on lateral view
(1) Increase in bulk of the anterior part of the heart.
(2) Localized increased convexity of the lower anterior border of the heart in hypertrophy.

Indirect signs

(1) Prominent right atrial border.
(2) Dilated pulmonary trunk.
(3) Signs of pulmonary arterial hypertension.

LEFT VENTRICULAR ENLARGEMENT

When the left ventricle enlarges, all its diameters increase, but particularly its long axis when dilatation is marked (*Figure 39*). The position of the aortic valve is largely fixed, and an increase in the long axis of the ventricle results in a downward displacement of its apex. As the ventricular border of the heart on the anterior view is formed by the lateral border of the ellipsoid left ventricle, the border elongates and moves downwards or outwards or both. This border forms a single long smooth curve (*Figure 40*). In the transverse heart the apex is normal in position, while in the vertical heart it is low, sometimes being below the diaphragm. As the left ventricle also enlarges posteriorly, it produces a prominent convexity

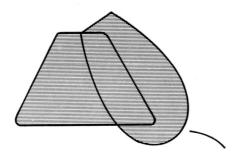

Figure 39. Left ventricle enlarged: normal right ventricle

of the lower half of the posterior border of the heart on the lateral view, and the left ventricle is usually projected well behind the posterior border of the inferior vena cava (*Figure 41*). This may, however, not be the case if left ventricular enlargement occurs mainly laterally or if the patient's left side is rotated forward enough to project the posterior left ventricular border in front of the inferior vena cava. It will be appreciated that the maximum convexity of the posterior left ventricular border is to the left of the midline and the inferior cava is to the right of the midline, and thus slight rotation of the patient will be enough to bring the posterior border of the left ventricle in front of the vena cava.

Prominence of the ascending aorta is often associated with enlargement of the left ventricle in aortic valve disease, coarctation, hypertension or aneurysm. Dilatation of the ascending aorta, however, is a characteristic feature of Fallot's tetralogy and pulmonary atresia, and in these diseases it must not be mistaken for indirect evidence of left ventricular enlargement. Pulmonary venous hypertension without left atrial enlargement is another valuable indirect sign that cardiac enlargement is due to the left ventricle. If the left atrium is enlarged, the diagnosis may be dominant mitral stenosis with right ventricular enlargement. When the left atrium is dilated, its appendix often obscures the upper part of the left ventricular border and makes differentiation between an enlarged right and left ventricle difficult. Nevertheless, an elongated left lower cardiac border may be apparent in conjunction with left atrial dilatation and will suggest the presence of mitral and/or aortic regurgitation.

In left ventricular hypertrophy, elongation of the ventricular border on the postero-anterior view, similar to that seen in dilatation, may be apparent (*Figure 42*). If the heart lies transversely the border may appear rounded, but still with a single rather long arc. An unusually convex lower posterior cardiac border, but without backward displacement of the contour, may be seen on the lateral view. Cardiac enlargement is present only in severe hypertrophy. Not infrequently both cardiac size and shape are normal in hypertrophy.

The causes of left ventricular enlargement are:

    (1) Mitral regurgitation (*see* Chapter 25).
    (2) Aortic obstruction and regurgitation (*see* Chapter 26).
    (3) Systemic hypertension.
    (4) Ischaemic heart disease (*see* Chapter 27).
    (5) Left-sided cardiomyopathy (*see* Chapter 28).
    (6) Aorto-pulmonary shunts (*see* Chapters 17 and 18).
    (7) Tricuspid atresia (*see* Chapter 23).

SUMMARY OF LEFT VENTRICULAR ENLARGEMENT

Dilatation of the left ventricle causes cardiac enlargement, often with a characteristic alteration in the shape of the heart. Hypertrophy of the left ventricle may not be associated with abnormality of cardiac size or shape; if severe, it may cause cardiac enlargement and the characteristic alteration in shape. The signs of left ventricular enlargement are as follows.

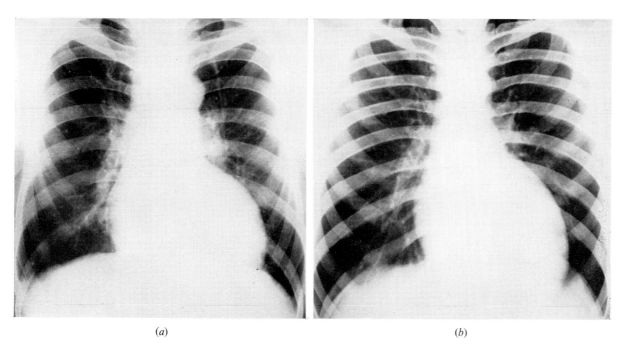

(a)   (b)

Figure 40. Left ventricular enlargement. (a) Normally placed apex. (b) Low apex

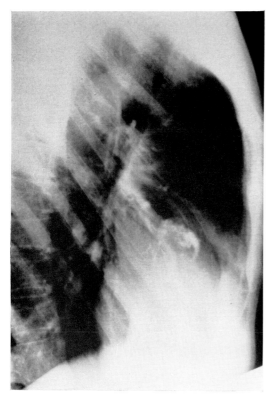

Figure 41. Left ventricular enlargement—posterior border projected behind inferior vena cava in lateral view

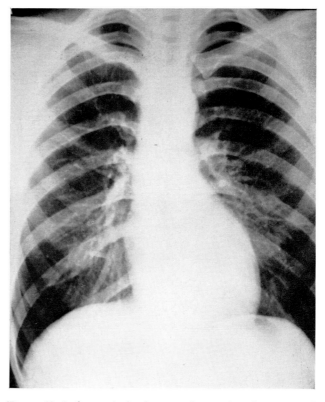

Figure 42. Left ventricular hypertrophy causing elongation of left border like dilatation (aortic stenosis)

Direct signs

Abnormal ventricular contour on anterior view
   (1) Downward and outward displacement of the ventricular border.
   (2) Depression of the apex.
   (3) A single long ventricular arc.

Abnormal posterior contour on lateral view
   (1) Prominent posterior convexity.
   (2) The posterior left ventricular border lying well behind the posterior border of the inferior vena cava.

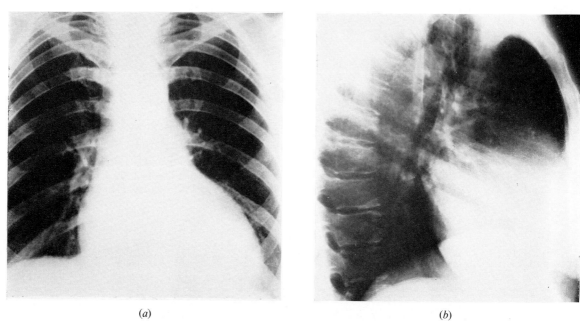

(a)   (b)

Figure 43. Biventricular enlargement (aortic and pulmonary stenosis). (a) Anterior view showing left ventricular enlargement. (b) Lateral view showing right ventricular enlargement

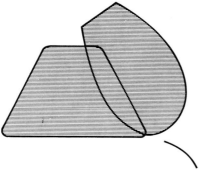

Figure 44. Combined ventricular enlargement

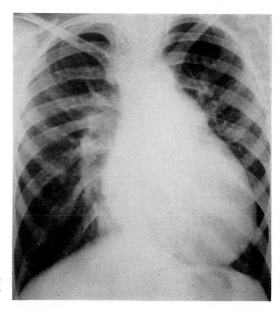

Figure 45. Biventricular enlargement (ventricular septal defect with pulmonary hypertension)—long ventricular contour with high apex

Indirect signs

    (1) Prominent ascending aorta.

    (2) Signs of pulmonary venous hypertension without important left atrial dilatation.

COMBINED VENTRICULAR ENLARGEMENT

If one ventricle is dominant, the cardiac shape may suggest enlargement of that ventricle. The lateral view may sometimes provide evidence that the other ventricle is also enlarged (*Figure 43*). If both ventricles are more or less equally enlarged, for example in ventricular septal defect and pulmonary hypertension, the left ventricular contour is both elongated and displaced upwards and outwards (*Figure 44*). The result is often a long ventricular contour and a high apex on the anterior view (*Figure 45*).

CHAPTER 4

The Great Vessels

PULMONARY TRUNK

On the anterior view the pulmonary trunk is border-forming for a short distance between the aortic knuckle and the left atrial appendix. In adults its contour may be straight, slightly concave or slightly convex. In infants it may be obscured by the thymus, but in children and adolescents, particularly females, it frequently has a convex contour which becomes less as age advances, reaching the adult pattern by the age of 20 years (*Figure 46*). Its left branch is usually identified just above and lateral to the pulmonary trunk as it arches over the left main bronchus; it then curves downwards and may merge with the shadow of the pulmonary trunk and so be confused with it. Its right branch cannot be identified since it lies within the mediastinum. On the lateral view the curved antero-superior contour of the pulmonary trunk is sometimes seen forming the lower posterior boundary of the retrosternal air space. The right branch is end-on, seen as an oval shadow in front of the tracheal bifurcation, and the left branch may be identified as it arches over the left main bronchus below and in front of the posterior part of the aortic arch (*Figure 47a*).

The following lesions may cause enlargement of the pulmonary trunk.

(1) Left-to-right shunts (*see* Chapters 16, 17 and 18).
(2) Pulmonary hypertension from any cause (*see* Chapters 9, 10 and 21).
(3) Pulmonary stenosis (*see* Chapter 24).
(4) Pulmonary regurgitation (*see* Chapter 24).
(5) Aneurysm in Marfan's syndrome (*see* page 119).
(6) Idiopathic dilatation.

When the pulmonary trunk dilates as a result of increased pressure or flow, it usually enlarges in a uniform manner. It is almost invariably dilated in left-to-right shunts at atrial and aorto-pulmonary levels, but in a ventricular septal defect with normal pulmonary pressures it is frequently normal in size. In any shunt with hyperkinetic pulmonary hypertension it is invariably enlarged. In the Eisenmenger syndrome (right-to-left or bidirectional shunts), pulmonary trunk dilatation is variable. In an atrial septal defect it is usually very large; in a ventricular septal defect it varies from normal to only moderate, whereas in ductus arteriosus it is often as large as in an atrial septal defect but shows considerable variation. The size of the pulmonary trunk, taken in conjunction with the pulmonary vascular pattern, is important in the differential diagnosis of communications at the atrial, ventricular and aorto-pulmonary levels when presenting as the Eisenmenger syndrome (*see* Chapter 21). In pulmonary hypertension due to emphysema, the heart is vertical in position and may not be enlarged; the pulmonary trunk dilatation often presents a not very impressive but long convex segment (*see Figure 117*). Hilar arteries often appear prominent because they contrast with the thin intrapulmonary vessels, and their enlargement does not necessarily indicate pulmonary hypertension. In obstructive airways disease due predominantly to bronchitis, pulmonary hypertension is more common than in emphysema; with the onset of congestive cardiac failure, the right heart, pulmonary trunk and pulmonary vessels dilate and the picture often resembles an atrial septal defect. After treatment, appearances may revert to normal. In pulmonary valve stenosis, the post-stenotic dilatation predominantly involves the roof of the pulmonary trunk and its high position is an important diagnostic feature; it may overlap the aortic knuckle (*see Figure 307*). This post-stenotic dilatation commonly extends into the left branch and can be identified on both anterior and lateral views (*see Figure 306*). Enlargement of the pulmonary trunk from any cause may be seen on the lateral view encroaching on the lower part of the retrosternal air space and in extreme cases coming into contact with the sternum.

The differential diagnosis of pulmonary trunk enlargement is:

(1) Left hilar mass or enlarged glands.

(2) Mediastinal tumour or cyst, especially thymic lesions and dermoid cyst.

(3) The ascending aorta in corrected transposition.

(4) Left pericardial defect.

Figure 46 (right). Convex pulmonary trunk in adolescent female

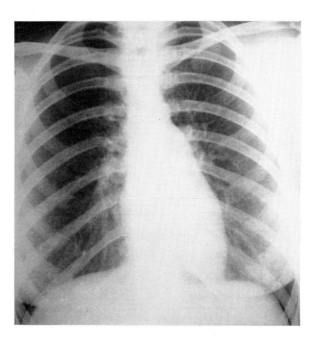

Figure 47 (below). Lateral view. (a) Normal right and left pulmonary arteries—right anterior to carina, left above carina below aortic arch. (b) Hilar mass below carina

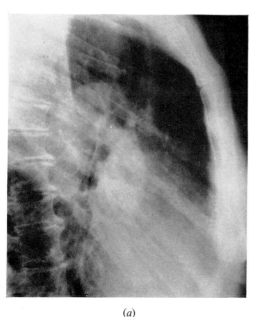

(a)

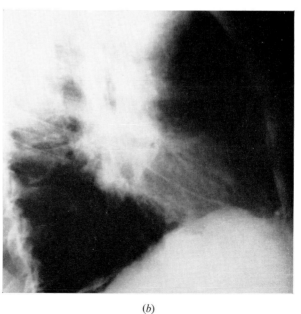

(b)

Glandular swellings may be indistinguishable from the pulmonary trunk (*Figure 48*), but are often lobulated and on the lateral view are seen in the middle mediastinum, where they lie around the tracheal bifurcation. On the lateral view the right pulmonary artery anterior to the tracheal bifurcation and the left pulmonary artery postero-superiorly must not be mistaken for glands, but any opacity below the bifurcation is highly suspicious (*Figure 47b*). Thymic tumours and dermoid cysts, although in the anterior mediastinum, may be closely related to the pulmonary trunk (*Figure 49*). The ascending aorta forms the left upper cardiac border in corrected transposition and may be mistaken for the pulmonary trunk if it is convex to the left, but its contour is usually too long (*see Figure 211*).

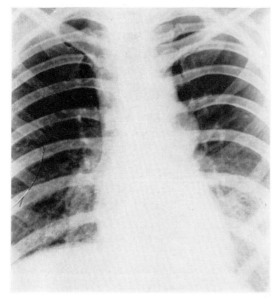

Figure 48

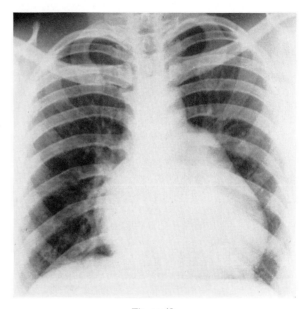

Figure 49

Figure 48. Enlarged lymph node simulating pulmonary trunk

Figure 49. Mediastinal cyst simulating pulmonary trunk

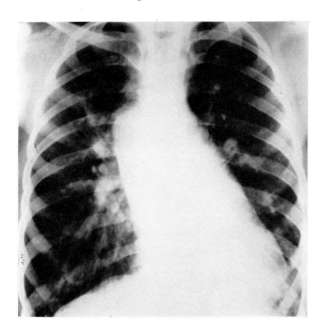

Figure 50

Figure 50. Large pulmonary trunk in complete transposition bulging to right

Failure to identify the pulmonary trunk on the anterior view suggests that it is either absent or small (*see Figure 251*), or that it lies in an abnormal position. When it is absent or small, the right ventricular outflow is usually hypoplastic and an obvious concavity is seen in the middle of the left cardiac border. An important exception is Ebstein's anomaly, in which the pulmonary trunk is small and invisible but the right ventricular outflow is dilated and may produce a long convex ventricular border (*see Figure 300*). In complete and corrected transposition, the pulmonary trunk occupies a posterior and central position and is invisible unless grossly dilated, when it may be seen bulging to the right or left of the midline (*Figure 50*).

ASCENDING AORTA

The ascending aorta forms the right upper cardiovascular border on the anterior view along with the superior vena cava. After the age of about 40 years, the aorta elongates and the ascending portion bulges to the right beyond the border of the superior vena cava. On the lateral view it is not well seen unless it is elongated or dilated, in which case it encroaches on the retrosternal air space and may reach the posterior border of the sternum.

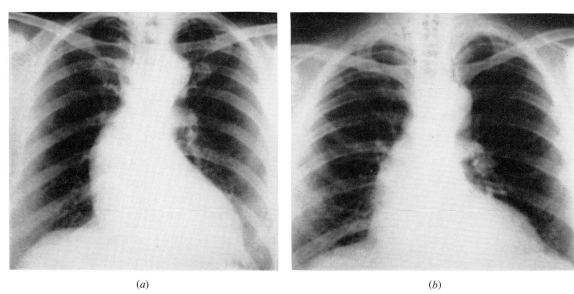

(a) (b)

Fig. 51 (above). Dilatation or elongation? (a) Elongated or unfolded aorta. (b) Dilated aorta in aortic regurgitation

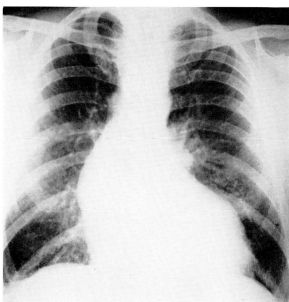

Figure 52 (right). Post-stenotic dilatation complicated by dissection

Causes of a prominent ascending aorta are:
(1) Aortic elongation (unfolded aorta).
(2) Aortic stenosis (*see* Chapter 26).
(3) Aortic regurgitation (*see* Chapter 26).
(4) Aneurysm; dissection, syphilis, Marfan's syndrome (*see* page 119), cystic medionecrosis, sinus of Valsalva, hypertension or atheroma.
(5) Coarctation with or without a bicuspid aortic valve (*see* Chapter 26).
(6) Fallot's tetralogy (*see* Chapters 19 and 20), pulmonary atresia (*see* page 182), truncus arteriosus (*see* page 208).

When the ascending aorta bulges to the right or anteriorly, it is often difficult to tell whether this is due to elongation or to dilatation (*Figure 51*). The reason is that in either projection, only one of its borders can be identified: in the anterior view its left border merges with the heart, and in the lateral view its posterior border does so. Elongation usually affects the whole of the thoracic aorta with prominence of the aortic arch and descending aorta, but occasionally it is confined to the ascending aorta and may then be misdiagnosed as dilatation. When there is doubt, the aorta is best described as prominent.

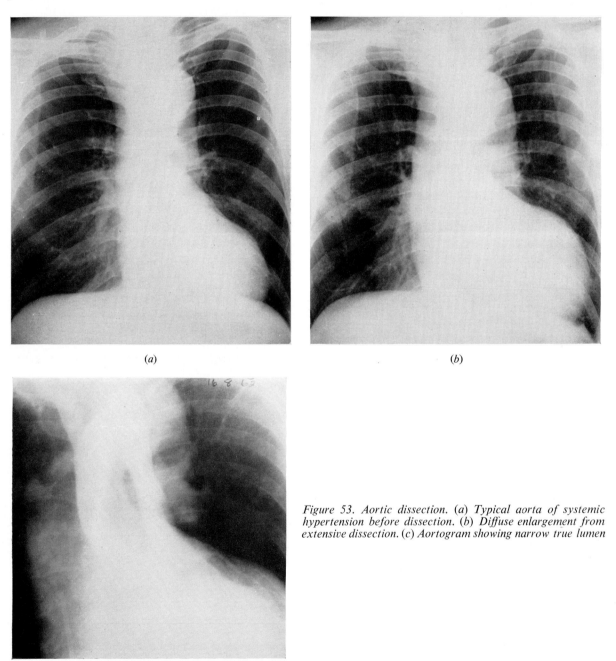

(a)

(b)

Figure 53. Aortic dissection. (a) Typical aorta of systemic hypertension before dissection. (b) Diffuse enlargement from extensive dissection. (c) Aortogram showing narrow true lumen

(c)

In aortic stenosis the only abnormality may be slight bulging of the ascending aorta beyond the superior vena caval border (*see Figure 322*). This is a particularly valuable sign in children and young adults, provided the patient is not rotated. Exposure of the film with slight rotation of the patient into the left anterior oblique position may render a normal ascending aorta prominent, and rotation into the right anterior oblique may hide a dilated aorta. Post-stenotic dilatation is slowly progressive and may attain a very large size suggesting the diagnosis of an aneurysm; indeed, aortic dissection is an occasional complication of post-stenotic dilatation (*Figure 52*). The latter occurs in fixed sub-aortic stenosis but less frequently than in valvar stenosis, and is therefore not an important differentiating point between the two. The ascending aorta is not dilated in hypertrophic obstructive cardiomyopathy, but it may bulge to the right due to lengthening of the long axis of the left ventricle with upward and outward displacement of the ascending aorta. In supravalvar stenosis the aorta is usually invisible.

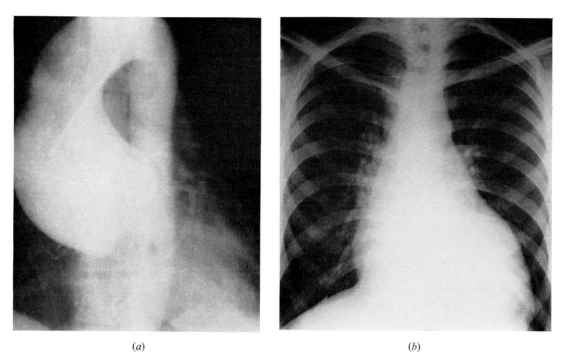

(*a*)　　　　　　　　　　　　　　　　　　　(*b*)

Figure 54. Marfan aorta. (a) Aortogram showing dilated aortic root. (b) Little or no aortic dilatation seen as aneurysm is intrapericardial

More diffuse dilatation of the ascending aorta is the rule in aortic regurgitation, sometimes with extension into the aortic arch (*see Figure 331*). In patients with aortic regurgitation and systolic hypertension, the descending aorta may be elongated (but not dilated). An unusually large ascending aorta is seen with congenital anomalies of the aortic root such as aorto/left ventricular tunnel, and this association is particularly important in children (*see Figure 332*). Gross diffuse aortic dilatation suggests disease of the aortic wall, in which case the regurgitation is primarily due to ring dilatation. Dissecting aneurysm usually begins above the aortic valve and causes regurgitation by involving the aortic ring and interfering with cusp closure. It may track downwards into the pericardium, spread to the entire aorta (*Figure 53*) (DeBakey type 1—DeBakey *et al.*, 1965), or remain confined to the ascending portion (DeBakey type 2). Aortic root aneurysm due to the Marfan syndrome (*see* page 119) or to cystic medionecrosis is usually dumbbell-shaped and rarely extends beyond the origin of the innominate artery (*see Figure 169*). A small aneurysm may cause aortic regurgitation while still occupying an intrapericardial position and producing no bulge on the chest x-ray (Keene *et al.*, 1971) (*Figure 54*). Calcification is seen most often in a syphilitic aneurysm, but is occasionally present in a chronic dissection or in a sinus of Valsalva aneurysm. Dilatation of the ascending aorta in systemic hypertension may be of sufficient severity, particularly in the West Indian population, to cause aortic regurgitation; in these patients the whole thoracic aorta is usually both elongated and dilated. In coarctation the ascending aorta is often dilated whether there is a bicuspid aortic valve or not, but dilatation is greater when there is haemodynamically significant valve disease.

In Fallot's tetralogy, pulmonary atresia and truncus arteriosus the whole ascending aorta is wide due to abnormal partitioning of the truncus by the spiral septum (*see Figure 251*). This is a valuable sign in the differential diagnosis from other causes of congenital cyanotic heart disease in which trunco-conal partitioning is normal, for example pulmonary stenosis and right-to-left shunt at atrial level.

AORTIC ARCH

The normal aortic arch crosses from right to left in front of the trachea and then arches over and behind the left main bronchus, passing backwards and downwards to the level of the body of T.4, where it lies just to the left of the midline. On the anterior view its distal part forms a rounded opacity which is termed the aortic knuckle or knob. Below the age of five years the knuckle may not be visible, lying within the contour of the mediastinum, but after this it gradually increases in prominence continuing after growth has ceased. After the age of 40 years the knuckle may be displaced upwards and to the left by general aortic elongation. Thus allowance for age must always be made when assessing the size and shape of the knuckle, particularly in the diagnosis of systemic hypertension (*see Figure 53a*). Calcified plaques are common and do not necessarily reflect the presence of atherosclerosis in other arteries. They tend to be situated in slight depressions of the aortic wall at the site of the ligamentum arteriosum and just below the origin of the left subclavian artery, from whence they spread in a circumferential fashion.

Causes of an enlarged aortic knuckle are:

(1) Systemic hypertension (elongation more than dilatation).

(2) Aneurysm; atheroma, dissection, syphilis, trauma; rarely Marfan's syndrome (*see* page 119) and cystic medionecrosis.

(3) Aortic regurgitation (*see* Chapter 26).

(4) Ductus arteriosus (*see* Chapter 18).

(5) Fallot (*see* page 180), pulmonary atresia (*see* page 182), truncus arteriosus (*see* page 208).

Systemic hypertension, if of sufficient severity and duration, produces marked aortic elongation with some dilatation. Although changes usually involve the entire thoracic aorta, they are often best appreciated in the aortic arch. Prominence of the aortic knuckle due to elongation is a normal age change and must not be confused with the hypertensive aorta (*see Figure 53a*): familiarity with the appearances of the normal aortic knuckle at all ages is essential (for appreciating not only its undue prominence but also its apparent smallness). Aneurysm of this part of the aorta is most frequently due to atheroma, syphilis, dissection or trauma, and is rare in Marfan's syndrome and cystic medionecrosis.

Dissection commonly begins just distal to the left subclavian artery, widening the aortic knuckle and a varying length of the descending aorta (DeBakey type 3—DeBakey *et al.*, 1965), often with an irregular contour (*Figure 55*). A left pleural effusion is common. Syphilis tends to affect the ascending aorta more than the arch.

Traumatic aneurysms most frequently involve the junction of the aortic arch and the descending thoracic aorta: they are deceleration injuries and the aortic tear occurs in the region of the ligamentum arteriosum, which is a relatively fixed point. The intima and media may be severed and the adventitia may be the only layer containing the blood. If rupture or surgery does not follow, the aneurysm may calcify (*Figure 56*). Marfan's syndrome and cystic medionecrosis usually involve the ascending aorta, the aorta beyond the innominate artery being normal, but the whole thoracic aorta sometimes dilates. Aneurysms involving the aortic arch may be exactly simulated by a malignant mass encircling the aorta (*Figure 57*).

In ductus arteriosus, funnel-shaped dilatation of the aorta (the infundibulum) occurs around the entry of the ductus, and the knuckle is broadened both laterally and downwards. This is best seen on the penetrated anterior view and can rarely be appreciated on the lateral (*see Figures 218–222*). It is not usually visible before 10 years but increases with age, being fairly constantly seen over the age of 20 years. Any adult patient who has a continuous murmur below the left clavicle without an identifiable infundibulum should be suspected of having some other cause for the murmur such as coronary or aortic sinus fistula. Very occasionally the ductus itself may be aneurysmal and produce a similar opacity, but this usually follows surgery.

In Fallot, pulmonary atresia and truncus arteriosus, the aortic knuckle and ascending aorta are wide due to uneven partitioning of the truncus, a knuckle of normal size being the rule in other types of

36

cyanotic congenital heart disease. Apparent smallness of the aortic knuckle is a constant feature of an atrial septal defect and helps in differentiating it from a ventricular septal defect, the latter usually showing a normal-sized knuckle and ductus arteriosus in which, particularly in adults, an infundibulum is seen.

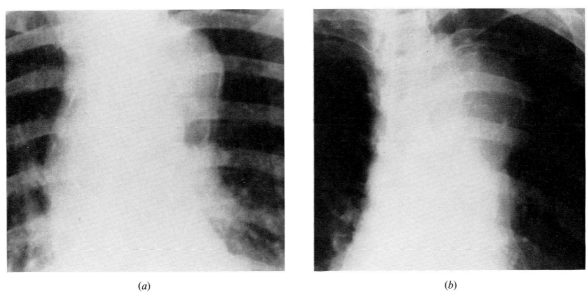

(a)   (b)

Figure 55. Aortic dissection. (a) Dilated aortic arch with calcified intima. (b) Dissection outside intimal calcification

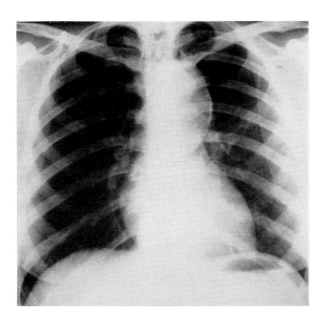

Figure 56. Calcified traumatic aneurysm

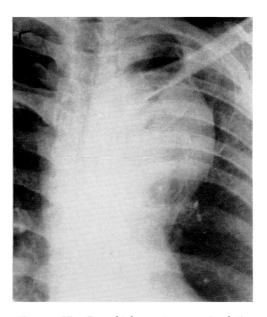

Figure 57. Bronchial carcinoma simulating aortic aneurysm

A small aortic knuckle is associated with severe mitral stenosis and reflects a severely limited cardiac output; the size of the aortic knuckle in general reflects the severity of mitral valve disease. An abnormal contour to the aortic knuckle is the most constant sign of coarctation (*see* Chapter 26) and is more often seen than rib notching. The following types are found (*see Figure 334*).

Double knuckle, in which the upper bulge is formed by the left subclavian artery and/or the aortic arch and the lower bulge by post-stenotic dilatation of the descending aorta.

High knuckle, formed by the left subclavian artery and/or the aortic arch without appreciable post-stenotic dilatation.

37

Low knuckle, formed by post-stenotic dilatation, but without prominence of the left subclavian artery or the aorta.

Flat knuckle, due to any combination of (*a*) absence of left subclavian artery, (*b*) small aortic arch, (*c*) narrow isthmus, (*d*) no post-stenotic dilatation.

Right aortic arch

A right aortic arch is present when the aorta arches over the right main bronchus to the right of the trachea. The majority of patients with a right arch have congenital heart lesions which usually involve abnormal development of the trunco-conal septum (Stewart *et al.*, 1966), and the following is the incidence of right arch in the various lesions.

(1) Truncus arteriosus—50 per cent (Keith *et al.*, 1967).

(2) Cyanotic Fallot's tetralogy and pulmonary atresia with ventricular septal defect—25 per cent (Hastreiter *et al.*, 1966; Jefferson *et al.*, 1972).

(3) Acyanotic Fallot's tetralogy—25 per cent (Nadas, 1963).

(4) Uncomplicated ventricular septal defect—2·6 per cent (Hastreiter *et al.*, 1966).

Most people with a right aortic arch have congenital heart disease, but some have a vascular ring. The ring may or may not cause symptoms.

There are two common types of right aortic arch.

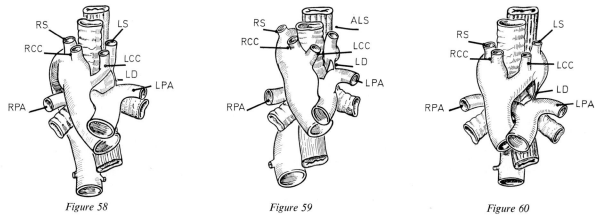

Figure 58   Figure 59   Figure 60

RCC = right common carotid artery.   RS = right subclavian artery.   ALS = anomalous left subclavian artery.   LPA = left pulmonary artery.
LCC = left common carotid artery.   LS = left subclavian artery.   RPA = right pulmonary artery.   LD = left ductus.

Figure 58. Right aortic arch with mirror image branching of the great vessels

Figure 59. Right aortic arch with anomalous left subclavian artery

Figure 60. Double aortic arch

Right arch with mirror image branching of great vessels (*Figure 58*)

Congenital heart disease is almost invariable. The right fourth arch and right dorsal aorta form the right aortic arch. The left fourth arch contributes to the left subclavian artery, and the left dorsal aorta distal to this is absent. The branching of the brachio-cephalic arteries is the mirror image of normal, the left innominate artery being the first branch and dividing into the left common carotid and left subclavian arteries. The ductus or ligamentum arteriosum may be on either side, but if on the left it connects the left subclavian artery to the left pulmonary artery. The descending aorta lies to the right of the midline. On the chest film the arch is seen as an opacity in the right tracheo-bronchial angle without any similar structure being detectable on the other side (*Figure 61a*). Because of its association with uneven trunco-conal septation, it is usually wide and often high, and on the penetrated anterior view the descending aorta is normally well seen on the right, approaching the midline as it descends to the diaphragm.

Right arch with anomalous left subclavian artery (*Figure 59*)

A vascular ring is much more common than congenital heart disease. The right fourth arch and right dorsal aorta form the right aortic arch in the same way as in the first type. The left fourth arch is absent; the first branch from the aortic arch is the left common carotid, and the left dorsal aorta persists, passing behind the oesophagus (*Figure 61b, c*) to give off the left subclavian artery, from which the ductus or ligamentum arteriosum may arise. The descending aorta may lie on either side of the midline. This arrangement may result in a vascular ring around the trachea and oesophagus formed by the aortic

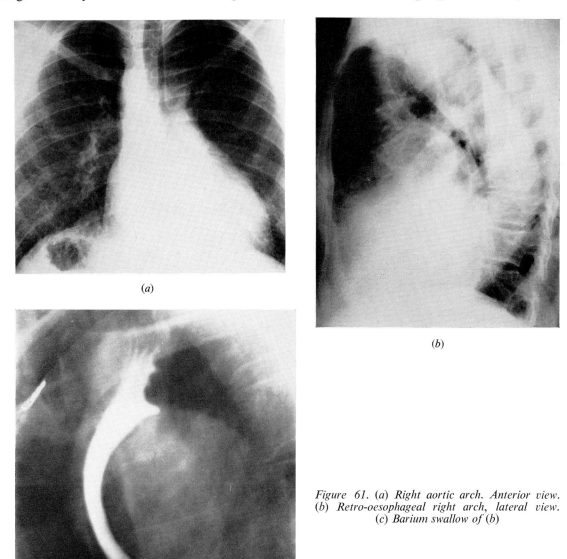

(a)

(b)

(c)

Figure 61. (a) Right aortic arch. Anterior view.
(b) Retro-oesophageal right arch, lateral view.
(c) Barium swallow of (b)

arch to the right, the left subclavian posteriorly, the ductus or ligamentum to the left and the pulmonary artery anteriorly. The appearances on the plain film differ from those of the first type in that the aortic knuckle is always normal in size as it lies in the right tracheo-bronchial angle, and there is a prominent retro-oesophageal component formed by the distal part of the right arch, the upper part of the descending aorta or the proximal bulbous portion of the left subclavian artery. An opacity is visible posteriorly in the upper mediastinum which indents the trachea and the barium-filled oesophagus.

Cervical aorta

Occasionally the aortic arch may lie so high that it presents as a pulsatile swelling in the neck. In a high proportion of cases, the arch is on the right and the descending aorta lies on the same side as the aortic arch until it reaches the mid-thorax, where it crosses to descend on the other side. This anomaly may not be associated with congenital heart disease, but there is often abnormal branching or atresia of the brachio-cephalic vessels.

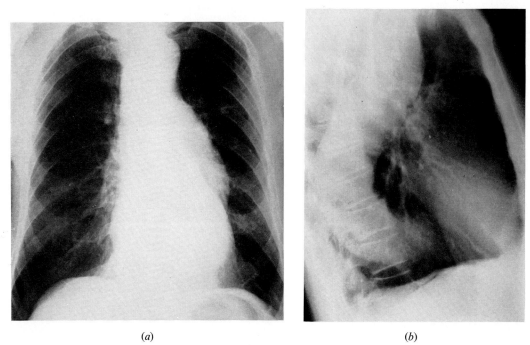

(a)   (b)

Figure 62. Aneurysm of descending aorta. (a) Anterior view—right side of descending aorta not visible, elongation only not excluded. (b) Lateral view—confirms aortic dilatation

Double aortic arch

The fourth arch and the dorsal aorta persist on each side to form a vascular ring around the trachea and oesophagus (*Figure 60*). The size of each arch varies, but the right is usually larger than the left, which may be atretic; only the right arch may be visible on the chest film, and the appearances may be mistaken for those of a single right arch. The common carotid and subclavian arteries arise separately on each side, and the descending aorta may lie on either side of the midline. This is usually an isolated anomaly which can cause symptoms of vascular ring, but if congenital heart disease is present, it is most commonly of the Fallot type. Barium swallow helps to identify each arch.

DESCENDING AORTA

The normal descending aorta begins at the level of the body of T.4 and lies on the anterior surface of the thoracic spine just to the left of the midline. Elongation of the aorta due to ageing causes progressive leftward displacement of the descending aorta, which, with excessive lengthening, may bulge so much that an aneurysm is simulated. Occasionally the lower half bulges to the right, presenting an increased density within the right heart border, which again resembles an aneurysm. Differentiation between aneurysm and unfolding is not possible unless both sides of the aorta can be seen on the postero-anterior and lateral views (*Figure 62*). Displacement of the descending aorta to the left can also result from left atrial dilatation, but differs from displacement due to elongation in that it is maximal at mid-thorax (at mid-atrial level) and that no elongation of the rest of the aorta is apparent (*see* page 19).

CHAPTER 5

Position of the Heart, Chambers and Great Vessels

POSITION OF THE HEART AND VISCERA

Situs solitus means a normal position of the thoracic and abdominal organs, namely the heart to the left, the larger lobe of the liver and the inferior vena cava on the right, and the stomach on the left (*Figure 63*).

The cranial part of the heart is termed the base and is formed by the aorta and the pulmonary artery. The caudal part comprises the atria and ventricles. The left lower cardiac border is normally formed by the left ventricle, the most convex portion of which is termed the apex. The right lower cardiac border, formed by the right atrium, is less convex. At the level of the apex, one-third of the heart lies to the right and two-thirds lie to the left of the midline. With very few exceptions the position of the apex indicates the side of the ventricles.

Almost invariably the larger lobe of the liver is on the same side as the right atrium because there is viscero-atrial concordance (*see* atrial localization, page 42). Thus in situs inversus, which is the mirror image of normal, the larger lobe of the liver and the right atrium are on the left and the apex of the heart is usually on the right. In some patients with asplenia or polysplenia, it may be impossible to determine the position of the right atrium and the larger lobe of the liver as there is a tendency to bilateral symmetry such as common atrium, transverse liver and bilateral venae cavae. There is also malrotation of the gastro-intestinal tract. The situs is then indeterminate and the rule of viscero-atrial concordance cannot be applied.

Whereas exceptions to viscero-atrial concordance are extremely rare, discordance between the side of the ventricular portion of the heart (the apex) and the viscero-atrial situs is not uncommon and takes two forms.

Dextroversion: apex on the right with situs solitus (*Figure 64*).

Laevoversion: apex on the left with situs inversus (*Figure 65*).

The third cardiac malposition is *dextrocardia*, in which the apex is on the right with situs inversus (*Figure 66*). Here there is ventricule-atrial concordance.

The relative height of the right and left leaves of the diaphragm is determined by the position of the cardiac apex and not by the larger lobe of the liver. In normal situs solitus the left leaf of the diaphragm is lower than the right, while in situs inversus with dextrocardia the opposite applies. In dextroversion and laevoversion, the diaphragm is also lower on the side corresponding to the apex (*see Figures 76* and *77*).

Malpositions of the heart are considered further on page 48.

POSITION OF CARDIAC CHAMBERS AND GREAT VESSELS

The term right atrium refers to the anatomical right atrium, into which drain the systemic veins whether it lies on the right or the left side of the left atrium. Similarly, the term left atrium means the anatomical left atrium, into which drain the pulmonary veins whatever its position. The terms right ventricle and left ventricle are used in the same way; amongst other characteristics, the right ventricle has a tricuspid valve and a crista supraventricularis separating the pulmonary from the tricuspid rings, and the left ventricle has a mitral valve with no conal muscle between the aortic and mitral valve rings (aortic/mitral continuity—*Figure 67*).

Normally in situs solitus the cardiac septa form an angle of about 45 degrees with the coronal plane, the anterior end (the ventricular septum) lying to the left and the posterior end (the atrial septum) to

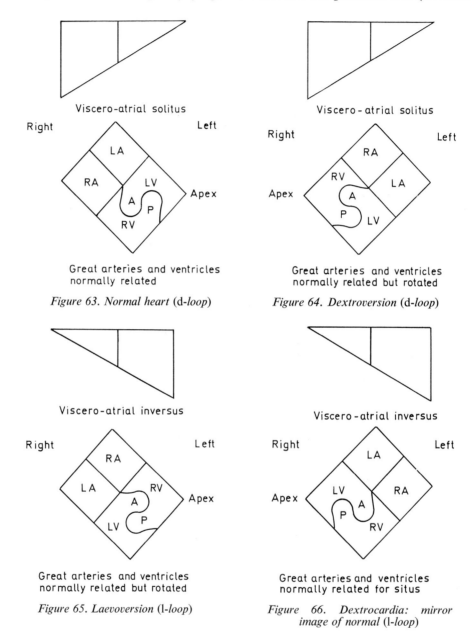

Figure 63. Normal heart (d-loop)

Figure 64. Dextroversion (d-loop)

Figure 65. Laevoversion (l-loop)

Figure 66. Dextrocardia: mirror image of normal (l-loop)

the right of the midline. Thus, the right ventricle lies to the right and in front of the left ventricle. The ventricles and great vessels form a 180 degrees spiral which is clockwise when viewed from above, so that the ascending aorta comes to lie to the right and anteriorly relative to the left ventricle, which is left and posterior, and the bifurcation of the pulmonary trunk is left and posterior relative to the right ventricle, which is right and anterior. This spiral relationship indicates normally related great vessels in contradistinction to all forms of transposition in which they lie parallel.

Atrial localization

During the third week of foetal life the left horn of the sinus venosus diminishes in size, ultimately to become the coronary sinus and drain into the right atrium. Through the disappearance of left-sided veins, the rest of the systemic venous return is diverted into the right horn of the sinus, which is absorbed into the right atrium. Events dictate, therefore, that the inferior vena cava will come to lie on the same side as the right atrium, and as its post-hepatic portion develops in relation to the larger lobe of the liver, the rule of hepato-cavo-atrial concordance is established. For practical purposes the rule may be extended to mean viscero-atrial concordance. By plain radiography of the upper abdomen, it is usually an easy matter to determine on which side the anatomical right atrium lies, but in practice it is only necessary to localize the gastric air bubble on the chest x-ray and assume that the right atrium lies on the opposite side. Thus the presence of viscero-atrial situs solitus or viscero-atrial situs inversus can be determined. If the liver is seen to lie transversely, polysplenia or asplenia should be suspected. If this is confirmed, it may be impossible to determine the situs on plain films (or even after catheterization and angiocardiography) because of bilateral symmetry.

Figure 67. Normal ventricular anatomy in lateral angiograms. (a) Right ventricle showing crista separating tricuspid and pulmonary valve rings. (b) Left ventricle showing aortic/mitral continuity

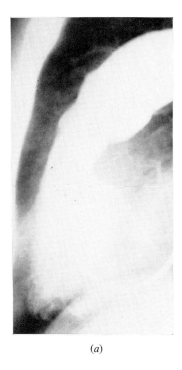
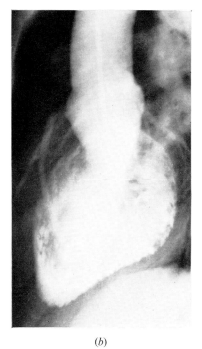

(a)   (b)

Ventricular and great vessel localization

About the twenty-third day of foetal life, the primitive heart tube normally bends anteriorly and to the right to form the bulbo-ventricular loop (dextro- or *d*-loop). As the truncus arteriosus and the right ventricle develop from the distal right anterior part of the loop and the left ventricle from the proximal left posterior part, the right ventricle lies to the right of and anterior to the left ventricle. Later, the trunco-conal septum divides the outflow tract of the ventricles and truncus in a 180 degrees spiral. This results in a complete cross-over between the main portion of each ventricle and its great vessel. The ascending aorta therefore occupies a position opposite to that of the left ventricle. It lies above and corresponds to the spatial position of the right ventricle (right and anterior). In later sections it will be seen that the ascending aorta indicates the position of the right ventricle whether the great vessels are normally related or transposed and whether the ventricles are normally situated or inverted.

ABNORMAL POSITION OF ATRIA

As there is viscero-atrial concordance, the right atrium is on the right side in situs solitus with or without dextroversion (ventricles rotated to the right) and on the left side in situs inversus with or without laevoversion (ventricles rotated to the left). The exceptions to the rule of viscero-atrial concordance are so rare as to be of little practical importance, but they have to be mentioned. They are as follows.

(1) The pre-hepatic portion of the inferior vena cava may lie on the left side with cross-over in the liver, the post-hepatic portion entering the right atrium on the right side.

(2) With absence of the post-hepatic portion of the inferior vena cava, a left pre-hepatic inferior vena cava may drain into a right superior vena cava via the hemiazygos and azygos systems.

(3) The visceral and atrial situs may be uncertain in asplenia and polysplenia.

ABNORMAL POSITION OF VENTRICLES AND GREAT VESSELS

If the side of the ascending aorta can be detected on the plain films, it provides information about the position of the right and left ventricles. It has been mentioned that, when the great vessels are normally related, they form a spiral of 180 degrees in such a way that the ascending aorta comes to lie opposite the left ventricle and on the same side as the right ventricle. When there is transposition of the great vessels, no such twist occurs because the trunco-conal septum develops as a straight partition between the aorta and the pulmonary artery, which lie parallel to each other.

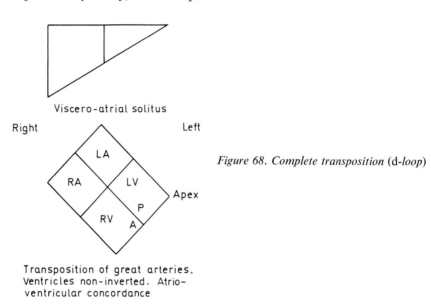

Figure 68. Complete transposition (d-loop)

In complete transposition (*Figure 68*) the heart tube bends normally to the right, forming a *d*-loop so that the right ventricle lies to the right of the ventricular septum. The great vessels are parallel. The aorta originates from the right ventricle and travels directly upwards from the base of the heart in the right anterior position, corresponding in spatial position to the right ventricle; the aortic valve lies to the right and in front of the pulmonary valve, and *d*-transposition is said to be present (*Figure 69*).

In corrected transposition (*Figure 70*), the heart tube bends to the left, forming an *l*-loop so that the right ventricle lies to the left of the ventricular septum and the ventricles are inverted. The great vessels are parallel. The aorta originates from the right ventricle and lies in a left anterior position, again corresponding to the position of the right ventricle; the aortic valve lies to the left and in front of the pulmonary valve, and *l*-transposition is said to be present (*Figure 71*).

The ascending aorta therefore corresponds to the position of the right ventricle relative to the septum, whether or not there is transposition or ventricular inversion (aortic localization of the right ventricle). The rule also applies in double outflow right ventricle. In single ventricle the ascending aorta indicates the right ventricular side of the ventricular complex. In truncus arteriosus, the truncus may be regarded as the equivalent of the ascending aorta and indicates the position of the right ventricle. There are only rare exceptions to this relationship between the great vessels and the ventricles (Van Praagh, 1967); for example, there may be a *d*-loop (right ventricle to the right) with an *l*-transposition (aorta to the left and anterior).

Two further points may be helpful in the diagnosis of transposition on the plain films. First, in *d*-transposition the aorta tends to be much more in front of the pulmonary artery than to its right side,

44

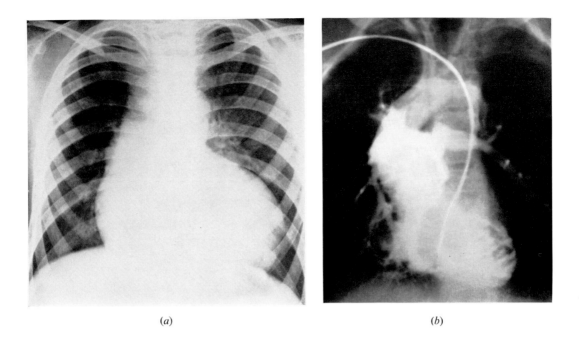

(a)   (b)

Figure 69. Complete transposition. (a) Anterior view. (b) Anterior angiogram—aorta to right of pulmonary trunk. (c) Lateral angiogram—aorta anterior to pulmonary trunk

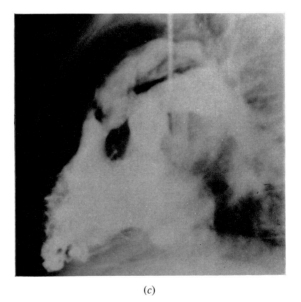

(c)

and thus a narrow vascular pedicle is common (*Figures 72* and *73*); but in *l*-transposition the aorta is usually quite far to the left of the pulmonary artery, and thus the vascular pedicle is often broad with a prominent aorta forming the left upper border of the base of the heart (*see Figure 71a*). Secondly, a *d*-loop is commoner with a left apex and an *l*-loop with a right apex, hence the common association of corrected transposition with dextroversion (*see below*).

It will be seen that in complete transposition with situs inversus and dextrocardia there is an *l*-loop, since the heart is a mirror image of the *d*-loop in complete transposition with situs solitus (*Figure 73*). Similarly, in corrected transposition with situs inversus and dextrocardia there is a *d*-loop, since the heart is a mirror image of the *l*-loop in corrected transposition with situs solitus (*Figures 74* and *75*). Dextroversion and laevoversion do not affect the type of loop in transposition.

45

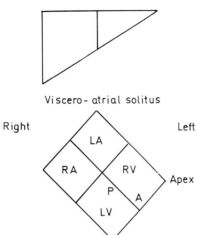

Viscero- atrial solitus

Right   Left

LA

RA   RV   Apex

P   A

LV

Transposition of great arteries.
Ventricles inverted. Atrio-ventricular
discordance

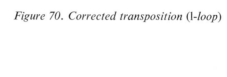

Figure 70. Corrected transposition (l-loop)

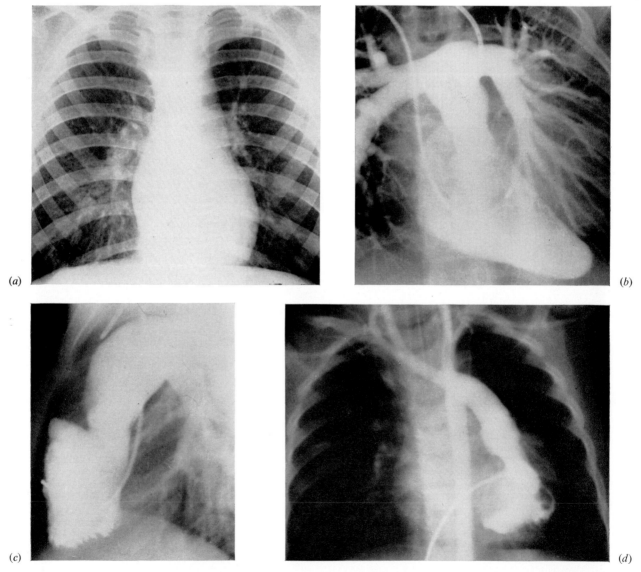

(a)   (b)

(c)   (d)

Figure 71. Corrected transposition. (a) Anterior view—left upper cardiac border formed by ascending aorta. (b) Anterior angiogram—central position of pulmonary trunk. (c) Lateral angiogram—pulmonary trunk relatively posterior. (d) Anterior angiogram—aorta to left. (Cont.)

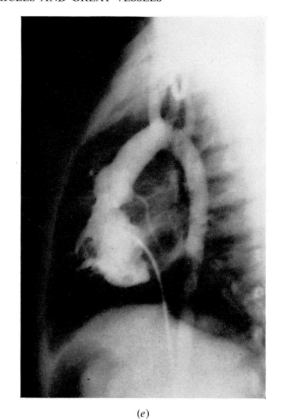

Figure 71. (e) Lateral angiogram—aorta relatively anterior

(*e*)

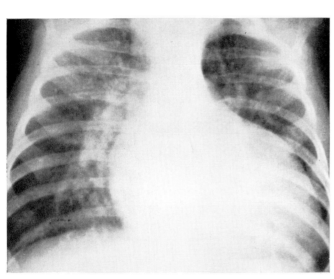

Figure 72. Complete transposition with narrow vascular pedicle

It must be emphasized that angiocardiography is essential in the diagnosis of transposition and associated defects. The basic angiocardiographic features of transposition are as follows (*see Figures 69b, c* and *71b–e*).

(1) A sub-aortic conus—the hallmark of transposition (Van Praagh *et al.*, 1967). Angiocardiographic diagnosis depends on establishing that:

    (*a*) The crista (conus) lies below the aortic valve.

    (*b*) There is discontinuity between the aortic and mitral valve rings and/or continuity between the pulmonary and mitral valve rings due to absence of sub-pulmonary conus.

    (*c*) The aortic valve lies cranial to the pulmonary valve.

(2) Evidence that the trunco-conal septum developed as a straight partition, shown by parallel great vessels.

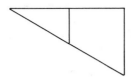

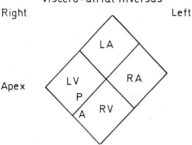

Transposition of great arteries.
Ventricles non-inverted. Atrio-
ventricular concordance

*Figure 73. Dextrocardia: complete
transposition (l-loop)*

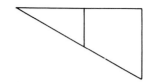

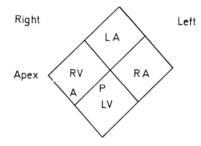

Transposition of great arteries
Ventricles inverted. Atrio-
ventricular discordance

*Figure 74. Dextrocardia: corrected
transposition (d-loop)*

ABNORMAL POSITION OF THE HEART

An abnormal position of the heart may result from developmental malposition or from displacement.

MALPOSITION

Three malpositions are recognized (Anselmi *et al.*, 1972).
Dextrocardia: apex on the right with situs inversus (*see Figure 66*).
Dextroversion: apex on the right with situs solitus (*see Figures 64* and *76*).
Laevoversion: apex on the left with situs inversus (*see Figures 65* and *77*).

Dextrocardia

In dextrocardia, the most common malposition, congenital heart lesions are rare (approximately 10 per cent), probably because the apex is appropriate to the situs. When present, the anomalies are usually simple and uncomplicated by transposition or ventricular inversion.

Dextroversion

In dextroversion the apex is inappropriate to the situs and complex congenital heart lesions with cyanosis are common (approximately 90 per cent). Transposition is found in about two-thirds and ventricular inversion in about half the cases. Pulmonary stenosis is common, and the following abnormalities of cardiac septation may be found.

Trunco-conal septum
   Failure to twist: transposition, double outflow right ventricle.
   Deviation: Fallot's tetralogy, pulmonary atresia.
   Failure to develop: truncus arteriosus.

Ventricular septum
   Ventricular septal defect.
   Single ventricle.

Atrial septum
   Atrial septal defect.

Laevoversion

In the least common malposition of laevoversion, again with an apex inappropriate to the situs, the incidence and types of congenital heart disease are similar to those found in dextroversion.

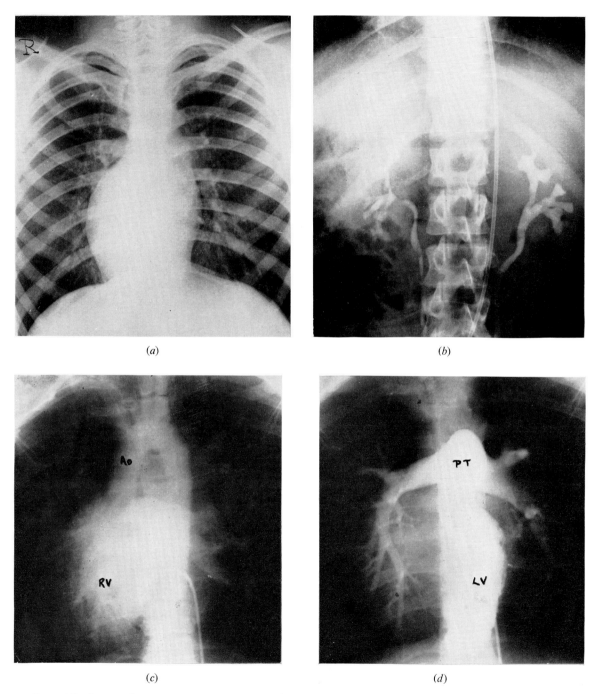

Figure 75. *Corrected transposition, situs inversus, dextrocardia. (a) Anterior view. (b) Abdomen showing liver on left, left kidney lower than right. (c) Anterior angiogram—aorta to right above right ventricle. (d) Anterior angiogram— central pulmonary trunk*

The side of the apex, and thus the ventricular portion of the heart, is usually determined without difficulty on the plain chest x-ray but may be confirmed in doubtful cases by palpation of the precordium, auscultation of the heart or study of the electrocardiogram.

49

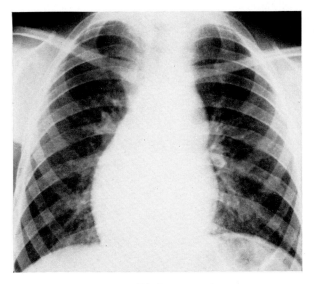
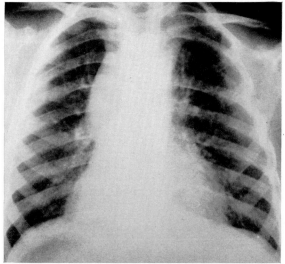

Figure 76. Dextroversion   *Figure 77. Laevoversion*

DISPLACEMENT OF THE HEART

The heart may be displaced from its normal position by:
(1) Eccentric cardiac enlargement.
(2) Pericardial defect (*see* page 288).
(3) Pulmonary collapse, fibrosis or hypoplasia.
(4) Pleural effusion, pneumothorax or pleural fibrosis.
(5) Thoracic deformity: scoliosis, flat chest, depressed sternum (*see* Chapter 13).
(6) Unilateral diaphragmatic elevation.

The commonest cause of eccentric cardiac enlargement is pure right atrial and right ventricular dilatation, as exemplified in atrial septal defect. Because the venae cavae are relatively fixed, the heart is displaced and rotated into the left chest. Tumours and cysts of the heart and pericardium are rare causes of eccentric cardiac enlargement and displacement. Unilateral pericardial defect is usually left-sided and the heart is deviated to the left. In pulmonary collapse, fibrosis or hypoplasia and in pleural fibrosis, the heart is pulled towards the side of the disease; in addition, there may be other signs of reduction in lung volume such as fissure displacement, compensatory emphysema, diaphragmatic elevation and narrowing of intercostal spaces. In pleural effusion or pneumothorax, the heart is pushed away from the abnormal side. Quite marked deviation of the heart may be caused by elevation of one or other leaf of the diaphragm, as seen in eventration or phrenic paralysis.

ASPLENIA AND POLYSPLENIA

Congenital absence of the spleen or the presence of multiple spleens is associated with abnormalities reflecting persistence of early foetal bilaterality. Although viscero-atrial situs can usually be established, it may be uncertain because of isomerism (bilateral symmetry such as transverse liver or bilateral vena cava) and abdominal heterotaxy (malrotation of the gut with gastric fundus on either side). Malposition of the heart is common (*Figure 78*).

Asplenia suggests bilateral right-sidedness because:
(1) Both atria may resemble the right atrium.
(2) Both lungs have three lobes.
(3) Both lobes of the liver resemble the right lobe.

Polysplenia (Moller *et al.*, 1967) suggests bilateral left-sidedness because:
(1) There is absence of a normal right-sided structure—the gall bladder.
(2) Both lungs have two lobes.
(3) There is an excess of a left-sided organ—2 to 9 spleens of equal size.

Congenital cardiac anomalies which have a high incidence in both asplenia and polysplenia are:
(1) Bilateral superior vena cava.
(2) Common atrium or atrial septal defect.
(3) Anomalous pulmonary venous drainage.
(4) Ostium primum or complete canal.
(5) Single ventricle or ventricular septal defect.
(6) Transposition—often corrected.
(7) Malposition—often dextroversion.

Cyanotic heart disease with pulmonary stenosis or atresia is common with asplenia, whereas with polysplenia there is usually a left-to-right shunt without cyanosis. In polysplenia the hepatic portion of the inferior vena cava may be absent, with caval blood draining via the azygos vein.

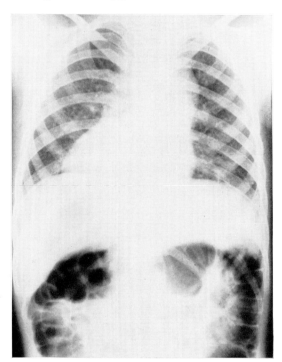

Figure 78. Asplenia with transverse liver and dextroversion

SUMMARY

If the heart occupies an abnormal position in the chest, the cause may be embryological malposition or physical displacement.

The position of the apex (the ventricular portion of the heart) and its relation to the situs indicate the type of malposition—dextrocardia, dextroversion or laevoversion.

Congenital heart disease is uncommon and simple in dextrocardia, but common and complex in dextroversion and laevoversion.

Whatever the position of the heart, two principles are applicable to the localization of the chambers and great vessels.

Viscero-atrial concordance: the right atrium lies on the side of the larger lobe of the liver (or opposite the gastric fundus).

Aortic localization of right ventricle: the right ventricle lies on the side of the ascending aorta whether or not there is transposition or ventricular inversion.

It is often impossible to diagnose transposition on the plain chest radiograph, but a narrow base to the heart is suggestive of complete transposition and a wide base suggests corrected transposition.

A transversely lying liver suggests asplenia or polysplenia. The lungs show oligaemia in asplenia and plethora in polysplenia. In both conditions there is often malposition of the heart. Occasionally the viscero-atrial situs cannot be determined.

CHAPTER 6

Calcification of the Cardiovascular System

INTRODUCTION

Cardiovascular calcification may be dystrophic or metastatic. In the former case, calcification occurs in degenerate or dead tissue with normal calcium metabolism, but it has been suggested that hypercalcaemia may accelerate dystrophic calcification (Gould, 1968). Cardiovascular calcification is nearly always dystrophic. In metastatic calcification there is or has been hypercalcaemia and calcium may be seen in the myocardium, systemic arteries or pulmonary arteries. It may also be deposited in tissues outside the cardiovascular system.

The following types of dystrophic calcification may be encountered on the plain radiograph.

Endocardium
Endocardial thrombus in ventricles or atria; endomyocardial fibrosis.

Myocardium
Ventricular: aneurysm, infarct, surgical trauma, post-inflammatory, following rheumatic fever, diphtheria, tuberculosis, spread from aortic and mitral valves or pericardium.
Atrial: rheumatic heart disease.

Pericardium
Constrictive pericarditis, adherent pericardium.

Valves
Aortic valve: congenital monocuspid or bicuspid valve, rheumatic endocarditis, syphilis, aortic sclerosis, ankylosing spondylitis, Reiter's syndrome, rheumatoid arthritis, post-homograft and rarely autograft valve replacement.
Mitral valve: rheumatic endocarditis, subvalvar and ring calcification.
Pulmonary valve: pulmonary stenosis and/or regurgitation, pulmonary hypertension with or without shunts, homograft valve replacement.
Tricuspid valve: associated with pulmonary stenosis, tricuspid regurgitation, shunts.

Coronary arteries
Atheroma, fistula, aneurysm.

Ascending aorta
Syphilis, dissection, Marfan, cystic medionecrosis, atheroma, sinus aneurysm.

Aortic arch
Age change, atheroma, dissection, syphilis, ductus arteriosus, ductus aneurysm, arteritis.

Descending aorta
Atheroma, dissection, arteritis.

Pulmonary trunk and pulmonary arteries
Pulmonary hypertension.

Tumours and rare causes
Myxoma and other tumours, hydatid cyst, intravascular thrombus.

ENDOCARDIUM

Endocardial calcification may occasionally be encountered in diseases where endocardial thrombus or thickening occurs. It is rarely demonstrated in thrombus overlying infarcted myocardium or in left ventricular aneurysm. It may be seen in the cardiomyopathies characterized by endocardial thrombosis and thickening, particularly endomyocardial fibrosis. Endocardial calcification typically lies well inside the outline of the heart.

MYOCARDIUM

Myocardial calcification results, with but few exceptions, from coronary artery occlusion. Aneurysm of the left ventricle is usually present. When the left ventricular wall is particularly thin, the calcium lies

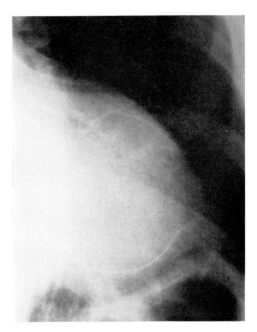

Figure 79. Calcified left ventricular aneurysm

peripherally and probably in the pleuropericardium rather than in the myocardium (*Figure 79*). Calcium is occasionally deposited in dead muscle with little chamber dilatation. The calcification is nearly always related to the antero-lateral part of the left ventricular wall, but may extend posteriorly. It is possible that rheumatic fever and other post-inflammatory states may rarely result in calcification of the ventricular myocardium. Calcification may spread from the aortic and mitral valve rings into the neighbouring left ventricular myocardium and ventricular septum, one result being heart block. Metastatic calcification is rare, but may be widespread (Testelli and Pilz, 1964). Patients are seen in whom myocardial calcification has no obvious cause (*Figure 80*). The distribution may then be unusual: Kirk and Russell (1966) reported two cases in which there was band-like calcification corresponding to the spiral muscles of the heart. One case had calcific aortic stenosis which may have acted as a starter for the myocardial calcification.

LEFT ATRIUM

Left atrial calcification, resulting from severe rheumatic involvement of the atrial wall, presents as straight or curved lines of calcification a few millimetres thick. It is usually most marked in the postero-superior aspect of the left atrium below the lower lobe bronchi, and may be confined to this area. If it is widespread, a complete ring of calcification is seen on the penetrated anterior view. On the lateral view, calcification appears C-shaped with the mitral valve lying in the open part of the 'C' (*Figure 81*). The mitral valve may or may not be calcified. The septal surface of the left atrium is usually free of calcium, but this cannot be appreciated on the anterior or lateral view as in both these views the atrial septum lies oblique to the x-ray beam. The appendix alone may show calcification; this is well seen on the left border on the anterior view, but may also be detected in the middle of the upper part of the heart on the

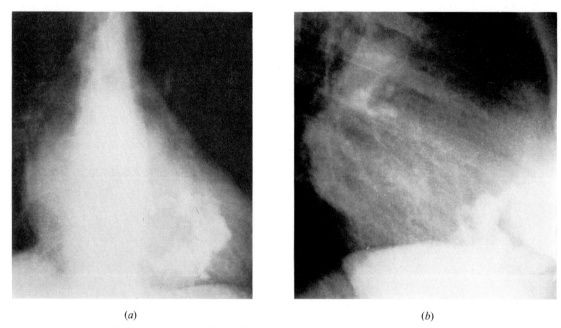

(a) (b)

Figure 80. Calcified myocardium of unknown cause. (a) Anterior view. (b) Lateral view

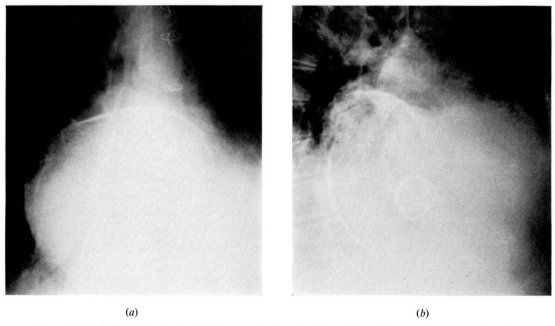

(a) (b)

Figure 81. Calcified left atrial wall. (a) Anterior view. (b) Lateral view (Starr valve in mitral orifice)

lateral view. Calcification rarely extends into the pulmonary veins. Thrombus, very often present within the calcified left atrium, may itself calcify and then thick laminated calcium may be detected (*Figure 82*).

The patient with calcification of the left atrium is usually female and middle-aged with severe mitral valve disease. Mitral stenosis is usually present, but there is evidence that some mitral regurgitation is always present and is important in the aetiology of wall calcification (Fuenmayor, 1959). The fact that calcification is most marked in the postero-superior part of the left atrium, the site of impact of the regurgitant jet, adds support to this. Most patients have other valves involved; atrial fibrillation is usually present, and a history of systemic embolism is common.

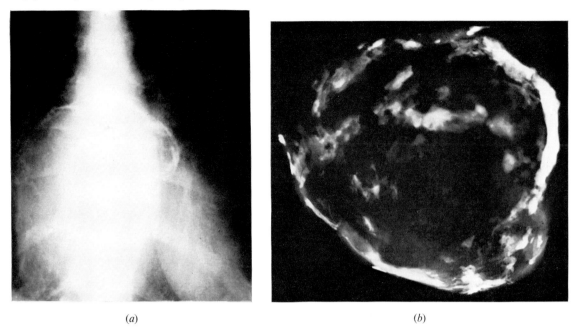

(a)   (b)

Figure 82. Calcified left atrial thrombus. (a) Anterior view. (b) Autopsy specimen

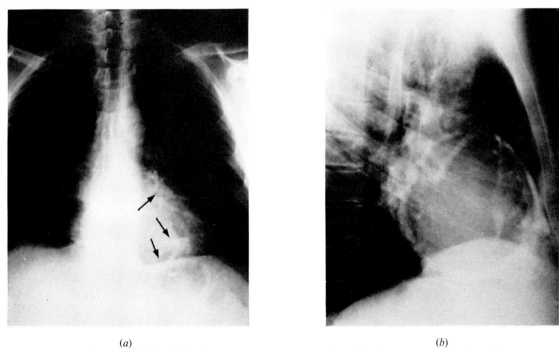

(a)   (b)

Figure 83. Pericardial calcification in constrictive pericarditis. (a) Anterior view. (b) Lateral view

PERICARDIUM

Pericardial calcification results from organization of blood or exudate in the pericardial sac and may or may not be associated with constrictive pericarditis. Constriction is most commonly caused by tuberculosis, but almost every type of pericarditis has been implicated. The calcium is most dense in the atrioventricular and interventricular grooves, and then shows as thick oblique circles or arcs of calcification

(*Figure 83*). From the grooves the calcium spreads over the surface of the atria and ventricles. Calcium localized in the posterior atrio-ventricular groove may lie in close relationship to the mitral valve and be mistaken for valve calcification. Single or multiple calcified pericardial plaques (calcified adherent pericardium) are seen in about 5 per cent of patients with chronic rheumatic heart disease, which is

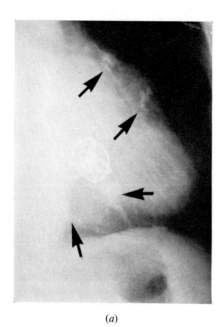 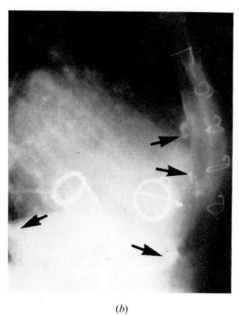

Figure 84. Pericardial plaques

(*a*) (*b*)

usually severe. The plaques are distributed in a haphazard way over the pericardium and do not cause constriction (*Figure 84*). The pericardial position of the calcium is diagnosed by showing its peripheral position in tangential views and by demonstrating its situation in the grooves between the atrial and ventricular chambers.

VALVES

Knowledge of the anatomy and relationships of the valves and fibrous skeleton of the heart is essential for understanding the localization of valve calcification.

Aortic valve and aortic root

The aortic valve lies in the base of the heart just to the right of its centre, facing upwards and to the

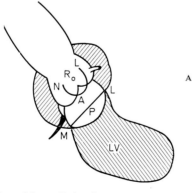

Figure 85. Aortic root and mitral valve—anterior view

Aortic root: L = left coronary sinus
N = non-coronary sinus
R = right coronary sinus

Mitral valve: A = anterior cusp
P = posterior cusp
L = antero-lateral commissure
M = postero-medial commissure
LV = left ventricle

right with a slight forward tilt following the direction of the proximal ascending aorta. The valve ring supports three cusps. The right coronary cusp is anterior, the left coronary cusp is left posterior, and the non-coronary cusp right posterior. Because of the inclined plane of the valve ring, the non-coronary cusp is always the lowest or caudal and the left coronary cusp the highest or cranial (*Figure 85*).

As the aortic valve lies just to the right of centre in the base of the heart, calcification in the valve overlaps the spine on the anterior view. If the heart is displaced to the left, it is seen just outside the spine below and medial to the segment formed by the left atrial appendix (*Figure 86*). On the lateral view it lies midway between the anterior and posterior cardiac borders just above the ventricular contours. Calcification in the aortic valve lies largely above a line drawn from the tracheal bifurcation to the anterior sterno-diaphragmatic angle, whereas mitral valve calcification is seen predominantly below this line

Figure 86. Calcified aortic valve—anterior view

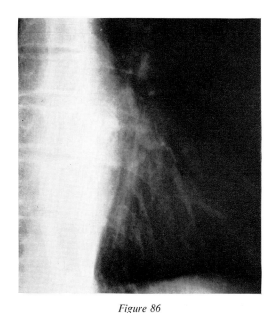

Figure 87. Calcified aortic valve—lateral view

Figure 88. Calcified aortic valve—commissure type

Figure 86

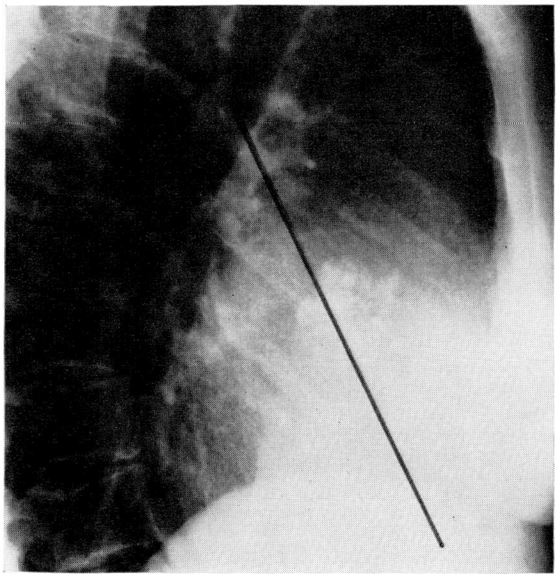

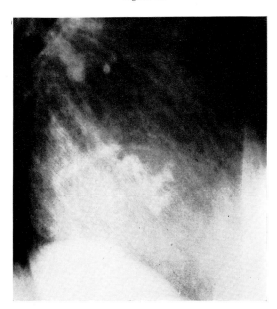

Figure 87

Figure 88

(*Figure 87*). The tracheal bifurcation is identified as a dark round or oval air shadow seen at the caudal end of the tracheal air shadow. As the two leaves of the diaphragm are not often projected at the same level, it is necessary to take a point midway between the two sterno-diaphragmatic angles as the anterior reference point of the line. The sign is reliable provided there is no deformity of the thoracic cage. On fluoroscopy the calcium is best seen in the left anterior oblique view. Movement is largely vertical but also in a counter-clockwise direction, being downward and forward in systole and upward and backward in diastole (Mercer, 1969).

Identification of the calcified aortic valve may also be possible by means of the pattern of calcium, which is of three types—commissural, ring or plaque-like. In the commissural type, one or two bands are seen representing calcification along the lips of a bicuspid valve. A smaller band may be identified at right angles, indicating calcium in the raphe of two fused cusps producing a T-shaped pattern (*Figure 88*). A complete or partial ring is quite common and reflects calcification in the bases of the cusps or in the ring itself (*Figure 89*). Neither the commissural nor the complete ring pattern is seen in mitral valve calcification. Aortic valve calcification may just appear as a plaque, indistinguishable from mitral calcification except for its position. The bicuspid valve is the commonest cause of aortic valve calcification, and the commissural and ring patterns are frequent. The valve is stenotic or predominantly stenotic with some regurgitation. A severely regurgitant bicuspid valve is most frequently the result of bacterial endocarditis, and calcification is rare. In about half the cases of bicuspid aortic valve, the valve orifice and its commissures lie in the sagittal plane with the two coronary arteries on either side. In the other half,

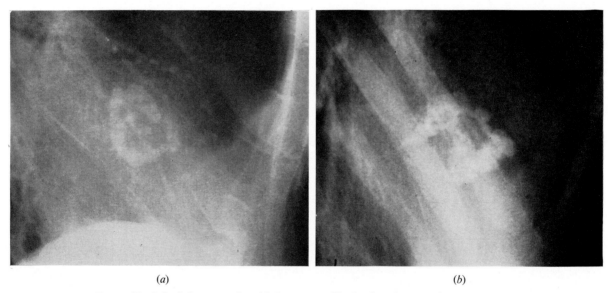

(a)   (b)

Figure 89. Calcified aortic valve. (a) Ring type. (b) Combined ring and commissure type

the commissures lie in the coronal place with the two coronary arteries arising anteriorly. In about half, a raphe is present; it lies to the right side of the sagittal orifice and anterior to the coronal orifice between the coronary arteries (*see Figure 320*). It may be possible to appreciate the type of cusp fusion by the direction of the calcified band on the lateral view, as the plane of the aortic ring is often abnormally vertical due to dilatation of the aortic root, so that an undistorted *en face* projection of the valve is achieved. If the ring pattern or a large plaque is seen, calcification has usually spread outside the confines of the valve into the ventricular septum (*see Figure 91*) and the anterior cusp of the mitral valve. A unicuspid valve is much less commonly seen as a cause of aortic stenosis and calcification. It takes two forms, one resembling pulmonary valve stenosis with an aperture in a dome, and the other having a single commissural orifice. It is not possible to make a diagnosis from the pattern of calcification on the plain films.

Rheumatic fever is the next most common cause of isolated calcification of the aortic valve. As with the congenital bicuspid valve, calcification is most commonly associated with dominant stenosis and rarely with pure regurgitation. The valve is tricuspid with commissural fusion, and calcification is usually plaque-like. If calcification of the aortic and mitral valves is present, rheumatic fever is always responsible with two rare exceptions: spread of calcification from the ring of a bicuspid aortic valve into the anterior cusp of the mitral valve, and senile calcification of the aortic and mitral valves. In syphilis, there may be cusp calcification with aortic regurgitation but never stenosis. The wall of the ascending aorta may also show calcification with or without aneurysm. Healed bacterial endocarditis causes aortic regurgitation, usually without calcification. Calcified aortic valves become infected much less frequently than uncalcified ones.

In patients in their sixties or beyond, calcium may be deposited in the depths of the sinuses of Valsalva, in the bases of the cusps and in the valve ring. The process is an age change probably akin to subvalvar mitral calcification (*Figure 90*). Rigidity of the cusps may result in an ejection systolic murmur, but without significant obstruction. If spread occurs centrally, splinting of the cusps may cause senile aortic stenosis. Some systemic diseases affecting collagen may be responsible for calcification of the aortic valve and aortic regurgitation. Ankylosing spondylitis is the most common, the disease process being limited to the cusps, the ring, the sinuses of Valsalva and the bundle of His. The incidence of calcification of homografts in the aortic orifice is not yet known, but it is much less frequent than in the pulmonary orifice. Existing early atheroma in the graft, so easily overlooked, is one predisposing factor. The calcification occurs in the base of the cusps, and centripetal spread to produce aortic stenosis appears to be rare.

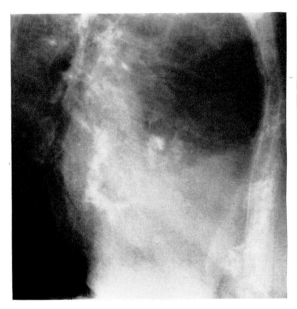
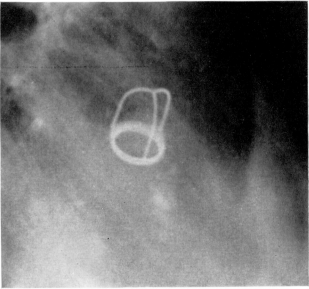

Figure 90. Senile calcification in aortic and mitral valves —lateral view

Figure 91. Spread of calcification from aortic valve into septum —aortic Starr valve replacement

If aortic valve calcification is heavy, heart block may occur by extension downwards from the region of the right and non-coronary cusps into the right fibrous trigone, the membranous ventricular septum (*Figure 91*) and the bundle of His.

Mitral valve

The mitral valve lies in the posterior wall of the left ventricular outflow tract immediately below, behind and to the left of the aortic valve (*see Figure 85*). Its orifice faces downwards, forwards and to the left towards the apex of the left ventricle. The upper antero-medial third of the ring gives origin to the larger anterior cusp, which forms the posterior wall of the left ventricular outflow. The lower postero-lateral two-thirds of the mitral ring lies in the posterior wall of the left ventricle and gives attachment to the smaller quadrilateral posterior cusp, which takes no real part in the formation of the left ventricular outflow tract. The anterior and posterior cusps are continuous with each other at the antero-lateral and postero-medial commissures, where small accessory cusps may be found. As the mitral orifice is oblique, the antero-lateral commissure lies higher than and lateral to the postero-medial commissure. Internal to each commissure, chordae from the corresponding antero-lateral and postero-medial papillary muscles are concentrated at two critical areas of tendon insertion, about 2·5 cm apart. In rheumatic fever the disease is concentrated at these two sites, where fusion and subsequent calcification are common (*see* page 230).

On the anterior view, calcification of the mitral valve is visible just to the left of the spine and lower than aortic valve calcification (*Figure 92a*). If the left atrium is enlarged, it is seen at the left inferior

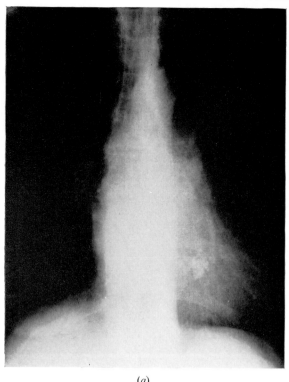

(a)

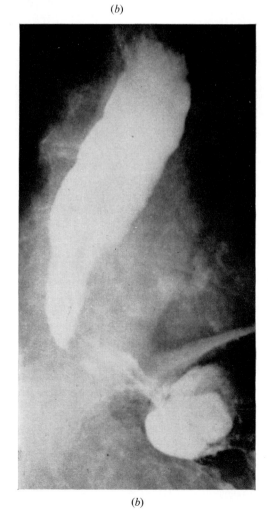

(b)

Figure 92 (above). Mitral valve calcification. (a) Anterior penetrated view. (b) Lateral view

Figure 93 (below and right). Mitral valve calcification. (a) Commissures—anterior view. (b) Senile subvalvular calcification—anterior view

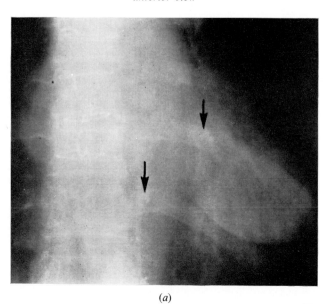

(a)

(b)

boundary of the increased chamber density. The larger the left atrium, the further leftwards and caudally lies the calcium. On the lateral view the mitral valve lies postero-inferior to the aortic valve, and calcium is seen at the junction of the middle and posterior thirds of the ventricular part of the heart. The calcium lies predominantly below the line drawn from the tracheal bifurcation to the anterior sterno-diaphragmatic angle, whereas aortic valve calcification lies mainly above this line (*Figure 92b*). On fluoroscopy in the right anterior oblique view, it is seen to have a more horizontal movement than the aortic valve.

Calcification of the mitral valve is nearly always caused by rheumatic heart disease. It is more common in men and its incidence increases with age. It is seen in mitral stenosis or in mitral stenosis and regurgitation, but is less common in pure or dominant mitral regurgitation. Nearly all men over the age of 50 years with mitral stenosis have a calcified mitral valve (Kitchen and Turner, 1967). It is frequently associated with adverse features such as atrial fibrillation, multiple valve lesions and a large heart. The calcium appears as one or more plaques. If on the anterior view it is in a low and medial position, it lies in or near the postero-medial commissure; if high and lateral, in or near the antero-lateral commissure (*Figure 93a*); and if between the two areas, in the main part of the cusps (*Figure 92a*).

The only other important mitral calcification is the subvalvar variety. Calcium accumulates in the acute angle between the posterior cusp of the mitral valve and the posterior left ventricular wall. The probable mechanism is stasis, deposition of platelets, organization and calcification in this relatively stagnant recess of the left ventricle. Subvalvar mitral calcification occurs in old age and is much more common in women. It is seen in Paget's disease, and may then be found in men. Diabetes and left ventricular hypertrophy are considered predisposing causes (Kirk and Russell, 1969). The calcification presents radiologically as a wide U, C or J-shaped band up to two centimetres thick and corresponding in position to part or all of the attachment of the posterior cusp to the ring (*Figures 90* and *93b*). It may spread round the ring into its antero-medial part, but rarely if ever completely encircles the valve. Occasionally the ring alone is calcified and the subvalvar angle is spared. Subvalvar calcification is usually asymptomatic and discovered unexpectedly on x-ray or autopsy. Very rarely it produces mitral stenosis or regurgitation by spreading into the cusps.

Calcification, whether rheumatic or subvalvar, may infiltrate in various directions. Involvement of the myocardium is important surgically as it may add to the difficulties of removing a valve prior to valve replacement. Spread into the membranous ventricular septum may involve the bundle of His or its branches to produce heart block; Harris *et al.* (1969) found mitral calcification as a cause of chronic heart block in 3 out of 65 cases.

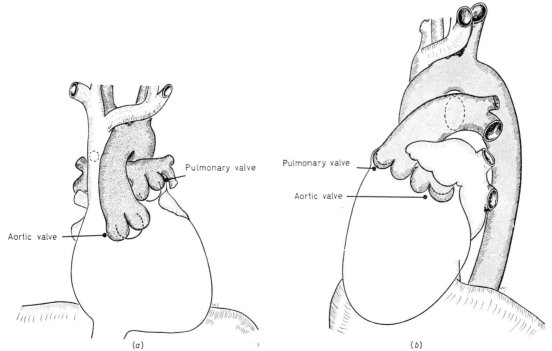

Figure 94. Pulmonary and aortic valves. (*a*) *Anterior view.* (*b*) *Lateral view*

Pulmonary valve

The pulmonary valve is anterior, cranial and to the left of the aortic valve, and faces mainly upwards and backwards. The cusps and sinuses are named posterior, right and left (*Figure 94*). Calcification, rarely heavy, is seen commonly in patients of middle age with pulmonary valve stenosis and Fallot's tetralogy, and occasionally in pulmonary hypertension with or without shunts or after bacterial endocarditis (Gabriele *et al.*, 1970). On the anterior view it lies below and medial to the pulmonary trunk border between the spine and the left atrial appendix. On the lateral view it is seen within the upper anterior part of the heart, close behind the sternum.

Homografts placed in the outflow tract of the right ventricle for severe Fallot's tetralogy or pulmonary atresia often acquire calcification, sometimes within three months of operation (*Figure 95*). The calcium appears to be unimportant haemodynamically as it lies mainly in the wall of the homograft and not in the cusps.

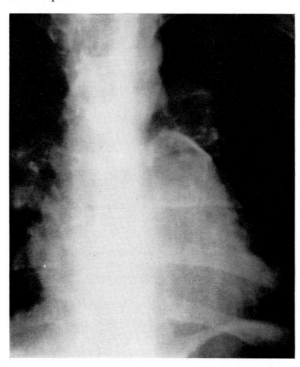

Figure 95. Calcified aortic homograft inserted in right ventricular outflow tract

Tricuspid valve

The tricuspid ring is wider than the mitral ring. It is situated in front, to the right of and a little below the mitral ring, facing to the left, forward and slightly downward towards the left inferior angle of the right ventricle. The ring supports three cusps, namely septal, anterior and posterior. Part of the ring supporting the septal cusp lies immediately below the right coronary and non-coronary sinuses of the aortic valve and separates the membranous septum in front from the atrio-ventricular septum behind (*Figure 96*).

Calcification may occur in the tricuspid valve with pulmonary stenosis in which it is subjected to a high right ventricular systolic pressure (*Figure 97*); this probably renders it more susceptible to rheumatic damage. It has been reported in atrial septal defect, presumably as a result of trauma from high flow, and may occur with lone tricuspid regurgitation (Clarke, 1972).

CORONARY ARTERIES

Coronary artery calcification appears as a plaque or double line and is most frequently seen in the proximal part of the left coronary artery on the penetrated anterior view of the chest (*Figure 98*). When in the anterior descending branch, it lies just within the cardiac border, but if in the main stem or the circumflex branch it appears well inside. It must not be mistaken for costal cartilage or bronchial wall calcification. Calcification is rarely seen in the right coronary artery because its incidence here is less than in the

VALVES

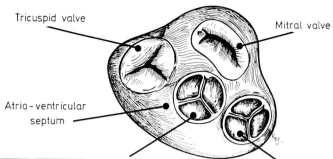

Figure 96. *Transverse plane diagram of valves seen from above*

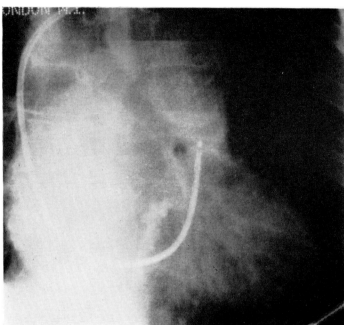

Figure 97. Calcified tricuspid valve in pulmonary stenosis

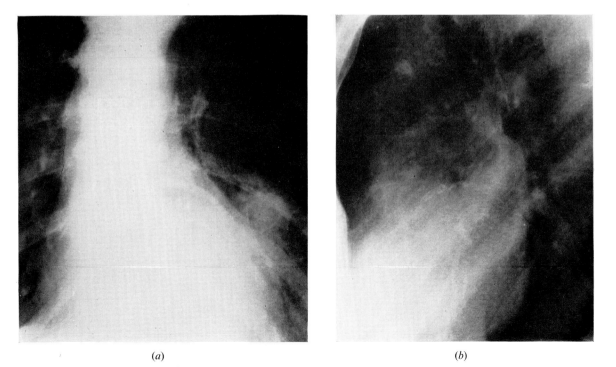

(a)   (b)

Figure 98. Calcified left coronary artery. (a) Anterior view. (b) Lateral view

left and because the spine may overlie the proximal part of the right coronary artery on the anterior view. On the lateral view, coronary calcification is less well seen, probably because of motional blur caused by

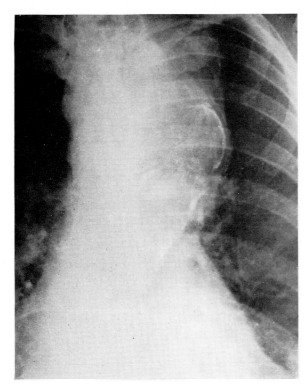

Figure 99. Calcified dissecting aneurysm

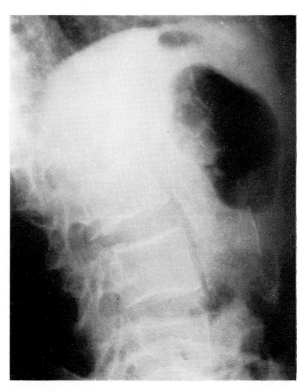

Figure 100. Calcified aorta in aortitis

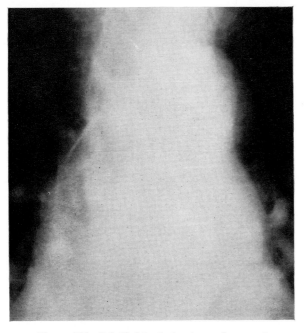

Figure 101. Calcified jet lesion in aortic stenosis

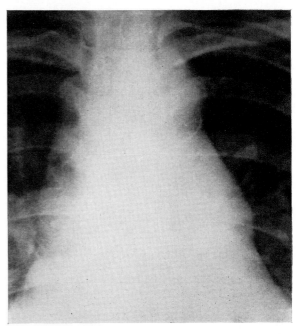

Figure 102. Calcified infundibulum in ductus arteriosus

the necessarily long exposure time. If calcification is present in a coronary artery, its wall is usually thickened but its lumen may not be significantly narrowed. The younger the patient, the denser the calcification, the greater its length and the more vessels involved, the more likely it is that the arterial lumen will be compromised. Calcium which is obvious in a patient under 50 years of age is highly suggestive of ischaemic heart disease, but calcification is quite commonly seen in patients aged over 65 years without symptoms.

THORACIC AORTA

Aortic calcification is most often seen in the arch in patients above the age of 40 years. It does not necessarily indicate atherosclerosis in other parts of the vascular system. The calcium is deposited as small plaques in two depressions, one at the site of the ligamentum arteriosum and the other a little further forward below the origin of the left subclavian artery (Dalith, 1961). Calcification spreads round the aortic wall from these sites. The plaques often overlap one another on the anterior view to appear as a dense arc 1–3 mm thick, but are not easily seen on the lateral view.

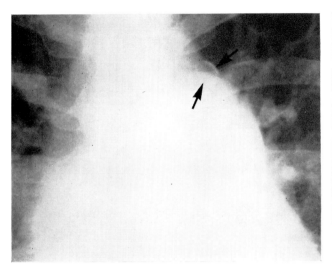 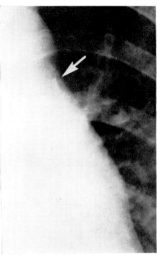

Figure 103. Calcified ductus arteriosus

Atheroma is usually responsible for calcified plaques in the arch other than the type mentioned above and in the descending aorta, but are seen in the ascending aorta when the disease is widespread. Similarly, aneurysm due to atheroma is largely confined to the arch and the descending aorta. Syphilis characteristically presents as calcification in the ascending aorta, usually but not invariably with aneurysm and aortic regurgitation; the aortic cusps may also calcify. Aortic sinus aneurysm may show calcification in relation to the aortic root. Healed dissecting aneurysm may cause calcification anywhere in the aorta (*Figure 99*). Unruptured traumatic aneurysms may also calcify (*see* page 36). The calcification of arteritis often involves the branches of the aorta as well as the aortic arch and the descending aorta (*Figure 100*). A jet lesion in aortic stenosis may occasionally show localized calcification in the ascending aorta (*Figure 101*).

DUCTUS ARTERIOSUS

Calcification of the ductus arteriosus tends to occur in middle-aged patients and in those with pulmonary hypertension. It is most frequently at the aortic end of the ductus in relation to the funnel-shaped aortic dilatation or infundibulum. Its position is identical with that of the common aortic arch plaque, but it appears thinner and more even (*Figure 102*). Less often it is confined to the ductus, and then shows as a short vertical line or arc and rarely as a circle (*Figure 103*). Calcification of the pulmonary artery may occur in a jet lesion from the duct or as a result of atheroma associated with pulmonary hypertension (Eisenmenger syndrome—*Figure 103*). A calcified aneurysm of the duct most commonly follows surgery. The ligamentum arteriosum may calcify, but this cannot be demonstrated without tomography.

PULMONARY TRUNK

The pulmonary trunk and proximal pulmonary arteries may show calcified atheroma. The plaques are thinner than in the systemic arteries. All cases have severe pulmonary hypertension, and the Eisenmenger syndrome is the most frequent cause (*Figure 104*). Widespread calcification of the pulmonary arteries may follow hypercalcaemia of infancy and may result in multiple pulmonary stenoses.

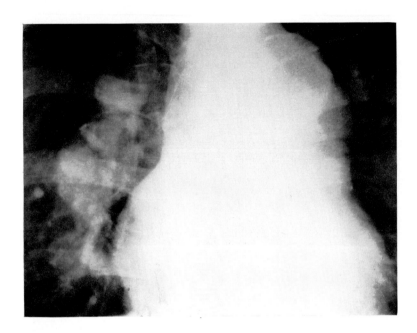

Figure 104. Calcified atheroma in pulmonary trunk and right hilar arteries

TUMOURS AND CYSTS

These are dealt with in Chapter 29.

Myxomas are benign pedunculated tumours arising from the atrial septum. Although three-quarters are seen in the left atrium, calcification appears more common in right atrial myxoma. If tumour calcification is slight, it may be invisible on plain films due to blurring because of its rapid movement, but detectable on fluoroscopy. Mobility of heavily calcified tumours distinguishes them from thrombus, which is adherent to the atrial wall. Calcified right atrial tumours may cause severe trauma to the tricuspid valve, resulting in tricuspid regurgitation and enlargement of the right atrium and right ventricle. Calcification is seen in benign tumours in childhood.

Hydatid cysts are a rare cause of intracardiac calcification. They are most commonly found in the left ventricular myocardium. After rupture into the blood stream or pericardium, the cyst inspissates and its wall may calcify and present as a thin curved density.

SECTION II
The Lungs

CHAPTER 7

Anatomy and Physiology

ANATOMY

For purposes of description the lungs on the anterior view of the chest are divided into zones. The upper zone lies above a horizontal line drawn through the lower border of the anterior end of the second rib; the middle zone lies between this line and one drawn through the lower border of the fourth rib, and the lower zone is below the line through the fourth rib. If a lateral view is available—and the radiological examination of the chest is incomplete without one—an attempt must be made to relate pathology to lobes or segments.

Structures in the lungs are rendered visible by virtue of their contrast density compared with air. The normal visible structures are fissures, bronchi, pulmonary arteries and pulmonary veins.

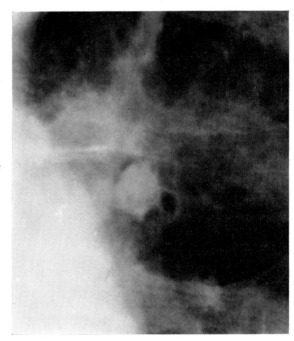

Figure 105. Left upper lobe artery with adjacent bronchus. The artery is dilated

Part or all of the middle fissure may be seen on the anterior and lateral views. The oblique fissures are normally visible only on the lateral view, and there may be difficulty in deciding to which side they belong. Two other fissures are occasionally visible: (1) the inferior accessory, which is seen on the anterior view and is usually part of the oblique fissure between the middle and right lower lobes, but occasionally represents an accessory fissure between the medial basal and the other basal segments of the right lower lobe; and (2) the sub-apical, seen on the lateral view lying between the apical and posterior basal segments of either lower lobe.

A bronchus forms a ring shadow if it runs for some distance parallel to the x-ray beam. The left upper anterior segmental bronchus is the one most frequently seen where it lies close to the segmental artery near the upper pole of the left hilum (*Figure 105*). Unless running parallel to the x-ray beam, intrapulmonary bronchi are invisible provided their walls are not thickened, so that the term 'bronchovascular markings' is meaningless. Neither should 'lung markings' be used. Description of intrapulmonary structures should be anatomical, although the term 'pulmonary vessels' is acceptable where arteries and veins are indistinguishable.

As the right pulmonary artery runs horizontally to the right within the mediastinum, it is invisible on the anterior view, but it can be seen on the lateral view as an oval opacity in front of the tracheal bifurcation. The left pulmonary artery is visible on the anterior view during its short antero-posterior course in the upper pole of the left hilum. It may sometimes be identified on the lateral view curving over the left main bronchus above and behind the right pulmonary artery (*see Figure 47a*).

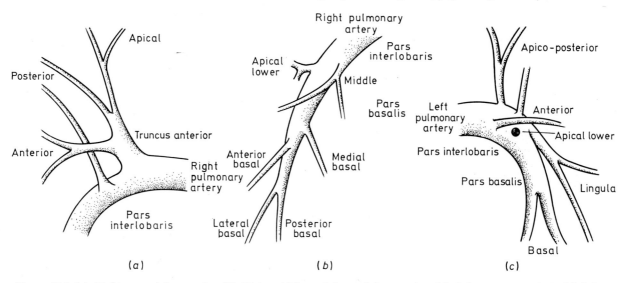

Figure 106. (a) Right upper lobe arteries. (b) Right middle and lower lobe arteries. (c) Pulmonary arteries of left lung

The intrapulmonary arteries are closely related to the bronchi, which together form the broncho-vascular bundles. The anatomy of the lobar and segmental arteries is illustrated in *Figure 106*, the terminology adopted being the same as that of the bronchial tree (Brock, 1950; Jefferson, 1965). Although the pulmonary arteries follow the same pathway as the bronchi, their origin is often different. This is most obvious in the left upper lobe, where there may be anything from two to seven segmental arteries in contrast to the three segmental bronchi (apico-posterior, anterior and lingular), which are anatomically constant. On the right side there is a constant upper lobe segmental artery, the truncus anterior (*Figures 106* and *107a*). On the anterior view this may be mistaken for an anomalous pulmonary vein entering the superior vena cava.

Pulmonary arteries taper towards the periphery. Branching appears slightly irregular and is of two types:

(1) Bifurcation into two branches of roughly equal diameter.
(2) Collateral branching, in which the larger vessel continues in the direction of the axial pathway and the smaller arises at right angles. The collateral branches supply the deep parts of the lung and are responsible for the even mottled or reticular pattern of the small vessels.

Structurally the proximal pulmonary arteries are elastic and the peripheral arteries muscular. The transition occurs along the segmental arterial pathways (Elliott and Reid, 1965). With allowance for magnification, the largest muscular arteries probably measure about 3 mm on the anterior view, and the smallest elastic arteries about 4 mm.

The course of the pulmonary veins is quite distinct from that of the arteries and bronchi. The peripheral veins drain the secondary lobules and run in the interlobular septa, and the larger veins are situated between segments where their position is variable. This is in contrast to the arteries, which have a constant intrasegmental distribution. The upper lobe veins are formed in the infraclavicular region by the junction of two veins, usually with a more caudal lateral tributary. They descend lateral to the upper lobe arteries and, crossing in front of the descending pulmonary artery in the hilum, enter the upper and outer portion of the left atrium (*Figure 107*). The upper lobe vein and artery are more easily differentiated on the right side because the truncus anterior and its apical division are constant (*Figure 107*); the left upper lobe arteries are variable in origin and number, so that arteries and veins are often indistinguishable. The right lower lobe veins can nearly always be distinguished from the segmental arteries as they

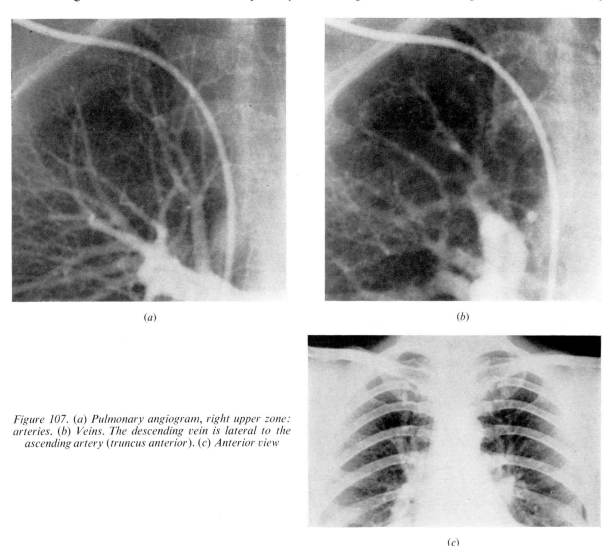

(a)

(b)

Figure 107. (a) Pulmonary angiogram, right upper zone: arteries. (b) Veins. The descending vein is lateral to the ascending artery (truncus anterior). (c) Anterior view

(c)

are more horizontal and cross in front of the arteries below the right hilum to form a single vein which enters the right lower portion of the left atrium (*Figure 108*). The veins of the left lower lobe are more vertical, their point of entry into the left atrium being higher, and run in a similar direction to the arteries. There are four main pulmonary veins, two upper and two lower. The middle lobe vein usually joins the right upper lobe vein, but may enter the left atrium separately. The right lower vein may show a dilatation close to its entry into the left atrium. This dilated venous confluence must not be mistaken for a tumour (*Figure 109*).

The width of the pulmonary vessels in a normal person is dependent on blood flow. In the erect position, flow diminishes progressively from the lower to the upper zones, being nil at the apex (Friedman and Braunwald, 1966; West, 1968). As vessel calibre reflects these flow patterns, in the erect position the vessels in the first anterior intercostal space rarely measure more than 3 mm, whereas those immediately above the diaphragm may be 6 mm or more; vessels above the clavicle are less than 1 mm or invisible. In the supine position, upper and lower zone vessels become approximately equal in width (*Figure 110*). It is important to bear this in mind when interpreting supine chest films, tomograms and pulmonary arteriograms.

There are six groups of lymphatics in the lungs: pleural, interlobular, perivenous, periarterial, peribronchial and anastomotic. All lymphatics have valves which direct flow towards the hila. The pleural lymphatics are larger, and are most numerous in the lower zones and scanty over the upper zones. In the lower zones they are approximately 1 mm in diameter and outline the interlobular septa on the surface of the lung. Lymph flows from the pleural into the interlobular lymphatics which lie between the

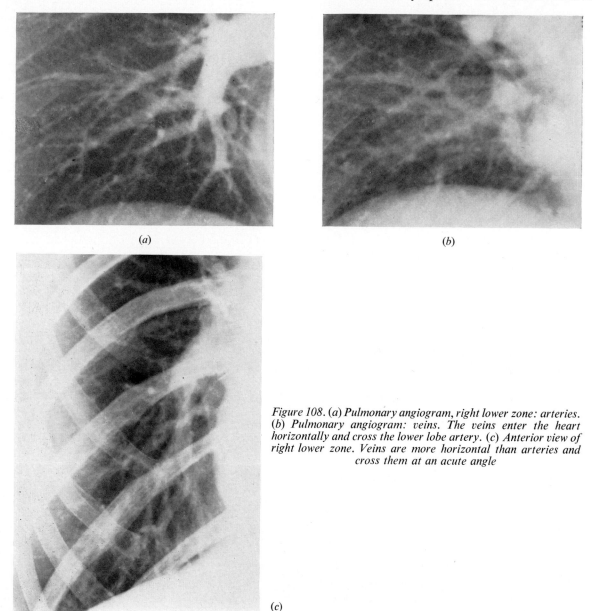

(a)

(b)

Figure 108. (a) Pulmonary angiogram, right lower zone: arteries. (b) Pulmonary angiogram: veins. The veins enter the heart horizontally and cross the lower lobe artery. (c) Anterior view of right lower zone. Veins are more horizontal than arteries and cross them at an acute angle

(c)

secondary lobules and drain the periphery of the acini. These join to form a perivenous lymphatic which may continue to the hilum or cross intervening lung to anastomose with peribronchial or periarterial channels. All lymphatic pathways ultimately pass through hilar glands and thence to the innominate or subclavian veins.

PHYSIOLOGY

In the following discussion, pressures in the pulmonary circulation are taken from a zero point corresponding to the middle of the anterior–posterior diameter of the chest at the level of the sternal end of the third intercostal space. At this point the normal mean right atrial pressure is about 5 mm Hg.

Right ventricular contraction generates a pulsatile flow in the pulmonary arteries, capillaries and veins, with a peak systolic pressure in the pulmonary artery of about 20 mm Hg ($\pm$ 5 mm Hg). Thereafter the pressure falls and in end-diastole approximates to the mean left atrial pressure at around 9 mm Hg ($\pm$ 3 mm Hg). At this point, left ventricular pressure (measured just before the onset of the left atrial A wave) equals left atrial pressure and corresponds fairly well with the mean pulmonary capillary venous

Figure 109 (right). Dilated venous confluence

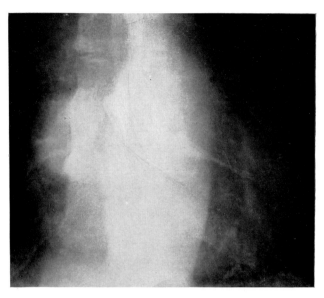

Figure 110 (below). Left upper zone vessels. (a) Erect. (b) Supine, showing dilatation of vessels to similar calibre to that of lower zones

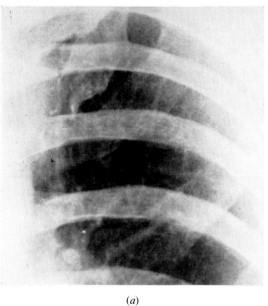

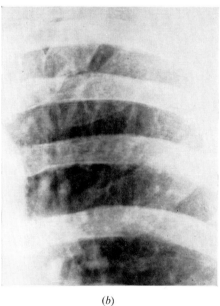

(a)

(b)

(PCV) or wedge pressure recorded through a catheter wedged in a small pulmonary artery. Mean pulmonary artery pressure for the whole cycle is around 15 mm Hg ($\pm$ 3 mm Hg). The pulmonary vascular bed is therefore a low resistance system with a pressure gradient of only about 6 mm Hg. The resistance to flow is dependent on the calibre of the arterioles and small muscular arteries, whose ratio of wall thickness to lumen is small compared with equivalent arteries in the systemic circulation. In adults the normal resting pulmonary flow ranges from 4 to 6 litres per minute. Exercise may increase the flow up to 15 litres. If the response to exercise is measured with the patient recumbent and working a bicycle as is customary during catheterization, a small immediate rise in pressure occurs on elevation of the legs to the thorax. A further rise occurs immediately exercise begins, but the mean pressure does not exceed 30 mm Hg. Some of the rise may be accounted for by increased venous return and slight elevation of the pulmonary venous pressure. Similar responses are seen after injection of contrast medium, and angio-cardiography may be considered as a modified exercise test. In the erect position, pulmonary pressures do not rise with exercise; although this fact is not completely explained, the absence of redistribution of blood from the legs to the thorax may be a factor.

The relationship between resistance, pressure and flow in the pulmonary circulation is complex be-cause the lungs contain a large volume of blood of variable viscosity at low pressure, flowing in a pul-satile fashion through highly distensible vessels suspended in the thorax, which is undergoing rhythmic changes in size and pressure (Harris and Heath, 1962). Nevertheless, for clinical purposes, calculation of the pulmonary vascular resistance remains a good practical guide to the state of the lungs in heart disease. This is done by the formula

$$R = \frac{P}{Q}$$

where R = resistance in units;

$\quad\quad P$ = pressure gradient in mm Hg across the pulmonary vascular bed, i.e. the difference between mean pulmonary artery and mean left atrial pressures;

$\quad\quad Q$ = blood flow in litres per minute.

The normal pulmonary vascular resistance does not exceed 3 units. For example, if the normal figures quoted above are used:

Mean pulmonary artery pressure = 15 mm Hg.
Mean left atrial pressure = 9 mm Hg.
Cardiac output = 4 litres per minute.

$$R = \frac{15-9}{4} = 1 \cdot 5 \text{ units.}$$

CHAPTER 8

Plethora and Oligaemia

PLETHORA

As stated in Chapter 7, the width of the pulmonary vessels depends on blood flow, provided the arterial and venous pressures are normal. Plethora means enlargement of pulmonary vessels primarily due to increased flow, and the term should be used specifically to indicate the presence of left-to-right shunt (*Figure 111a–d*). It denies important pulmonary stenosis. Cyanosis is present only if there is veno-arterial mixing with bidirectional shunting. The following lesions are associated with plethora.

Left-to-right shunt only (*see* Chapters 16, 17 and 18)
    (1) Partial anomalous pulmonary venous drainage.
    (2) Secundum atrial septal defect.
    (3) Primum atrial septal defect.
    (4) Atrio-ventricular canal.
    (5) Left ventricular–right atrial defect.
    (6) Ventricular septal defect.
    (7) Aortic sinus fistula.
    (8) Coronary artery fistula.
    (9) Aorto-pulmonary septal defect.
  (10) Ductus arteriosus.

Bidirectional shunt (*see* Chapters 20, 22 and 23)
    (1) Inferior vena caval type of atrial septal defect.
    (2) Atrial septal defect with absent coronary sinus and left superior vena cava connected to left atrium.
    (3) Single atrium.
    (4) Total anomalous pulmonary venous drainage.
    (5) Double outflow right ventricle.
    (6) Single ventricle.
    (7) Complete transposition.
    (8) Tricuspid atresia with large ventricular septal defect.
    (9) Pulmonary atresia with large systemic supply to lungs.
  (10) Truncus arteriosus.

The easiest artery to assess when considering the pulmonary vessel pattern is that to the right lower lobe. The upper limit of normal width is stated to be 16 mm in adult males and 15 mm in adult females (Chang, 1962). Enlargement of the right lower lobe artery is seen in 90 per cent of patients with an increased pulmonary flow, and there is a strong correlation between the degree of enlargement and the size of the shunt expressed as pulmonary to systemic flow ratio (*see* Appendix C). A normal-sized artery with increased flow is most often encountered with ventricular septal defect, seen in about 20 per cent of the patients with a flow ratio under 2:1.

With increased flow, the segmental arteries and veins also appear enlarged. However, this change may only be convincing in the lower zones in small shunts, possibly because appreciable increase in flow is confined to the dependent parts of the lungs. With large shunts, flow increases in the upper zones

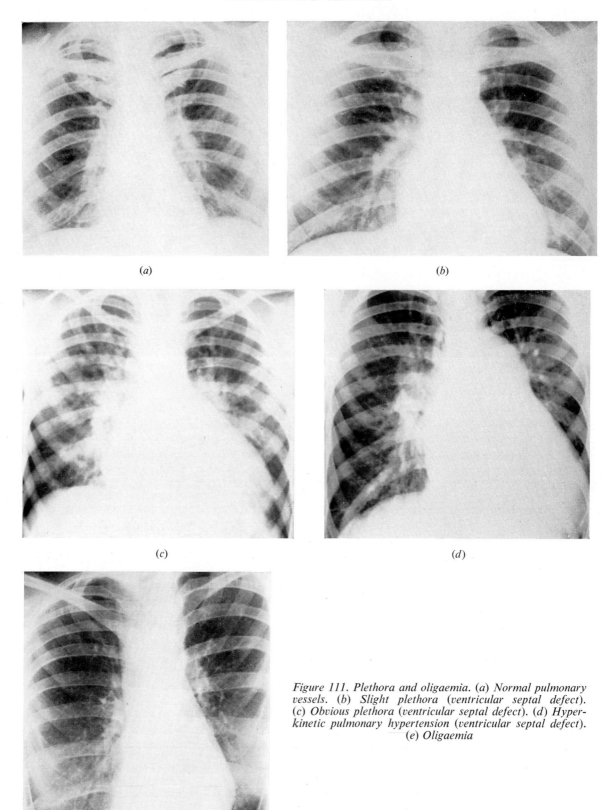

(a)

(b)

(c)

(d)

Figure 111. Plethora and oligaemia. (a) Normal pulmonary vessels. (b) Slight plethora (ventricular septal defect). (c) Obvious plethora (ventricular septal defect). (d) Hyperkinetic pulmonary hypertension (ventricular septal defect). (e) Oligaemia

(e)

and approaches that in the lower zones (Dollery *et al.*, 1961), so that on the chest radiograph the differential between upper and lower zone vessel size is lost. Interpretation of changes in the peripheral vessels is difficult, particularly as radiographic underexposure may cause an apparent increase in their size and number. On the whole it is best to ignore them when trying to decide whether or not plethora is present.

With moderate degrees of plethora, vessels taper evenly towards the periphery, but if the shunt is very large the limit of distensibility of the muscular arteries is reached and the pressure rises because of torrential flow (hyperkinetic pulmonary hypertension). Plethora is then always gross, but the tapering may be more abrupt so that the hilar and proximal segmental vessels are wider relative to the more distal vessels: anterior bowing of the sternum is commonly present (Davies *et al.*, 1962) (*Figure 112*). In infants and young children there may also be generalized mottling from overperfusion pulmonary oedema, as the high pressure is directly transmitted to the capillary bed without the protective vasoconstriction of the small muscular arteries (*Figure 113*).

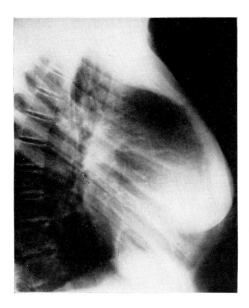

Figure 112. Sternal bowing

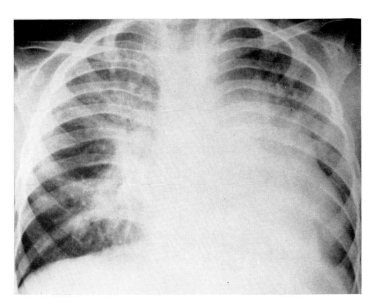

Figure 113. Overperfusion pulmonary oedema

When the vascular resistance is very high, the left-to-right shunt is small or reversed (Eisenmenger syndrome). The radiological picture is that of pulmonary arterial hypertension (*see* Chapter 10) and the term plethora should not be used.

Table 4 is a guide to the interpretation of the chest radiograph in terms of haemodynamics, and represents the findings in a mixed group of 400 shunts in which pressures and flows have been measured (*see* Appendix C). It serves to outline the general trend and also shows that exceptions do occur. For example, in young adults with atrial septal defect the flow ratio may be 4:1 with only slight plethora and no cardiac enlargement.

TABLE 4

Haemodynamics	Heart				Plethora			
	Normal	*+1*	*+2*	*+3*	*0*	*+1*	*+2*	*+3*
Small shunt (P/S < 2:1); normal PA pressure	30%	50%	20%	0	10%	50%	40%	0
Large shunt (P/S > 2:1); normal PA pressure	20%	40%	30%	10%	0	25%	50%	25%
Large shunt with hyperkinetic pulmonary hypertension	0	40%	40%	20%	0	25%	25%	50%

The chances of a shunt being above or below 2:1 with a normal or slightly enlarged heart are about equal, but with a larger heart the shunt will exceed 2:1 in at least two-thirds of cases, and in more if the enlargement is gross. The chance of a shunt being under 2:1 with no plethora is almost 100 per cent; with slight plethora the chance is 60 per cent under 2:1, and with obvious plethora it is 70 per cent over 2:1. In general, therefore, the correlation of flow with plethora is closer than with heart size.

OLIGAEMIA

Oligaemia refers to a general reduction in width of the pulmonary arteries and veins and indicates a pulmonary blood flow below normal (*see Figure 111e*). The causes are listed below.

Obstruction to right ventricular outflow with a right-to-left shunt
Fallot and its differential diagnosis (*see* Chapters 19 and 20).

Obstruction to right ventricular outflow without a shunt (*see* Chapter 24)
Pulmonary valve stenosis; infundibular stenosis; pulmonary atresia with intact septum (*see* page 182); pulmonary artery stenosis; massive pulmonary embolism (*see* page 99); extrinsic pressure from tumour, aneurysm of aorta, mediastinitis, constrictive pericarditis.

Obstruction to right ventricular inflow (*see* Chapter 23)
Tricuspid atresia; tricuspid stenosis and regurgitation; Ebstein's anomaly; right atrial myxoma (*see* page 281); underdeveloped right ventricle.

Failure of right ventricle as a pump
Right ventricular failure; Uhl's anomaly (*see* page 219).

Although pulmonary blood flow is reduced in the Eisenmenger syndrome (right-to-left shunt with pulmonary hypertension), this is not included as a cause of oligaemia because the radiological picture is dominated by the changes of pulmonary arterial hypertension: the proximal vessels are dilated, and oligaemia is evident only in the peripheral parts of the lungs.

Fallot's tetralogy is the commonest cause of oligaemia. Although ventricular systolic pressures are equal, pulmonary flow is low due to the right-to-left shunt at ventricular level caused by outflow obstruction to the lungs. There is a fairly close correlation between the size of the right-to-left shunt, as indicated by the systemic oxygen saturation, and the degree of oligaemia (*see* Appendix C). Oligaemia is less often seen in pulmonary stenosis with intact ventricular septum because the right ventricular hypertension (up to 300 mm Hg systolic pressure) maintains a normal pulmonary flow. When oligaemia is seen it means severe obstruction, often with shunt reversal across the atrial septum and hence a low pulmonary flow.

In tricuspid atresia, where the obstruction is to right ventricular inflow, oligaemia may exactly resemble Fallot but the heart shadow is different (*see* page 220). Severe tricuspid stenosis or regurgitation can cause oligaemia, and in particular the signs of pulmonary venous hypertension due to severe mitral valve disease may be masked.

The diagnosis of oligaemia is often made with uncertainty because some normal people have small pulmonary vessels. As with plethora, it is better to concentrate on the larger vessels, especially the right lower lobe pulmonary artery. The normal lower limit of width is stated to be 10 mm in adult males and 9 mm in adult females (Teichmann *et al.*, 1970).

CHAPTER 9

Pulmonary Arterial Hypertension

Pulmonary arterial hypertension is said to be present when the pulmonary artery systolic pressure (measured at the mid-chest) exceeds 30 mm Hg. The level of the pressure is determined by the relationship between the pulmonary blood flow and the vascular resistance (*see* page 73). Pulmonary arterial hypertension may be primarily due to abnormalities involving the pulmonary arterial wall or lumen, or may be secondary to pulmonary venous hypertension or a central shunt. Arterial changes in pulmonary hypertension are reversible if due to vasoconstriction; they may be organic, but a vasoconstrictive element is often present with organic changes. The muscular arteries develop medial hypertrophy and constriction, the arterioles acquire a muscular wall, and later the intima thickens. The elastic arteries show a variable degree of dilatation.

The basic radiological changes (*Figure 114*) are:

(1) Dilatation of the pulmonary trunk and proximal pulmonary arteries (the elastic arteries).
(2) Narrowing of distal pulmonary arteries (the muscular arteries).

The transition varies in level, but is usually in the segments and may be abrupt or gradual. The small peripheral vessels often appear reduced in number and size, but this may be difficult to appreciate. Other changes include tortuosity of segmental arteries and calcified atheroma in the pulmonary trunk and its lobar branches (*Figure 115*). The plaques are thinner than those seen in systemic arteries.

CAUSES OF PULMONARY ARTERIAL HYPERTENSION

Excluding pulmonary arterial hypertension secondary to venous hypertension or central shunts, which are discussed in Chapters 10 and 21, the causes are as follows.

Embolism: thrombus, tumour, parasite.
Arteritis: polyarteritis, lupus.
Drugs and poisons: aminorex, cobalt.
Hypoxia: high altitude, respiratory infection in children.
Respiratory disease: cor pulmonale.
Primary pulmonary hypertension.

It may be impossible on clinical or radiological grounds to separate primary from thrombo-embolic pulmonary hypertension, and recourse to catheterization and angiography is usually necessary. In both conditions the basic changes of central vessel dilatation and peripheral vessel narrowing are present, but in thrombo-embolism there may be evidence of uneven vascular obliteration, infarct scars and pleural thickening (Chrispin *et al.*, 1963) (*Figure 116*). Similar appearances may occur with polyarteritis nodosa and systemic lupus.

Tumour emboli may also cause pulmonary hypertension. Of particular interest is malignant trophoblastic disease, in which the radiological appearances may revert to normal spontaneously or as a result of treatment (Evans *et al.*, 1965). Impaction of Schistosoma parasites in the pulmonary arteries is responsible for the pulmonary hypertension of bilharzia (Garcia-Palmieri, 1964), and it has recently been suggested that the high incidence of pulmonary hypertension in Ceylon may be due to the filarial worm in the pulmonary arteries (Obeyesekeve and de Soysa, 1970).

Drugs and poisons may also cause pulmonary hypertension, although the mechanism is obscure. Aminorex fumarate, taken to reduce appetite and weight in European countries during 1966–68 (Foliath *et al.*, 1971), and the addition of cobalt to beer in Canada (Morin *et al.*, 1967) have both been shown with little doubt to cause pulmonary hypertension; it is probable that other chemicals will be found to be a cause of so-called 'primary' pulmonary hypertension.

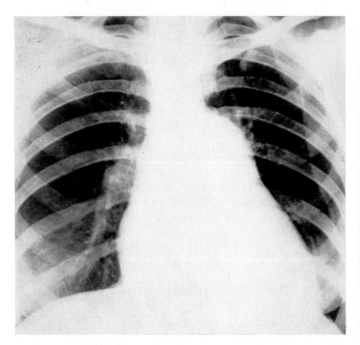

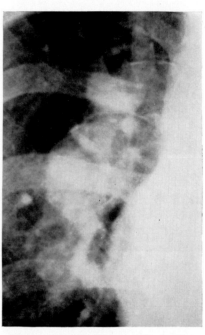

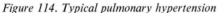

Figure 114. Typical pulmonary hypertension

Figure 115. Calcified atheroma of pulmonary arteries with tortuosity of segmental branches

The low alveolar oxygen tension at high altitudes induces vasoconstriction in the small muscular pulmonary arteries, causing pulmonary hypertension which becomes manifest between 5,000 and 10,000 feet. Chronic mountain sickness (Monge's disease—Monge, 1948) is due to loss of acclimatization to high altitude and presents with the features of severe pulmonary hypertension. High altitude pulmonary oedema occurs after rapid ascent to heights over 11,000 feet, particularly if combined with exertion in a cold dry atmosphere. The lungs show ill-defined opacities in all zones. The pulmonary artery pressure is high, but the wedge pressure is normal (Roy *et al.*, 1969), a fact difficult to explain in conjunction with alveolar oedema. Hypoxic pulmonary hypertension and congestive cardiac failure are also seen in children with upper respiratory tract obstruction with enlarged tonsils and adenoids, usually between the ages of two and six years when lymphoid hyperplasia is at its greatest. Pulmonary oedema and pleural effusion are also seen and are equally difficult to explain (Bland *et al.*, 1969).

COR PULMONALE

The definition of cor pulmonale has for long been controversial. In 1961 the World Health Organization defined chronic cor pulmonale as 'hypertrophy of the right ventricle resulting from disease affecting the function and/or structure of the lung, except when these pulmonary alterations are the result of diseases that primarily affect the left side of the heart or of congenital heart disease'. Right ventricular hypertrophy was defined as an outflow measuring over 5 mm in thickness. As cor pulmonale (if this expression is to be used at all) is usually a clinical diagnosis, right ventricular hypertrophy can only be diagnosed by clinical palpation of the precordium, electrocardiography and plain radiography. The definition excludes all causes of pulmonary venous hypertension as well as pulmonary arterial hypertension associated with central shunts, but includes such conditions as kypho-scoliosis and obesity

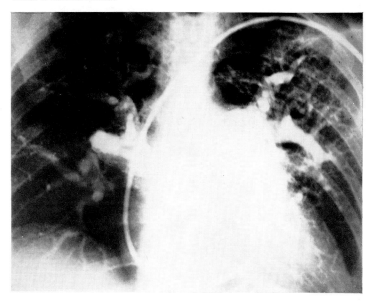

(a)

Figure 116. Thrombo-embolic pulmonary hypertension. (a) Angiogram—tortuous vessels, uneven vascular obliteration. (b) Anterior view —large central arteries, uneven vascular obliteration, raised right hemidiaphragm

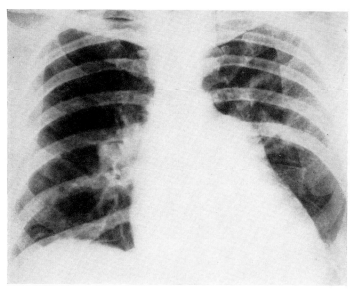

(b)

which have a secondary effect on respiratory function. Using this definition, but excluding pulmonary arterial disease which is considered above, the causes are as follows.

Diseases of the respiratory pathways
    Chronic obstructive airways disease: emphysema, bronchitis.

Diseases of the lung parenchyma
    Diffuse lung disease: fibrosis, granuloma, infiltration, cystic disease.

Diseases of the pleura
    Diffuse pleural thickening.

Conditions affecting the thoracic cage and diaphragm
    Kypho-scoliosis, thoracoplasty, obesity.

Unresponsive respiratory centre

There are three main types of chronic airways obstruction (Burrows *et al.*, 1966).

Emphysema type or 'pink puffer', which has:
    Radiological evidence of emphysema.
    Little sputum.
    Total lung capacity increased.
    Diffusing capacity reduced.
    No heart failure.

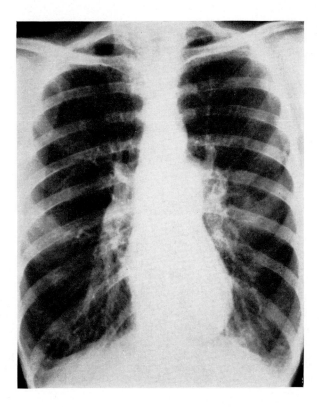

Figure 117 (left). Emphysema (pink puffer)—vertical heart, low flat diaphragm, central vessels large, peripheral vessels sparse

Figure 118 (below). Chronic bronchitis (blue bloater)— large hilar vessels, uneven vascular obliteration. (a) In failure. (b) After treatment

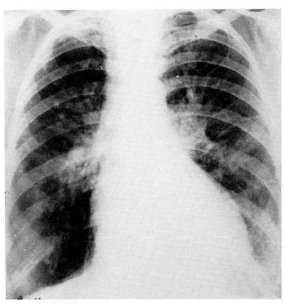

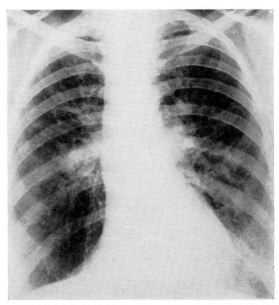

(a)   (b)

Bronchial type or 'blue bloater', which has:
No radiological evidence of emphysema.
Much sputum.
Total lung capacity reduced.
Diffusing capacity normal.
Recurrent heart failure with cyanosis and oedema.

Mixed type with features of both

The patient with emphysema ('pink puffer'—*Figure 117*) usually shows obvious evidence of air trapping (low diaphragm, vertical heart, large retrosternal air space) and emphysema (narrow straight sparse intrapulmonary vessels, flattening of diaphragm in frontal and lateral projections). The hilar vessels appear enlarged in contrast to the narrow pulmonary vessels, and although this combination suggests pulmonary hypertension, it should not be diagnosed on these grounds as the hilar enlargement is apparent rather than real. Pulmonary hypertension is rare in emphysema and is difficult to assess radiologically. It can be diagnosed with confidence only when the pulmonary trunk or the heart is enlarged; even this may be difficult, as the large pulmonary trunk may present merely as a long but unimpressive convexity, and with the typical vertical heart the right ventricle may be enlarged despite a cardiothoracic ratio of well under 50 per cent.

The chronic bronchitic or 'blue bloater' (*Figure 118*) may present, when not in heart failure, with a normal chest radiograph. Sometimes the lungs show scarring and irregular vascular obliteration, and changes of air trapping may be present, but the specific features of emphysema are absent. With the onset of congestive failure, there is a sudden increase in heart size and the pulmonary trunk and pulmonary arteries dilate. Dilatation extends further down the arterial pathway than in other forms of pulmonary hypertension and the picture resembles a left-to-right shunt, particularly an atrial septal defect. After treatment the heart, pulmonary trunk and pulmonary vessels quickly revert to normal, but eventually the typical changes of pulmonary hypertension may become established. Patients with cor pulmonale due to obesity are clinically and radiologically similar.

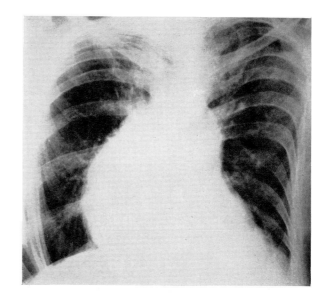

Figure 119. Scoliotic pulmonary hypertension (pulmonary artery systolic pressure 80 mm Hg) showing small hilar and intrapulmonary arteries

Proximal vessel dilatation indicative of pulmonary hypertension may be obscured in diffuse lung or pleural disease. It is not seen in association with scoliosis because of vascular hypoplasia (*Figure 119— also see* page 110).

CHAPTER 10

Pulmonary Venous Hypertension

VENOUS HYPERTENSION

When there is an increase in resistance to flow beyond the pulmonary capillaries, pressure rises in the pulmonary veins with the production of post-capillary or pulmonary venous hypertension; the pulmonary capillary venous pressure then measures 15 mm Hg or more. There is a corresponding slight rise in pulmonary arterial pressure, which is purely passive provided the pulmonary vascular resistance remains normal. The causes of pulmonary venous hypertension may lie in the pulmonary veins or in the left heart, but the effect on the pulmonary circulation and the resulting radiological changes in the lungs are similar.

Pulmonary venous hypertension may be due to lesions in the following sites.

Pulmonary veins
Total anomalous pulmonary venous drainage with stricture or below diaphragm.
Atresia.
Veno-occlusive disease.
Thrombosis.
Mediastinitis.
Tumour infiltration.

Left atrium
Cor triatriatum.
Tumour (myxoma, rarely others).

Mitral valve
Mitral stenosis.
Mitral regurgitation.

Left ventricle
Ischaemic heart disease.
Cardiomyopathy.
Aortic stenosis.
Aortic regurgitation.
Hypertension.
Coarctation.
Constrictive pericarditis.

PLEURO-PULMONARY CHANGES

The pleuro-pulmonary changes of pulmonary venous hypertension are considered under six headings:
(1) Upper zone vessel dilatation.
(2) Interstitial oedema.
(3) Pleural effusion.
(4) Alveolar oedema.
(5) Haemosiderosis.
(6) Ossific nodules.

It is possible broadly to relate these changes to the height of the pulmonary venous pressure, but to give a numerical figure to a subjective impression is always liable to error. For proper comparison of radiological changes with haemodynamics, the film should be taken within 24 hours of cardiac catheterization and preferably before the examination if angiocardiography is to be performed, as injection of large doses of contrast medium may adversely affect the haemodynamics for at least 24 hours in patients with heart disease. A short period of bed rest may cause regression of interstitial oedema, and comparison of films of ambulant patients with catheter data is a potential source of error. Discrepancies will be encountered unless pressures are recorded not only at rest but also in response to exercise. It is not uncommon to find normal or only slightly elevated pressures under basal conditions but a steep rise on straight leg raising in patients who have clear radiological evidence of an elevated pulmonary venous pressure. With these provisos in mind, the general principles which apply are set out in Table 5.

TABLE 5

Pulmonary venous pressure (mean mm Hg)	Chest radiograph
Up to 19 at rest, *or* normal at rest but rising on exercise	Upper zone vessels dilated Lower zone vessels normal
Over 19 at rest	Upper zone vessels wider Lower zone vessels normal Interstitial oedema Small effusions
Over 30 at rest	Alveolar oedema Large effusions

Upper zone vessel dilatation

In pulmonary venous hypertension the earliest change on the chest radiograph is dilatation of the upper zone vessels (*Figure 120*), the lower zone vessel calibre remaining normal with a normal vascular resistance. The size of the upper zone vessels roughly parallels the height of the pulmonary venous pressure and reflects the degree of blood diversion to the upper zones (Friedman and Brauwald, 1966). Occasionally the upper lobe veins may be the only obviously dilated vessels, but more often both veins and arteries are widened so that all vessels above the hilum are a little wider than those at a comparable level below. Vessels in the first anterior interspace rarely measure more than 3 mm in diameter; if they are wider, the diagnosis of an elevated pulmonary venous pressure is almost certain. Occasionally vessels in the upper and lower zones appear equal in calibre, and then the changes may be mistaken for plethora.

The statistical relationship of the pulmonary venous pressure to upper zone vessel dilatation in patients with chronic valve disease is as follows. With normal upper zone vessels the resting pressure is normal in 80 per cent of cases; with slightly dilated vessels the pressure is raised in 75 per cent, and with obvious dilatation it is raised in 95 per cent. Analysed the other way, with a normal pressure the vessels are normal in 75 per cent of cases, with a pressure up to 20 the vessels are slightly or obviously enlarged in 85 per cent, and with a pressure over 20 they are enlarged in almost 100 per cent. The correlation is thus very strong, and the discrepancies are no doubt due to the numerous sources of possible error discussed above (*see* Appendix C).

Where the pressure rise is acute as in left ventricular failure, the degree of dilatation may change quite quickly, but in some patients, for an unknown reason, dilatation may be absent despite obvious interstitial oedema. Lung disease may profoundly affect the picture. Healed tuberculosis in the upper zones may prevent vessel dilatation because of vascular obliteration even though visible scarring is minimal (*Figure 120c*). Emphysema has a similar effect when present in the upper zones, and when confined to the lower zones it can cause upper zone blood diversion in the absence of pulmonary venous hypertension.

The mechanism of blood diversion to the upper zones is not clear, and it has been suggested that the hydrostatic increment of pressure in the lower zones in the erect position is a factor. This is unlikely to be the whole story, because evidence of blood diversion can be seen in infants with high pulmonary venous pressure who do not assume an erect posture. Perivascular oedema of lower zone vessels has also been suggested as a cause.

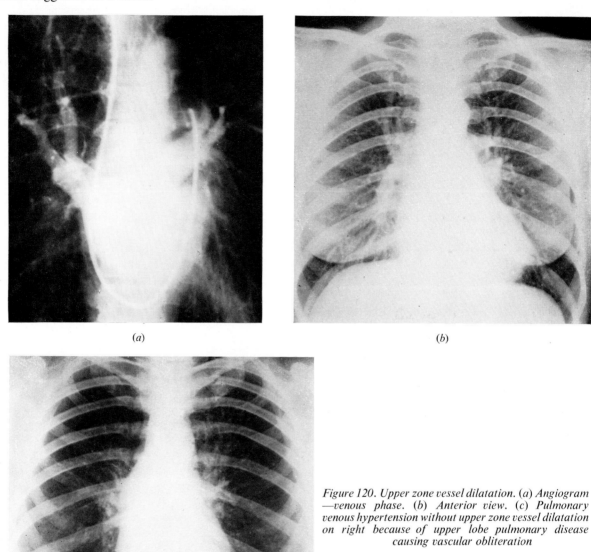

(a)

(b)

(c)

Figure 120. Upper zone vessel dilatation. (a) Angiogram —venous phase. (b) Anterior view. (c) Pulmonary venous hypertension without upper zone vessel dilatation on right because of upper lobe pulmonary disease causing vascular obliteration

Interstitial oedema

When the capillary pressure exceeds the normal plasma osmotic pressure of 25 mm Hg, fluid including fibrin and red cells escapes into the interstitial tissues of the lung. Lymph flow is increased and all lymphatics dilate. There are many signs of interstitial oedema on the chest radiograph and they all reflect the presence of oedema fluid, dilated lymphatics and the deposition of haemosiderin in the interstitial tissues.

The statistical relationship of the measured pulmonary venous pressure to signs of interstitial oedema in patients with chronic valve disease is as follows. If the pressure is normal, oedema is absent in 99 per cent; with a raised pressure up to 19 mm Hg, oedema is present in 20 per cent; with a pressure over 19 mm Hg, oedema is present in 70 per cent. In a given patient with interstitial oedema, there is an 80 per cent chance of the pulmonary venous pressure being over 19 mm Hg (*see* Appendix C).

Septal lines (*Figure 121*)

These are also termed Kerley B lines (Kerley, 1933) or basal septal lines. They are dense, short, straight, horizontal lines most commonly seen in the costo-phrenic angles; occasionally they extend into the middle zones, but never into the upper zones. They may be so fine as to be barely visible, or as much as 4 mm wide. They result from thickening of the interlobular septa and therefore represent a tissue plane about 1 cm in depth (Heitzman *et al.*, 1967). Their density is thus much greater than that of any neighbouring vessel, and this is an important diagnostic point. Also unlike vessels, they do not branch. Most are seen to reach the lateral pleural surface, but they may appear to stop short if they do not meet the part of the pleura which is tangential to the x-ray beam. In children they are often better seen on the lateral view in the anterior portions of the lungs. Septal lines usually disappear rapidly after reduction of venous pressure by medical or surgical treatment, but occasionally they persist due to fibrous replacement of oedema fluid and deposition of haemosiderin, in which case they become thinner and more clear-cut.

Deep septal lines (*Figure 122*).—Two other types of line shadow are seen, caused by oedema of deep tissue planes probably around the anastomotic lymphatics. The first is the Kerley A line. This is a straight or slightly angled line, up to 4 cm in length, and dense and fairly uniform in thickness. It may be seen

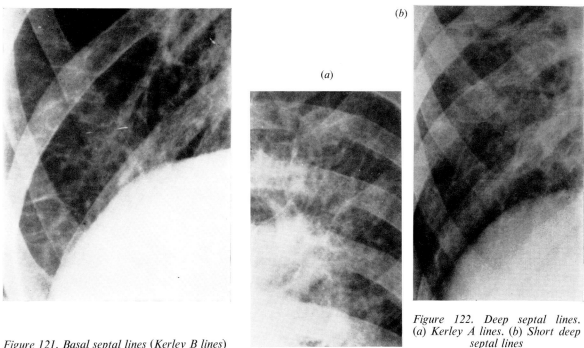

Figure 121. Basal septal lines (Kerley B lines)

Figure 122. Deep septal lines. (a) Kerley A lines. (b) Short deep septal lines

in any zone, but always runs towards the hilum. The second type is less well recognized. The lines are much finer and shorter, run in any direction, and are most frequently seen in the lower zones. If looked for carefully they are seen more often than A lines but less often than B lines.

Lobular pattern

Harley (1961) has described a lobular pattern in the lower zones which he ascribes to oedema of the interlobular septa seen *en face*. The authors are not convinced that they have recognized this appearance.

Perivascular and peribronchial oedema (Figure 123)

Oedema of the perivascular loose connective tissue blurs the edges of the segmental vessels. It may contribute to the apparent widening of the upper zone vessels and, as mentioned above, may be a causative factor in upper zone blood diversion. It may also be responsible for the fact that the lower zone

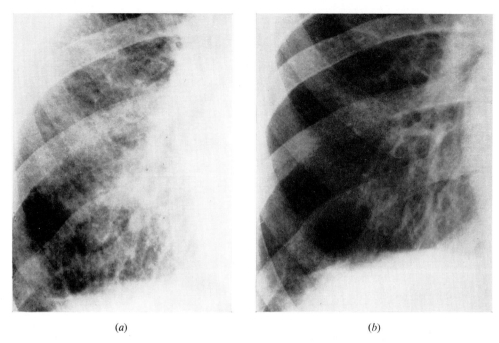

(a)   (b)

Figure 123. (a) Perivascular oedema. (b) After treatment

vessels may not appear narrow despite a lower than normal blood flow. Peribronchial oedema can be appreciated when a bronchus seen end-on has an abnormally thick wall, an appearance most often present in the left upper zone.

Hilar oedema (Figure 124)

Oedema fluid often collects in the loose connective tissue around the hilum. The outline of the vessels becomes indistinct (hilar haze) and the whole hilum is larger than normal.

Mottling (Figure 125) and loss of translucency (Figure 126)

The lung fields may show a generalized loss of translucency with or without the presence of fine mottling. These appearances are difficult to detect on a single film, but are easily appreciated in retrospect if compared with a film taken when the venous pressure was normal. They result from summation in depth of all the waterlogged interstitial tissues of the lung.

Pleural effusion

Pleural effusion (*Figure 127*) is common with pulmonary venous hypertension. Small effusions up to a few millimetres thick, running vertically into the depths of the costo-phrenic angles, are common but easily missed. Equally common, and well seen on the lateral view, are thin effusions in the fissures. These small effusions occasionally occur without septal lines and may be the only sign of interstitial oedema. Some of the fluid lies between the lung and the visceral pleura, a tissue plane continuous with the interlobular septa, while some lies in the pleural space. Larger effusions are usually associated with a higher venous pressure and are commoner in left ventricular failure than in mitral valve disease. They occasionally become loculated and may remain for weeks or months. A persistent effusion may be due to pulmonary infarction even though no infarct shadow is visible, and in mitral valve disease it may rarely be due to pulmonary venous thrombosis.

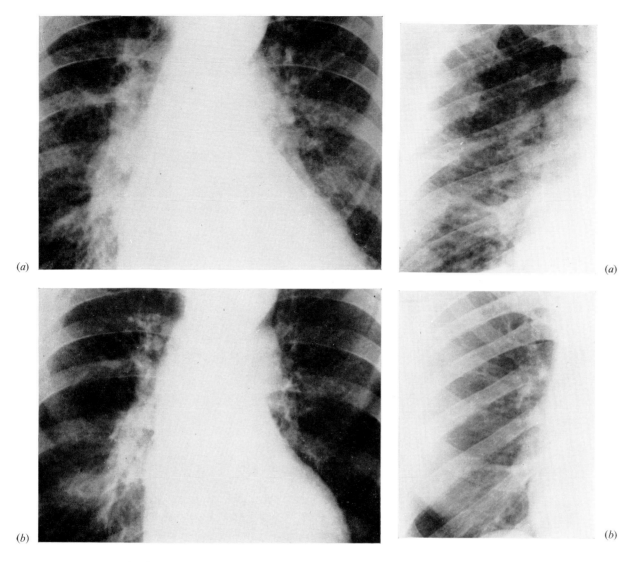

(a)

(a)

(b)

(b)

Figure 124. (a) Hilar oedema. (b) After treatment

Figure 125. (a) Mottling. (b) After treatment

Alveolar oedema

When the pulmonary venous pressure reaches 30 mm Hg, oedema fluid may be no longer contained within the interstitial tissues but escape into the alveoli (*Figure 128*). Radiologically this appears as an ill-defined semi-confluent shadowing which may lie in any part of the lungs, appear or disappear quickly, and change its distribution from day to day. On the other hand, if the oedema fluid contains fibrin so that organization occurs, clearing may be very slow. Signs of interstitial oedema and pleural effusion are frequently associated. The commonest appearance is the 'bat's wing' shadow in which the oedema apparently has a perihilar distribution. However, if a lateral view is taken, it shows that the fluid has a lobar distribution and lies in the base of the upper lobe or the apex of the lower lobe (Gleason and Steiner, 1966). On the anterior view there is usually a clear area between the edge of the oedema and the lateral pleural surface. The bat's wing shadow is occasionally unilateral and may be related to posture. It was at one time thought to be specific to uraemia, but is now known to occur in heart failure with normal renal function. The distribution of alveolar oedema is occasionally bizarre; for instance, it may be confined to a lobe, or may be entirely peripheral and indistinguishable from pneumonia and infarction. Oedematous lung is liable to become infected, but specific radiological signs are usually absent.

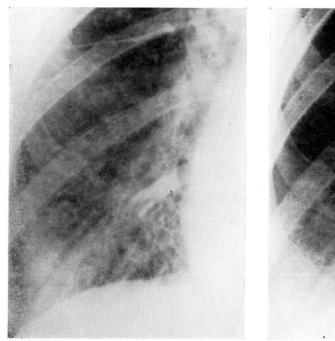

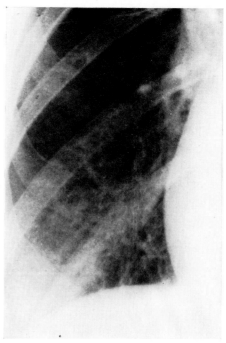

(a)   (b)

Figure 126. (a) Loss of translucency. (b) After treatment

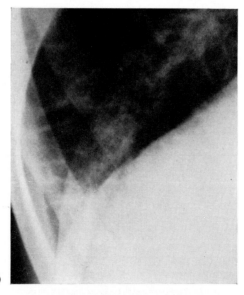

*Figure 127. Pleural effusion.
(a) Parietal effusion in costo-
phrenic angle with septal lines.
(b) Thin effusion in horizontal
fissure. (c) Loculated effusion in
oblique fissure*

(a)

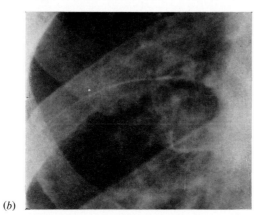

(b)

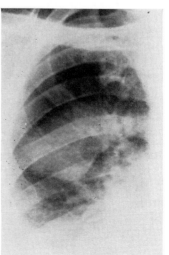

(c)

Pulmonary haemosiderosis

Pulmonary haemosiderosis (*Figure 129*) is due to focal deposition of haemosiderin in groups of alveoli and is associated with chronic pulmonary venous hypertension, but not necessarily with a high pulmonary vascular resistance. It must be distinguished from the idiopathic variety, in which there is a normal pulmonary venous pressure but which is occasionally associated with myocarditis and dilatation of the heart (Murphy, 1965). The lungs show diffuse mottling in all zones which may be fine or coarse, but the individual foci are roughly equal in size. The mottling may exactly resemble that of generalized interstitial oedema, but shows no change following medical or surgical treatment.

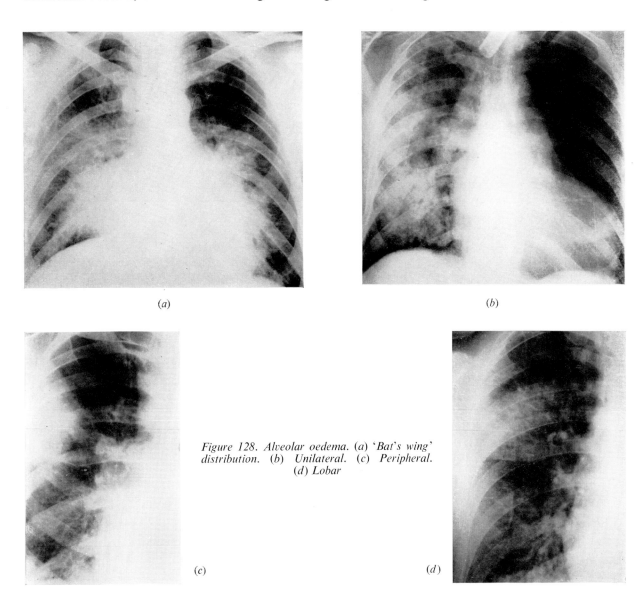

(a)

(b)

Figure 128. Alveolar oedema. (a) 'Bat's wing' distribution. (b) Unilateral. (c) Peripheral. (d) Lobar

(c)

(d)

Pulmonary ossific nodules

Ossific nodules in the lung (*Figure 130*) are also associated with chronic pulmonary venous hypertension and are due to heterotopic bone formation following organization of intra-alveolar oedema. They are most commonly seen in mitral valve disease, but may rarely occur with left atrial myxoma or chronic left ventricular failure. The nodules are dense and irregularly round or oval, and rarely a small central medullary space may be visible within. They vary in size from 1 to 10 mm, are larger and denser in the lower zones, and are not often seen in the upper zones. They tend to increase slowly in number and size. They can be distinguished from calcified tuberculosis by their lower zone distribution and their round or oval shape, but they may be confused with histoplasmosis or chickenpox pneumonia. They are said to be more common in males.

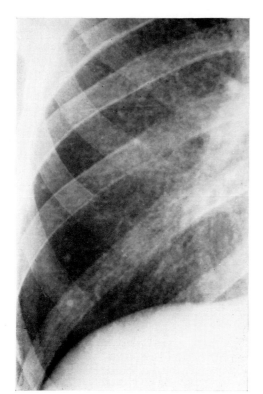

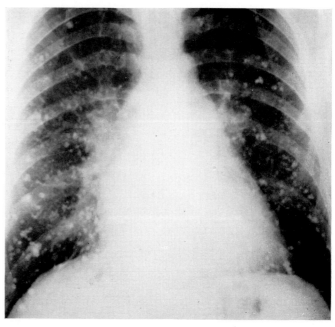

Figure 129 (left). Haemosiderosis

Figure 130 (below). Pulmonary ossific nodules

MIXED VENOUS AND ARTERIAL HYPERTENSION

Sustained pulmonary venous hypertension may cause obstructive changes in the small pulmonary arteries leading to an increase in pulmonary vascular resistance. There is a disproportionate rise in pulmonary arterial pressure compared with venous pressure, and the cardiac output is usually reduced.

TABLE 6

Pulmonary vascular resistance	*Radiological changes (per cent)*	
Normal	Upper zone vessels dilated	55
	Lower lobe artery large	1
	Lower segmental vessels narrow	2
	Pulmonary trunk dilated	4
3–9 units	Upper zone vessels dilated	95
	Lower lobe artery large	40
	Lower segmental vessels narrow	50
	Pulmonary trunk dilated	40
	and obviously so	5
Over 9 units	Upper zone vessels dilated	99
	Lower lobe artery large	80
	Lower segmental vessels narrow	95
	Pulmonary trunk dilated	85
	and obviously so	55

The pulmonary hypertension is both venous (post-capillary) and arterial (pre-capillary). The typical haemodynamics may be illustrated by using the formula $R = P/Q$ (*see* page 74) where R = resistance, P = pressure gradient across the lungs, and Q = pulmonary blood flow. If the mean pulmonary artery pressure is 50 mm Hg, the mean left atrial pressure is 25 mm Hg and the cardiac output is 2·5 litres per minute, then $R = (50 - 25)/2·5 = 10$ units.

The radiological changes are veno-arterial narrowing and dilatation of the pulmonary trunk and lobar arteries (*Figure 131*). A statistical guide to their haemodynamic significance is shown in Table 6, based on a study of 300 cases of chronic valve disease (*see* Appendix C).

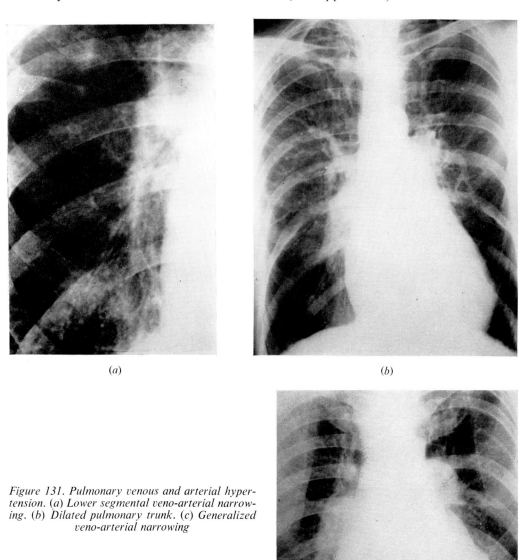

(*a*)

(*b*)

(*c*)

Figure 131. Pulmonary venous and arterial hypertension. (a) Lower segmental veno-arterial narrowing. (b) Dilated pulmonary trunk. (c) Generalized veno-arterial narrowing

The first recognizable evidence of an elevated pulmonary vascular resistance is narrowing of both arteries and veins and in the lower zones. The basal segmental arteries become narrow, irregular and a little tortuous, and it is often impossible to identify a lower lobe vein. The narrow lower zone vessels contrast with the normal or dilated lower lobar artery, which is well seen on the right side. The appearances reflect progressive reduction in blood flow throughout the lower zones.

A later change is dilatation of the pulmonary trunk which, when obvious, almost always means a resistance greater than 10 units and a pulmonary artery systolic pressure at or near systemic level. With a very high resistance at 15 units and above, veno-arterial narrowing is seen higher in the lungs and may finally involve the upper zones. Interstitial oedema tends to disappear and such cases may radiologically resemble primary pulmonary hypertension, in which proximal pulmonary artery dilatation is accompanied by uniform peripheral vessel narrowing. Indeed, the cardiac output may be so low that the mitral diastolic murmur is inaudible, the left atrium may not be large, and the presence of underlying mitral valve disease may be missed.

CHAPTER 11

Uneven Pulmonary Vascularity

Uneven pulmonary vascularity means the presence of vessels of unusual size in a lung or a part of a lung. They are either too small or too large. Discussion will be limited to the cardiovascular causes of uneven vascularity, and it should be helpful to read Chapter 7 on the normal pulmonary vascular pattern before proceeding (*see* page 70).

UNILATERAL DIFFERENCE IN VESSEL PATTERN

Arteries and veins in one lung are smaller or larger than normal. The commonest finding is of small vessels in one lung associated with large vessels in the other. The lung containing the small vessels may be hypertranslucent or may show evidence of reduction in volume such as mediastinal shift, elevated diaphragm and narrow intercostal spacing.

The cardiovascular causes are:

(1) Congenital absence of one pulmonary artery.

(2) Congenital pulmonary artery stenosis (*see* page 228).

(3) Surgical ligation, stricture or kinking, e.g. shunt operation, slipped pulmonary artery band.

(4) Extrinsic pressure from right aortic arch, aneurysm, tumour, mediastinitis, aberrant left pulmonary artery.

(5) Massive embolism (*see* page 99).

(6) Abnormal right ventricular ejection in Fallot's tetralogy, pulmonary valve stenosis and transposition.

(7) Hemitruncus arteriosus.

(8) Central shunts.

Emanuel and Pattinson (1956) have shown that when the right pulmonary artery is absent, the heart is either normal (*Figure 132*) or there are lesions involving the great vessels, particularly coarctation and ductus arteriosus. When the left pulmonary artery is absent or unconnected to the pulmonary trunk, Fallot and pulmonary atresia are common (*Figure 133*), and the incidence of right aortic arch is 60 per cent (as opposed to 25 per cent if these lesions are uncomplicated).

Alteration in vessel pattern is common after surgery. Increase in vessel size is to be expected after a shunt operation, and the change is most often unilateral after a Waterston anastomosis. The difference between the two sides may be accentuated if the right pulmonary artery is kinked at operation so that blood from the anastomosis is prevented from reaching the left lung. Ipsilateral increase in vessel size is uncommon after a Blalock shunt; indeed, occasionally the upper lobe vessels on the side of the anastomosis may actually be narrower than normal due to surgical interference. A pulmonary artery band may sometimes become displaced distally and obstruct one pulmonary artery more than the other.

Unilateral asymmetry may result from extrinsic pressure. The commonest cause is carcinoma of the bronchus, but a rare cause has been reported in Fallot's tetralogy in which the right pulmonary artery was compressed by a large right-sided aorta (Porstmann *et al.*, 1967).

An aberrant left pulmonary artery arises from the right pulmonary artery to the right of the midline and passes to the left between the trachea and the oesophagus. As the artery is compressed, it results in smaller left lung vessels. The anomaly presents like a vascular ring in infants with compression of the trachea, right main bronchus or oesophagus. On the lateral view the left pulmonary artery may be seen to indent the posterior wall of the trachea. The diagnosis is confirmed by anterior indentation of the barium-filled oesophagus (Philp *et al.*, 1972).

95

In the normal, the blood flow to the left upper lobe is a little greater than to the right because of the slight inclination of the right ventricular outflow and the pulmonary trunk in that direction (Davies and Dow, 1971). In Fallot's tetralogy with marked distortion of parietal and septal bands, the outflow tract is inclined towards the right. The deformity results in early and greater filling of the right lung,

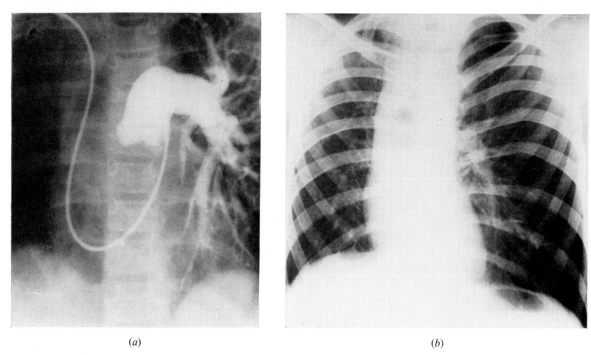

(a)   (b)

Figure 132. Absent right pulmonary artery. (a) Angiogram. (b) Anterior view—small right lung vessels with mediastinal shift to the right

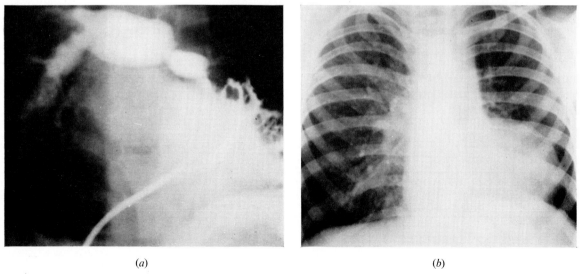

(a)   (b)

Figure 133. Absent left pulmonary artery in Fallot's tetralogy. (a) Angiogram. (b) Left pulmonary vessels smaller than right

which may show wider vessels than the left lung. Tilting of the right ventricular outflow is also seen in some cases of transposition (*Figure 134*), particularly with single ventricle (Davies and Dow, 1971). Pulmonary stenosis with transposition further encourages elective right-sided filling. Better filling of the left lung is seen in pure pulmonary valve stenosis (*Figure 135*). The jet is directed towards the roof of the pulmonary trunk and the left pulmonary artery, resulting in proximal vessel dilatation, well seen in the left lower lobe artery. Rarely, similar appearances are seen in Fallot's tetralogy, where the outflow tract is directed slightly towards the left (Wilson and Amplatz, 1967) and when important valve stenosis is present.

Systemic arterial supply to one lung may result from a congenital anomaly of the trunco-conus which is termed hemitruncus arteriosus or aortic origin of the pulmonary artery (*Figure 136*). One lung, usually

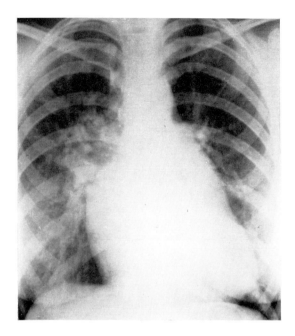

Figure 134. Corrected transposition showing vessel asymmetry

Figure 135 (below). Pulmonary valve stenosis. Post-stenotic dilatation extending into left segmental branches. (a) Angiogram. (b) Anterior view

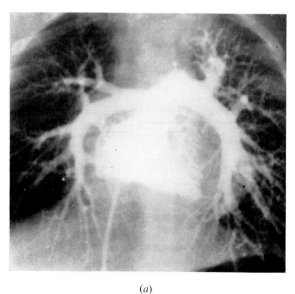

(a)

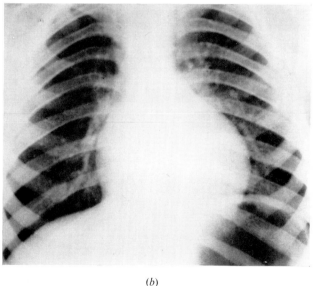

(b)

the right, is supplied by a large vessel arising from the ascending aorta, and the right lung is plethoric. The left lung is connected to the right ventricle, but there may be stenosis or atresia, which accentuates the vessel asymmetry.

In left-to-right shunts at the atrial, ventricular and aorto-pulmonary levels, vessels in the left lung may appear smaller and less numerous than in the right lung. The change may be seen throughout the lung or only in the upper zone. It is more frequently reported in ductus arteriosus (27·8 per cent) than in ventricular septal defect (10 per cent) and atrial septal defect (6·7 per cent) (Rosenbaum *et al.*, 1966).

In the authors' experience it is present in about 5 per cent of all shunts, most commonly in atrial septal defect (*Figure 137*). Angiography excludes unilateral pulmonary stenosis and shows narrower and less numerous intrapulmonary vessels.

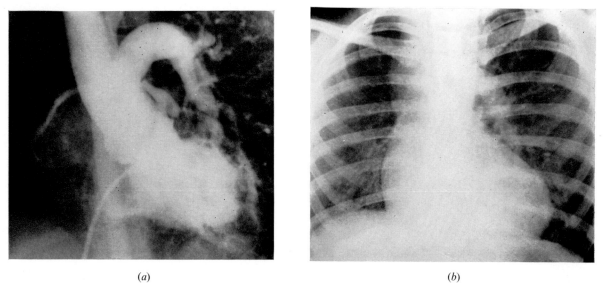

(a) (b)

Figure 136. Hemitruncus. Left lung supplied from ascending aorta. Right lung supplied from right ventricle via stenotic outflow and small pulmonary artery. (a) Angiogram. (b) Anterior view showing vessel asymmetry

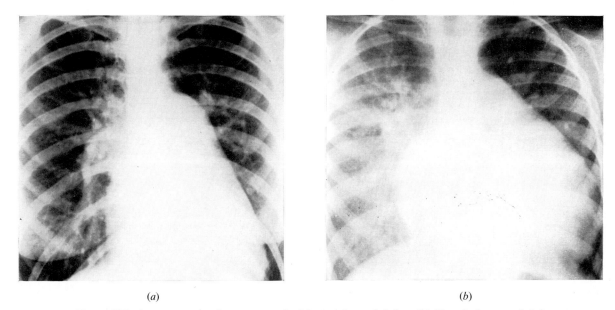

(a) (b)

Figure 137. Asymmetrical pulmonary vessels. (a) Atrial septal defect. (b) Ventricular septal defect

UNEVEN VASCULARITY OF A PATCHY NATURE

This is due to irregular perfusion of the lungs, either by the pulmonary arteries or by a systemic arterial supply from the thoracic aorta or its branches. The conditions which may cause this appearance are considered in other chapters, but are listed here for the sake of completeness.

(1) Peripheral pulmonary arterial stenosis (*see* page 228).
(2) Multiple pulmonary arteriovenous fistulae (*see* page 210).
(3) Multiple pulmonary emboli (*see* page 99).
(4) Pulmonary atresia (*see* page 182).

CHAPTER 12

Pulmonary Thrombo-embolism and Infarction

Air, fat, tumour, parasites and amniotic fluid may embolize to the lungs, but this chapter is concerned with embolism of thrombus originating in the systemic veins or the right heart. The clinical presentation and radiological appearances vary depending on the size and number of emboli and the presence or absence of infarction. If large emboli lodge in the pulmonary trunk and the main pulmonary arteries, the clinical picture is one of collapse, dyspnoea, tachycardia and hypotension. Emboli in lobar arteries may present in a similar way. In contrast, small emboli in the periphery of the lung often produce no immediate clinical signs or symptoms. If they are multiple and recurrent, the patient presents later with chronic pulmonary hypertension.

Infarction is not invariable with embolism, as an alternative arterial supply to the lung is available from the bronchial circulation; it is most likely to occur in the presence of chronic pulmonary venous hypertension. An infarct if small is often clinically silent, but when it involves half a segment or more it may cause fever, tachypnoea, haemoptysis, and pleurisy with or without effusion.

ACUTE PULMONARY EMBOLISM

The following classification (Chang, 1967b) relates both to the clinical picture and to the radiological appearance.

(1) Central
(2) Lobar and segmental ⎫ with or without infarction.
(3) Peripheral ⎭

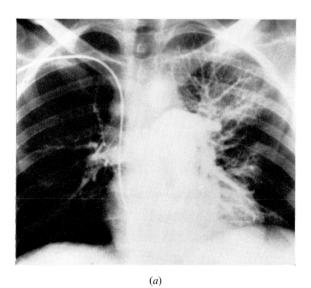 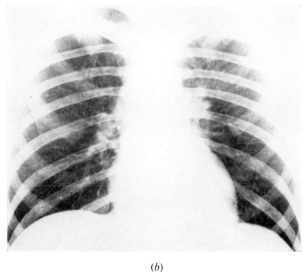

(a)   (b)

Figure 138. Massive pulmonary embolism. (a) Angiogram. (b) Anterior view—oligaemia in right lung and left lower zone

99

Central pulmonary embolism

One or more large emboli may lodge in the pulmonary trunk or the right and left pulmonary arteries (*Figure 138*) and cause ischaemia of the lung as first described by Westermark (1938). The affected areas

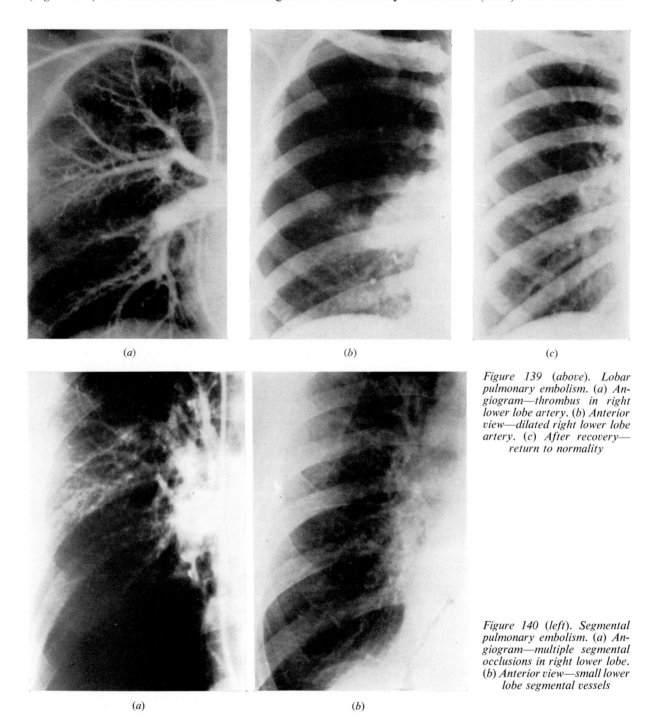

(a)   (b)   (c)

Figure 139 (above). Lobar pulmonary embolism. (a) Angiogram—thrombus in right lower lobe artery. (b) Anterior view—dilated right lower lobe artery. (c) After recovery—return to normality

(a)   (b)

Figure 140 (left). Segmental pulmonary embolism. (a) Angiogram—multiple segmental occlusions in right lower lobe. (b) Anterior view—small lower lobe segmental vessels

are abnormally radiolucent, with absent or small vessels; the changes are widespread and patchy when obstruction is incomplete. Compensatory dilatation may be seen in unobstructed areas (Kerr *et al.*, 1971). The diaphragm is raised as a result of decreased lung volume. There is no dilatation of the pulmonary trunk, the hilar arteries remain small, and there is no widening of the right lower lobe pulmonary artery (upper limit of normal 16 mm in men, 15 mm in women). The right atrium and ventricle dilate slightly, but this may be difficult to assess because only portable films may be available. Infarction is rarely seen, probably because effective treatment or death usually occurs before it has time to develop.

Lobar and segmental embolism

Medium-sized emboli are usually multiple and obstruct lobar and segmental arteries (*Figures 139* and *140*), most commonly in the lower lobes. Ischaemia with absent or small vessels is patchy, and the artery containing the embolus may have an amputated appearance just proximal to the ischaemic area. Compensatory dilatation in unaffected parts of the lung is more obvious than with central pulmonary embolism and is occasionally accompanied by overperfusion pulmonary oedema. Diaphragmatic elevation may be present if an embolus lodges in a lower lobe. In contrast to central pulmonary embolism, there is often dilatation of the pulmonary trunk and the right lower lobe artery, but the heart rarely enlarges much unless the obstruction is widespread. Infarction may occur, particularly in the presence of an elevated pulmonary venous pressure.

Peripheral embolism

Small emboli which obstruct the pulmonary arteries beyond the segmental arteries usually produce no detectable ischaemic changes or diaphragmatic elevation. They may present as small infarcts (*Figure 141*), usually without pleural effusion, but it is thought that many are radiologically as well as clinically silent. Widespread obliteration of the pulmonary vascular bed by small emboli eventually causes chronic pulmonary hypertension (*Figure 142*).

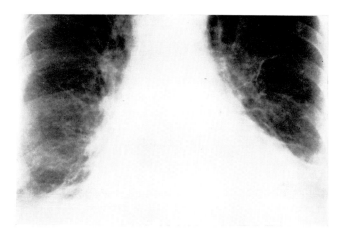

Figure 141. Pulmonary infarcts—small, basal, symptomless   *Figure 142. Chronic thrombo-embolic pulmonary hypertension*

PULMONARY INFARCTION

Infarcts (*Figure 143*) are a complication of pulmonary embolism and occur when a portion of embolized lung receives an insufficient collateral blood supply from the bronchial and neighbouring pulmonary circulations. The lung is consolidated from effusion of blood and fluid into the alveolar spaces. Infarcts may be reversible (Hampton and Castleman, 1940) or complete. When they are reversible, the alveolar walls remain intact and the radiological shadows are transient. When complete, the alveolar walls may be destroyed and the shadows persist. An infarct may develop immediately after embolization or be delayed for five days (Fleischner, 1962), but there is no time lag between the formation of an infarct and its appearance on the x-ray.

The radiological features of pulmonary infarction are:
    (1) The infarct shadow.
    (2) Pleural effusion.
    (3) Diaphragmatic elevation.

Infarcts are commonest in the lower zones and rare in the upper zones except with chronic pulmonary venous hypertension. They vary in size from just visible to 10 cm (Fleischner, 1962). The lung is consolidated and slightly reduced in volume. If the infarct is reversible, clearing may occur in a day or two. If it is complete, the consolidation is initially ill-defined, but after about two or four days it becomes better demarcated. It had been thought theoretically that an infarct should be cone-shaped with its base

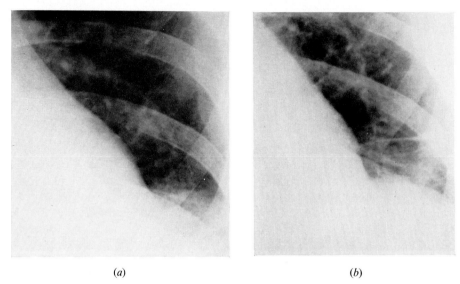

(a)   (b)

Figure 143. Pulmonary infarction. (a) Fresh infarct. (b) Healed infarct

on the pleura until Hampton and Castleman (1940) showed that only the basal half or third of the cone was actually infarcted. This is why a triangular shadow with its base on the pleura is never seen. An infarct may be almost any shape from a band to a circle, depending on its position relative to the projection, but it can always be shown to be contiguous with a pleural surface on an appropriate tangential view. During healing it contracts in size and finally ends up as a linear or band-like scar. Very rarely, an infarct cavitates as a result of avascular necrosis or secondary infection.

Pleural effusion is absent with small peripheral infarcts, but often occurs early with infarcts in the lower lobe. It tends to be larger and more persistent with pulmonary venous hypertension, when it may hide the infarct shadow so that the effusion is the only sign of underlying infarction. Basal infarcts may be clinically silent in the presence of pulmonary venous hypertension and blood diversion to the upper zones, presumably because the pulmonary circulation is very little compromised. Rapid accumulation of fluid may prevent pleuritic pain, and the effusion may become chronic and loculate. On resolution, the fluid either absorbs completely or leaves basal pleural thickening.

Infarcts have to be differentiated from infection, collapse due to sputum retention, and contusion of the lung at surgery. An early pleural effusion and diaphragmatic elevation are useful points in favour of infarction.

LATE CHANGES OF EMBOLISM

Emboli may lyse and a normal circulation may be re-established in under two weeks. Recanalization of blocked arteries may occur, but often the perfusion is poor because of displacement of thrombus into the distal branches. This may show radiologically as permanent areas of ischaemia. Thrombus may slowly acquire calcium so that the hilar arteries become abnormally dense and clear-cut. Widespread occlusion of the vascular bed results in chronic thrombo-embolic pulmonary hypertension; uneven pulmonary vascularity, infarct scars and pleural thickening may suggest the diagnosis (*see Figure 116*).

SECTION III
Other Systems in Heart Disease

CHAPTER 13

The Bony Thorax

NOTCHING OF THE RIBS

In 1928 Roesler described notching of the ribs as a sign of coarctation of the aorta. The erosions are caused by dilatation, tortuosity and increased pulsation of the aortic or posterior intercostal arteries (*Figure 144*). Notching does not involve the inferior border of the rib but the antero-inferior surface in the intercostal groove. Notches are not seen in the anterior parts of the ribs because the subcostal grooves are absent and the anterior intercostal arteries run between the ribs. They are also absent from the first two ribs as the first and second posterior intercostal arteries arise not from the aorta but from the superior intercostal branch of the costo-cervical trunk of the subclavian artery, and so do not form part of the distal collateral pathway into the aorta. The notches may be shallow and scalloped or deep and round. They are surrounded by a rim of thin but well-defined bone sclerosis, an appearance which distinguishes them from such conditions as hyperparathyroidism and tuberose sclerosis (*Figure 145*). They are usually bilateral but asymmetrical.

Unilateral notching suggests that the intercostal arteries on the side without the erosions are not being subjected to a high perfusion pressure from the ipsilateral subclavian artery. Unilateral right-sided notching occurs when the left subclavian artery is obstructed or when the coarctation lies proximal to its origin, and left-sided notching when there is an anomalous right subclavian artery arising from the low pressure portion of the aorta distal to the coarctation. Prominent notching of the last three ribs suggests that the obstruction is lower down in the thoracic or upper abdominal aorta, and that the diagnosis is more likely to be aortitis with obstruction than coarctation. Notching does not develop in pre-duct coarctation, when the collateral supply to the descending aorta comes from the pulmonary artery. It is also absent in pseudo-coarctation, in which the aorta is kinked but not obstructed; the aortic configuration on the anterior view exactly resembles true coarctation. Development of notching is related to the severity and duration of the obstruction. It has been reported in infants aged under 1 year (Martelle and Moss, 1962) but is very rare below the age of 5 years.

For many years after Roesler's description, rib notching was considered diagnostic of coarctation. It is now known that enlargement of any of the three structures lying on the subcostal groove (intercostal artery, vein or nerve) may cause pressure erosion of bone. Of the arterial causes other than coarctation, aortitis with obstruction may provoke an intercostal collateral circulation. The lesion is often more distally situated than coarctation and erroneously referred to as coarctation at an unusual site.

Unilateral rib notching following Blalock's subclavian/pulmonary artery anastomosis was first described by Kent (1953) (*Figure 146*). The posterior intercostals form the major collateral circulation from the aorta to the arm via the scapular anastomosis, and intercostal blood flow is in a direction opposite to that in coarctation. Development of notching is in no way related to the patency or otherwise of the Blalock anastomosis, but probably relates to the absence of other important collateral pathways to the arm. Collateral circulation from the brain via the vertebral artery, the subclavian steal syndrome, is prevented as the vertebral artery is ligated at operation. It is worth noting that notching usually takes about three years to develop after Blalock's operation, but may be visible within six months (Kent, 1953). It may regress within one to two years after correction of the coarctation.

Notching of the ribs is rarely seen in arteritis or atheroma of the subclavian artery as only the first part of the artery is commonly involved and the vertebral collateral system operates in preference to the posterior intercostal. The intercostal arteries occasionally take part in the collateral supply to the lung if there is deficient pulmonary blood flow as in pulmonary atresia (*Figure 147*) and multiple pulmonary

105

artery stenosis, but these vessels can only cross the pleura through adhesions caused by infection or surgical trauma; otherwise they enter the lung via the hilum from anastomosis with mediastinal arteries anteriorly. Rib notching may be related to an arteriovenous fistula of the lung or chest wall if intercostal

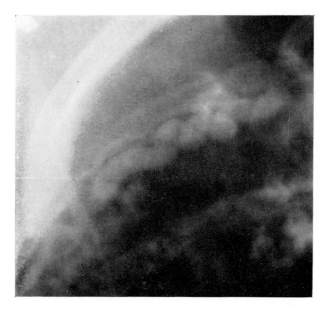

Figure 144. Dilated and tortuous intercostal artery in subcostal groove. Angiogram

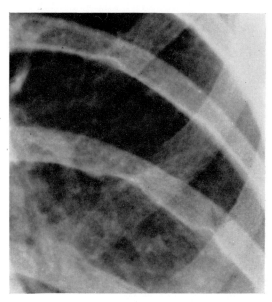

Figure 145. Rib notching. Coarctation

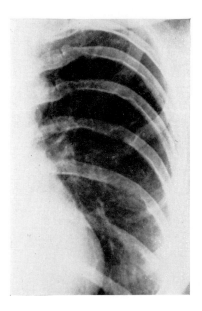

Figure 146. Rib notching after Blalock's operation

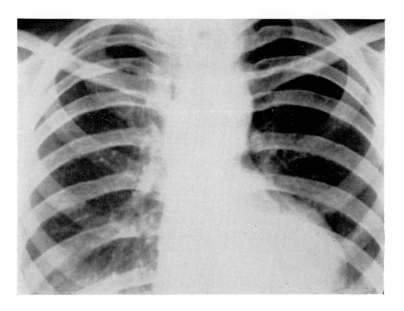

Figure 147. Notching of right upper ribs in pulmonary atresia

arteries are involved. Although dilated non-pulsatile venous collaterals might not be expected to erode bone, notching does occur as a result of chronic obstruction to the superior vena cava. Fibrosing media-stinitis, with its long clinical course, is the chief cause rather than malignant disease. Intercostal neuro-fibromas in Von Recklinghausen's disease (*Figure 148*) may produce notching indistinguishable from coarcation, but an extrapleural soft tissue mass or other evidence of neurofibromatosis may be evident within the thorax (Boon *et al.*, 1964). Notching is considered to be very rare without a definite underlying cause.

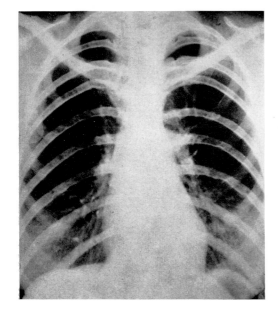

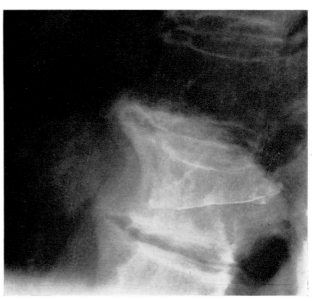

Figure 148. Rib notching in neurofibromatosis

Figure 149. Vertebral erosion from aortic aneurysm (artefact over spine)

OTHER CARDIOVASCULAR CAUSES OF BONE EROSION

Aneurysms of the ascending aorta may erode sternum, costal cartilage or rib and present under the skin as a pulsating mass. Those involving the descending aorta may cause erosion of vertebral bodies, but the intervertebral discs remain largely intact; the anterior vertebral surfaces thus appear scalloped (*Figure 149*). Very rarely an enlarged left atrium causes pressure erosion of the thoracic spine (Ashworth and Morgan-Jones, 1946).

STERNAL DEPRESSION

Pectus excavatum, funnel chest and depressed sternum are terms meaning backward displacement of the lower part of the sternum. Unlike the flat chest (*see* straight back syndrome), antero-posterior narrowing is confined to the lower part of the chest, the maximum depression usually being at the junction of the body of the sternum and the xyphoid process (*Figure 150*). In 1946 Evans published a paper in which he described 16 adults with depressed sternum who had been referred because of abnormal physical signs in the cardiovascular system. The relationship between the thoracic deformity and the cardiac signs had not been previously appreciated and the patients suffered from enforced restriction which in some cases had materially affected life and livelihood. Evans' thesis, now universally accepted, was that depressed sternum is not a cause of cardiac symptoms but only of signs. The authors have found only one case in the literature with abnormal haemodynamics: the right ventricular pressure curve showed a pronounced diastolic dip and plateau suggesting restriction of right ventricular filling (Lyons *et al.*, 1955).

Patients are usually of slender build. If a depressed sternum is present in a short fat female with large breasts, it may be missed clinically. The apex beat is displaced to the left due to cardiac displacement or compression, and an ejection systolic murmur is heard along the left sternal edge. On the anterior view the heart shows apparent enlargement or displacement to the left or both (*Figures 150* and *151*); the pattern does not appear to depend on the degree of antero-posterior narrowing of the chest, contrary to Evans' opinion. An ill-defined area of loss of translucency is frequently seen in the right cardiophrenic angle due to the increased antero-posterior depth and thickness of the chest wall in the region

107

of the right border of the sterno-costal depression and may suggest consolidation (*Figure 51*). The anterior portion of the ribs may be abnormally vertical. Evans mentioned that the lower part of the heart shadow may appear unusually translucent and the right atrial border elevated. Angiography shows that the pulmonary trunk lies abnormally vertically and near the anterior chest wall, suggesting that its superficial position is responsible for the audible ejection systolic murmur. Depressed sternum is not commonly associated with congenital heart disease except atrial septal defect; it is present in 16 per cent of fossa ovalis defects.

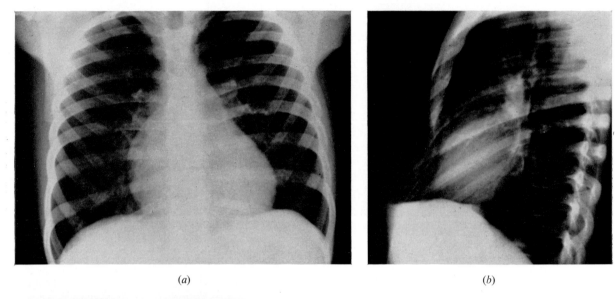

(a)

(b)

Figure 150 (above). Sternal depression causing apparent cardiac enlargement on the anterior view. (a) Anterior view. (b) Lateral view

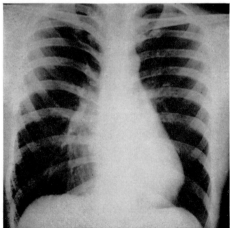

Figure 151 (left). Sternal depression causing cardiac displacement and loss of translucency in the right cardio-phrenic angle

DEFICIENT STERNAL SEGMENTATION

Ossification centres in the cartilaginous sternum are first visible in the sixth month of foetal life in the manubrium and the upper part of the body. Ossification does not appear in the lower part of the body until after birth, and in the xyphoid it appears still later. Normally there is one centre for the manubrium, three or four centres for the body and one for the xyphoid. Fusion of the ossific centres occurs in the opposite order to their appearance. The lower two segments of the body unite in early childhood, and the upper two between the ages of 16 and 25 years. Bony union across the manubrio-sternal joint is seen in only 10 per cent of normal adults, and the xyphoid fuses with the body in 30 per cent (*Figure 152*). Premature union of centres leading to deficient segmentation may be anticipated shortly after birth by demonstration of abnormally narrow sternal sutures (Currarino and Silverman, 1958) (*Figure 153*).

Sternal segments including the manubrium may unite in the first years of life to form a bone of one or two segments. Premature fusion leads to an abnormally short sternum, which may be bowed or angled forward to produce an unusual form of pigeon chest (Andren and Hall, 1961) (*Figure 154*). Occasionally

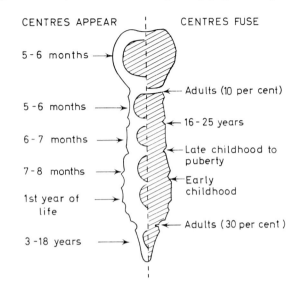

CENTRES APPEAR   CENTRES FUSE

5 - 6 months →

← Adults (10 per cent)

5 - 6 months →

← 16 - 25 years

6 - 7 months →

← Late childhood to puberty

Figure 152. Sternal development

7 - 8 months →

← Early childhood

1st year of life →

← Adults (30 per cent)

3 - 18 years →

the sternum is abnormally thick, a feature which may be appreciated at surgery during splitting of the sternum. After the age of 16 years, when the sternal segments are normally fused, the diagnosis of deficient segmentation is suggested by a short bowed, angled or thick sternum.

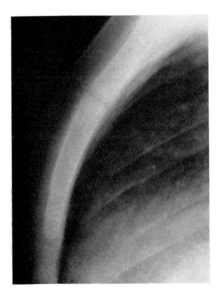

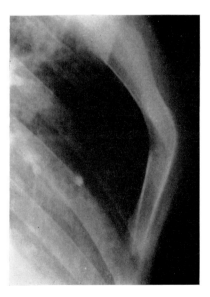

Figure 153 (left). Deficient sternal segmentation

Figure 154 (right). Deficient sternal segmentation causing pigeon chest

It is important to recognize early closure of sternal sutures because it is not often an isolated anomaly and congenital heart disease is the most common association (Gabrielson and Ladyman, 1963). Deficient segmentation is not helpful in diagnosis as it has been reported in all the usual forms of congenital heart disease and some of the rare lesions. Nevertheless, in the authors' material it was most frequently seen with ventricular septal defect, being present in 25 per cent of cases; just over half had pulmonary hypertension, and most of these had bowing as well as shortening of the sternum. It was found in 5 per cent of patients with atrial septal defects, two of whom had the Holt–Oram syndrome. It is associated with cardiac enlargement in 85 per cent. Sternal deformity was not found among 300 patients of all ages with acquired heart disease, but it has been reported in rheumatic heart disease at an early age. No satisfactory explanation for premature sternal fusion has been suggested. There is no evidence that it is genetic; it is possible that mechanical stress exerted by an abnormal heart may affect sternal ossification before and after birth.

STERNAL BOWING

The term bowing of the sternum should be reserved for a symmetrical deformity of the chest in which the sternum bulges forward with indrawing of the lower ribs (*see Figure 112*). It is specifically associated with the combination of high flow and high pressure in the pulmonary circulation, and ventricular septal defect, being the commonest cause of hyperkinetic pulmonary hypertension, is most frequently associated (Davies *et al.*, 1962). Increased flow and pressure decrease the compliance of the pulmonary vascular tree to produce stiff lungs. Increased force of contraction of the accessory muscles of respiration, especially the diaphragm, causes indrawing of lower ribs and anterior bulging of the sternum. Respiratory infections may contribute to lung stiffness. Closure of the communication or banding of the pulmonary artery may reduce or cure the deformity before the sternal segments unite. This specific type of sternal bowing must be distinguished from the short, curved or angled sternum resulting from deficient segmentation which is seen with all types of congenital heart disease. Marked right ventricular enlargement may cause generalized sternal prominence without indrawing of the lower thorax.

SCOLIOSIS

Scoliosis means curvature of the back due to deviation of the spinal column from the midline in the coronal plane. Structural scoliosis is not correctable by voluntary effort and is always associated with rotation of the vertebrae towards the convexity of the curve. The ribs on the convex side of the curve are rotated backwards, giving a false impression of kyphosis. Structural scoliosis is usually progressive until cessation of spinal growth, an event conveniently indicated by fusion of the apophysis of the iliac crest.

Cardio-respiratory complications are encountered only in patients with curves of more than 60 degrees. The prognosis is related to the aetiology of the scoliosis, the age of onset and the height of the curve. Severe congenital scoliosis is due to major abnormality of spinal segmentation, and curvature may progress disastrously during active growth. Prognosis is bad in poliomyelitis when muscular paralysis is extensive. When the aetiology of the scoliosis is a generalized tissue fault, the systemic manifestations of the disease may be more important than the scoliosis. Structural scoliosis may be associated with congenital heart disease (Table 7).

TABLE 7

Scoliosis and Congenital Heart Disease in 116 Patients

Atrial septal defect	40
Ventricular septal defect	30
Fallot's tetralogy and pulmonary atresia	30
Ductus arteriosus	11
Others	5

Infantile scoliosis usually resolves completely (James *et al.*, 1959), but a small percentage of cases progress to severe deformity and cardio-respiratory complications. After infancy, the later the onset of the scoliosis and the slower its progression, the better the prognosis.

High curves between T.1 and T.6 carry a poor prognosis and may progress to severe deformity. Low curves between T.9 and L.4 are compatible with a long life with no symptoms except backache, while middle curves between T.4 and T.10 have an intermediate prognosis. Breathlessness is a rare complaint in young patients and should arouse the suspicion of heart disease. Murmurs are no more common in scoliotics than in normal people, and their significance is the same.

If the chest radiograph is exposed in the conventional way with both shoulders touching the cassette, the spinal curve may obscure much of one lung and the heart. Simon (1969) has shown that if the film is taken after rotating the patient until the spinous process at the point of maximum curve lies centrally at the back of the chest, the lungs and heart are seen more clearly (*Figure 155*). The lung vessels are small and reflect the restricted pulmonary flow secondary to deficient alveolar growth where lung is

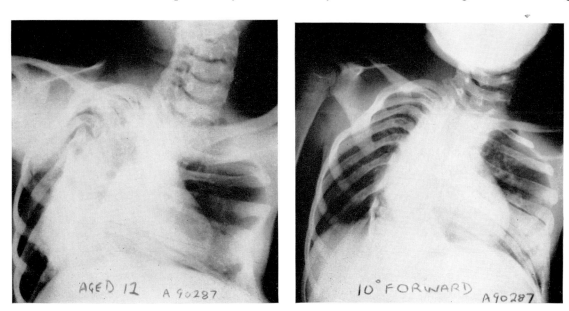

Figure 155. Straight and rotated chest radiographs in scoliosis

compressed. Simon (1969) found a good correlation between the diminution in vessel size and the degree of spinal curvature. The heart is seen to be normal in size on the rotated film unless there is associated congenital heart disease, cardiomyopathy or congestive failure.

Little has been written on the incidence of pulmonary hypertension. It does not occur unless the spinal deformity is severe, and is rare before adult life. Towers and Zorab (1969) reported normal pulmonary

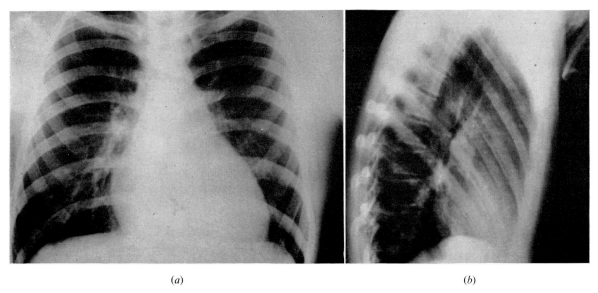

(a)   (b)

Figure 156. The flat chest. (a) Anterior view. Apparent cardiac enlargement. (b) Lateral view

artery pressures in ten severe scoliotics at rest and on exercise, but Fishman (1965) stated that the pressure rose in his severe cases on exercise, although it was normal or near normal at rest. He mentions that this level of pulmonary hypertension is usually well tolerated, but that acute hypoxia may precipitate a high pulmonary artery pressure and congestive cardiac failure. However, congestive failure may not always be associated with a very high pressure (Towers and Zorab, 1969); it may develop quite rapidly and for no clear reason. The immediate prognosis is usually good, but survival for more than two years after the first attack is unusual. Radiologically proximal vessel dilatation, the usual sign of pulmonary arterial hypertension, may not be seen because of the vascular hypoplasia (*see Figure 119*).

STRAIGHT BACK SYNDROME (FLAT CHEST)

In the straight back syndrome the dorsal spine is less kyphotic than normal, being straight or even lordotic. The sternum is vertical and often parallel to the spine. The result is a flat chest, a better name for this deformity. The whole vertical length of the mediastinum may be compressed between the spine and the sternum. On the anterior view the heart may show apparent enlargement or be displaced to the left (*Figure 156*). The ascending and descending portions of the thoracic aorta may be abnormally prominent because they are squeezed outwards. Left atrial dilatation may displace the descending aorta laterally, the point of maximum deviation corresponding to the middle of the left atrium, and even minor atrial enlargement may cause aortic displacement (*see* page 19). Displacement must not be confused with aortic unfolding, which usually shows a maximum convexity above or below the level

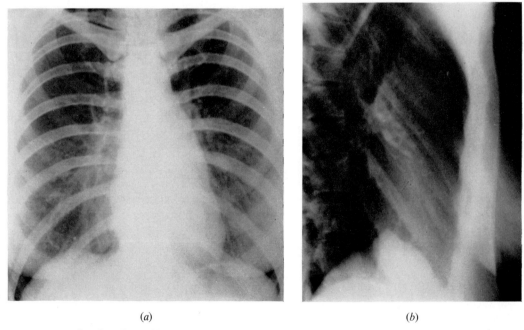

(a)   (b)

Figure 157. The flat chest. (a) Anterior view. Prominence in region of pulmonary trunk and left atrial appendix. (b) Lateral view

of the left atrium. The pulmonary trunk and the hila may be so prominent as to appear pathological (*Figure 157*). An ejection systolic murmur along the left sternal edge, sometimes quite loud, brings these patients to the cardiologist. The murmur usually diminishes on sitting up and on inspiration (Datey *et al.*, 1964). It is likely that the murmur is merely the physiological ejection murmur more easily heard because of the close proximity of the right ventricular outflow tract to the anterior chest wall.

CHAPTER 14

Inherited and Allied Syndromes with Heart Disease

DOWN'S SYNDROME (MONGOLISM)

Down's syndrome usually results from trisomy of autosome 21, is the commonest generalized dysplasia found with congenital heart disease and is usually recognizable at birth by external features, particularly of the face and palm. Diagnostic difficulty is occasionally encountered in the neonate, when skeletal radiology may be helpful.

Changes in the pelvis are the most characteristic. The iliac bones are flared outwards and the acetabular roofs are flat. In 1956 Caffey and Ross expressed these changes quantitatively. The angle between a line drawn through the lateral edge of the ilium and the horizontal they termed the iliac angle, and that through the acetabular roof and the horizontal they termed the acetabular angle. The sum of these two angles they called the iliac index (*Figure 158*). Astley (1963) suggested that if this index was less than 60 degrees, Down's syndrome was very probable; if the index was more than 78 degrees, it was improbable.

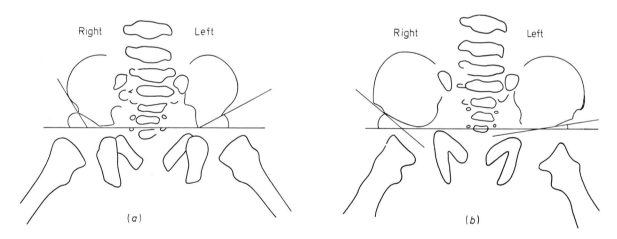

Figure 158. Iliac index. Iliac angle on right side; acetabular angle on left side. (a) Normal. (b) Down's syndrome

The skull is small and short with thin bones. The facial bones are hypoplastic with a short, hard palate. Absent frontal sinuses and a persistent metopic suture are commoner than in the normal population. The orbital roofs are abnormally high and slope upwards and outwards. The middle phalanx of the fifth finger is quite frequently small, but this is seen in other diseases. Two ossification centres are present in the manubrium sterni in 90 per cent of mongols, but also in 20 per cent of normals. In some patients there may be 11 pairs of ribs and tall lumbar vertebrae.

Polani (1968) found that the incidence of congenital heart disease in Down's syndrome was 23 per cent when the diagnosis was clinical, but 53 per cent in a necropsy series of 300. The cardiac defect was single in 74 per cent of cases; atrio-ventricular defect (endocardial cushion defect) was found in 25 per

113

cent, fossa ovalis atrial septal defect in 20 per cent, and ventricular septal defect in 15 per cent. Atrio-ventricular defects tend to be complex, and complete canal is common. Ductus arteriosus and Fallot's tetralogy were also seen, but other types of congenital heart disease were rare.

EDWARD'S SYNDROME (TRISOMY 18)

Trisomy 18 results from an extra autosome in the 18 position of the karyotype. Infants rarely survive more than a few months because of severe somatic and mental defects. They show a pitiful expression with a short upper lip, a small triangular mouth, low-set ears and a prominent occiput. The hands are thought to be characteristic with flexed fingers, adduction of the thumb and the index finger over-lapping the ring finger. The feet show short great toes with a 'rocker bottom' configuration.

Radiological features suggesting the diagnosis are seen in the hands, feet and pelvis. The phalanges and metacarpal of the thumb are short, the fingers show ulnar deviation, and a space is present between the bases of the second and third fingers. The plantar surface of the foot tends to be convex (rocker bottom), the distal phalanges are short and triangular, and the fourth and fifth toes are deviated laterally. The pelvic configuration is opposite to that in Down's syndrome: the iliac bones are rotated forward, and the acetabular roofs are short and oblique (anti-mongoloid pelvis).

Congenital heart disease of various types is present in over 90 per cent. Ventricular septal defect, ductus arteriosus and pulmonary valve stenosis are common. Malposition of the heart is not seen.

PATAU'S SYNDROME (TRISOMY 13–15)

Trisomy 13–15 results from an extra chromosome in the 13–15 or D group of the karyotype. As in trisomy 18, survival beyond infancy is exceptional because of severe generalized somatic and mental defects. Patients have a grotesque facial appearance; cleft lip and other severe midline facial clefts are characteristic. The eyes and ears may be hypoplastic. Haemangiomas of the face and upper trunk are seen. The limbs show polydactyly, retroflexed thumbs, tapering digits with convex nails, and prominent heels.

Radiological features suggesting the diagnosis are seen in the skull: the orbits are poorly formed and there is hypertelorism, widened sutures with poor ossification, sloping frontal bones, cleft palate, and absence of other midline structures. The interpedicular distances in the cervical spine may be increased, with associated clavicular and thoracic cage deformities. The hands show syndactyly, polydactyly and narrow terminal phalanges.

Congenital heart disease is present in over 90 per cent and almost all types have been encountered, but ventricular septal defect, ductus arteriosus, aortic valve disease and dextrocardia predominate.

TURNER'S AND ULLRICH'S SYNDROMES

In 1938 Turner described the combination of dwarfism, cubitus valgus, webbing of the neck and absent secondary sexual characteristics in seven females over the age of puberty. Four years later it was dis-covered that the ovaries were maldeveloped (Albright *et al.*, 1942; Varney *et al.*, 1942), and in 1944 Wilkins and Fleischmann described the condition as ovarian agenesis.

In 1930, eight years before Turner's publication and unknown to Turner, Ullrich described similar somatic features in children and young adults of both sexes without relating them to underdevelopment of the gonads. It was not until 1952 that Caflisch clearly separated Turner's syndrome as ovarian agenesis in post-pubertal girls from Ullrich's syndrome, which is seen in girls and boys with normal secondary sexual development. Some of the males with the latter condition, however, have evidence of abnormal sexual development such as hypospadias or undescended testes, and these are referred to as cases of Turner's syndrome in the male (Flavell, 1943).

The Turner and Ullrich phenotypes are similar and the differential diagnosis may be uncertain before the age of 16 years, when secondary sexual characteristics normally manifest themselves, but help may be obtained from sex chromatin and chromosome studies. Ninety per cent of females with Turner's syndrome have only one X-chromosome (45XO) and are chromatin negative; the rest show structural chromosome abnormalities or are mosaics. Patients with the Ullrich and male Turner syndromes have normal chromosomes. Noonan and Ehmke (1963) described pulmonary stenosis as a feature of the Ullrich and male Turner syndromes, and these disorders are sometimes referred to as Noonan's syndrome.

The Turner/Ullrich phenotype has many features which were not described in the original papers. Mentality is normal or only slightly impaired in Turner's syndrome, but may be more seriously affected in Ullrich's syndrome. Patients are dwarfed, but those with Ullrich's syndrome may be normal in height. Webbing of the neck and a low posterior hair line are common in each. The facial abnormality varies in degree and includes a prominent brow, a depressed nasal bridge and rather low ears. The chest tends to be broad with widely spaced nipples. Lymphoedema on the dorsum of the fingers and toes may sometimes be detected. Renal abnormalities such as horseshoe kidney and skeletal anomalies are sometimes found in Turner's but not in Ullrich's syndrome. The type of congenital heart disease associated with each is an important diagnostic feature.

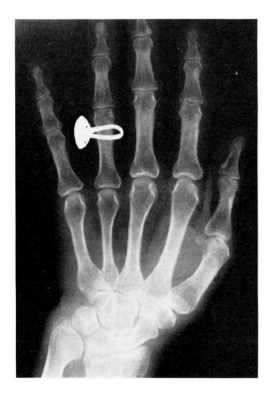
Figure 159. Turner's syndrome. Hand

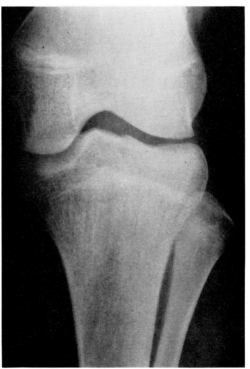
Figure 160. Turner's syndrome. Knee

As skeletal maturation in Turner's syndrome is normal up to the age of 16 years, epiphyses appear at a normal age, but epiphyseal fusion is delayed beyond 20 years. Osteoporosis may be evident, particularly in the hands and spine of severely affected patients. Although a great variety of skeletal abnormalities has been described in the literature, they are variable and individually non-specific. The most characteristic is metacarpal shortening, commonly involving the fourth metacarpal (*Figure 159*). Normally a line drawn tangentially through the distal articular cartilages of the fourth and fifth metacarpals extends distal to the third metacarpal head. When the fourth metacarpal is short, the line passes through the third metacarpal and the metacarpal sign is said to be positive. The sign is a little more frequent on the left side and in older children. It is, however, seen in other bone dystrophies, particularly pseudohypoparathyroidism, and infrequently as a familial condition in otherwise normal people. The proximal row of carpal bones may form an abnormally acute angle with a sloped distal radial articular surface, an appearance resembling Madelung's deformity (*Figure 159*). In older patients there may be overgrowth of the medial femoral condyle with depression of the medial portion of the tibial epiphyses and prominence of the inner part of the metaphysis (*Figure 160*). Increase in the carrying angle is much more apparent clinically than radiologically, but a radial tilt of the articular surface of the trochlea may be apparent. Astley (1963) noted that the forearm bones may curve in an ulnar direction and partly compensate for the increased carrying angle. He also reported, in 7 out of 15 patients, maldevelopment of the clavicles in which there was thinning of the lateral ends with abnormal curvature or modelling. The ribs may also be uneven due to abnormal modelling. Webbing of the neck is usually associated with a normal cervical spine, but anomalies at the C.1 and C.2 levels may be present, especially hypoplasia of C.1 (Finby and Archibald, 1963).

The most important difference between Turner's syndrome and Ullrich's syndrome is the different incidence of congenital heart disease. Coarctation and aortic stenosis comprise over 75 per cent of congenital heart disease in Turner's syndrome. Characteristically the aortic valve is thick and an ejection sound is absent. Siggers and Polani (1972) analysed 44 Ullrich and male Turner cases from the literature and 22 of their own, all with congenital heart disease. Pulmonary stenosis was by far the most frequent lesion, being present in 75 per cent of the patients in the literature and in 55 per cent of their own. It was either isolated or combined with other lesions, most commonly atrial septal defect. Other defects more frequent than in a matched control group with congenital heart disease were ductus arteriosus, coarctation of the aorta, anomalous pulmonary venous drainage and hypertrophic obstructive cardiomyopathy. Coarctation was found in only 18 per cent. Ventricular septal defect, either alone or with other lesions, occurred in 18 per cent, a lower incidence than in the controls. Aortic stenosis, Fallot's tetralogy and transposition of the great arteries were not found. The overall incidence of congenital heart disease in the Ullrich and male Turner syndromes was 47 per cent compared with 22 per cent in Turner's syndrome.

THE MUCOPOLYSACCHARIDOSES

The mucopolysaccharidoses are a group of diseases characterized by infiltration of fibroblasts and parenchymal cells by mucopolysaccharide, resulting in abnormalities of many systems including the skeleton and the heart. Seven types of mucopolysaccharidoses are distinguished, and the diagnosis is made by clinical, radiological and genetic studies and by the pattern of mucopolysaccharide excretion in the urine.

Patients usually appear normal at birth. Hurler's syndrome (Hurler, 1919) may be considered the prototype mucopolysaccharidosis, as many features common to the other types are seen. One or all of the following may be present during infancy or early childhood: mental retardation, dwarfism, large head with coarse features, lumbar gibbus, joint stiffness, rhinitis, corneal clouding, and hepato-spleno-megaly. Death from respiratory or cardiac disease usually occurs before the age of 10 years. The clinical features of Hunter's syndrome (Hunter, 1917) are similar, but the course of disease is milder: mental deterioration is slower to develop and there is no obvious lumbar gibbus or corneal clouding, but deafness is common. Although death often occurs in early adult life, survival to the age of 40 years or over is well documented. In both the Hurler and Hunter syndromes, mucopolysaccharide infiltration causes valve disease and cardiomyopathy; mitral regurgitation is the single commonest lesion. The Morquio syndrome (Morquio, 1929) is characterized by normal mentality but severe dwarfism with spinal shortening and barrel chest. The joints are stiff and genu valgum is common. The teeth have thin enamel leading to early caries. Aortic regurgitation is found, but its incidence is uncertain (McKusick, 1966). All mucopolysaccharidoses show a recessive inheritance, autosomal in all except Hunter's syndrome, which is sex-linked.

There are many radiological features common to all the mucopolysaccharidoses. The long bones are shortened and show deficient modelling, resulting in abnormal diaphyses which are more often too wide than too narrow. The tubular bones of the hands and feet are short and wide, and the bases of the metacarpals tend to be pointed. Metaphyses may be deformed and epiphyses irregular (*Figure 161*). The hands and sometimes other bones are osteoporotic. The ribs are wide anteriorly and narrow posteriorly. All patients have kyphosis, and there may be enlargement of the lower spinal canal.

Important features allow differentiation of the Hunter–Hurler group from Morquio's syndrome. In the Hunter–Hurler syndrome the vertebral bodies are normal or ovoid in the lateral view, and one or two in the upper lumbar region show a characteristic antero-inferior beak. The beaked vertebra is smaller than the rest, is displaced posteriorly and forms the apex of the kyphos (*Figure 162*). The spinal

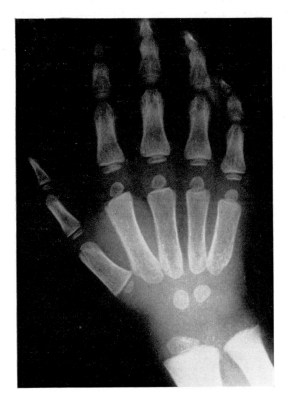

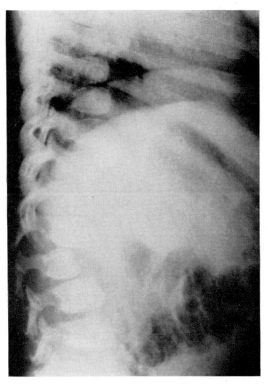

Figure 161. Mucopolysaccharidosis. Hand

Figure 162. Hunter's syndrome. Lateral spine

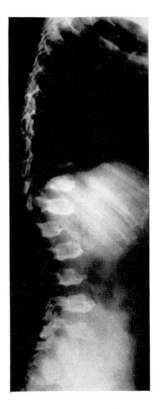

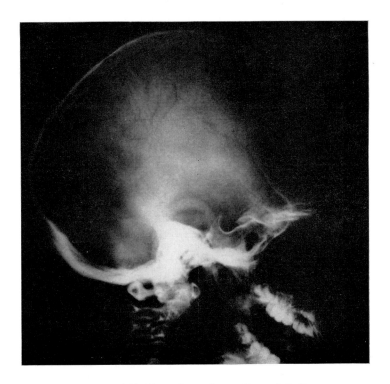

Figure 163. Morquio's syndrome. Lateral spine

Figure 164. Hunter's syndrome. Lateral skull

changes are different and more striking in the Morquio syndrome. There is universal vertebra plana, which results in considerable reduction in the length of the trunk and a barrel-shaped chest (*Figure 163*). Beaking is seen at the centre of one or many of the vertebrae, but as in the Hunter–Hurler syndrome, an upper lumbar vertebra may be displaced posteriorly with an antero-inferior beak (Langer and Carey, 1966). Scoliosis as well as kyphosis may be marked. Sometimes there is abnormal segmentation in the upper cervical spine with anomalies of the first and second cervical vertebrae.

In the Hunter–Hurler syndrome the skull is large and the sella is elongated and J-shaped due to abnormal growth of the sphenoid (*Figure 164*). In Morquio the skull is normal. The pelvis also differs in the two conditions. In Hunter–Hurler each iliac bone tapers towards a shallow acetabulum, but in Morquio the ilium is flared and there is a deep acetabular fossa with an irregular slanting roof. Diaphyseal abnormality—shortening, widening or constriction—occurs in both, but changes in the ends of the bones are more prominent in Morquio. The epiphyses show progressive irregularity of texture and contour with fragmentation and sometimes disappearance, a sequence of events typically seen in the capital femoral epiphyses. The metaphyses are often enlarged, cup-shaped and slanting, whereas the Hunter–Hurler metaphyseal deformity is usually confined to angulation. Coxa valga is a feature of both but is constant in Morquio.

The other mucopolysaccharidoses are too rare to merit description.

ELLIS–VAN CREVELD SYNDROME

In 1940 Ellis and Van Creveld established the existence of chondrodystrophy, polydactyly and ectodermal dysplasia as a clinical syndrome. It is inherited as an autosomal recessive trait and has a better prognosis than the mucopolysaccharidoses, many patients reaching adult life. Chondrodystrophy is the most constant feature, with shortening of the tubular bones, especially the distal bones of the limbs and the distal phalanges (*Figure 165*). Dwarfism is seen at birth, unlike the mucopolysaccharidoses. Other skeletal findings are hypoplasia and a medial position of the proximal tibial epiphysis leading to genu

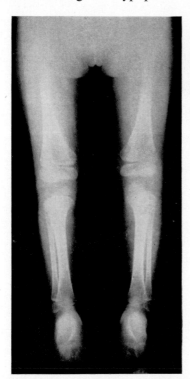

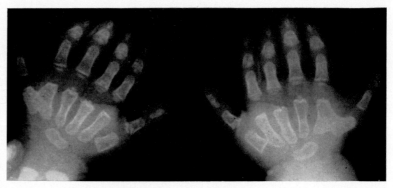

Figure 165 (above). Ellis van Creveld. Hands

Figure 166 (left). Ellis van Creveld. Legs

valgum (*Figure 166*), fusion of the capitate and hamate bones and acceleration of maturation. The polydactyly involves the ulnar side of the hand with the addition of a sixth digit, and the fifth and sixth metacarpal shafts are partially fused. Similar changes may be seen in the feet. The skull, spine and pelvis develop normally, but the acetabular roofs may show a curious trident deformity at birth which later disappears without residual deformity. The ribs are short, but otherwise the axial skeleton is normal. Ectodermal dysplasia is present in 70 per cent of patients and includes sparse hair, small finger nails and deformed teeth. Intelligence is usually normal. Nearly 60 per cent of patients have congenital heart disease, particularly single atrium. Giknis (1963) reviewed 36 cases and found congenital heart disease in 20; 11 of these came to autopsy, and single atrium was found in 7.

THE MARFAN SYNDROME

The Marfan syndrome (Marfan, 1896) is an autosomal dominant trait, often phenotypically incomplete but characteristically showing the triad of long slender bones and arachnodactyly, lens dislocation and cardiovascular abnormality. Other important features are poor muscular development and ligamentous laxity leading to kypho-scoliosis and early degenerative arthropathy. Skeletal abnormality is most obvious in the extremities, but evidence of increase in the length of the bones may also be appreciated in the axial skeleton; for example, the typical high arched palate merely reflects overgrowth of the palatal bones. A firm diagnosis of the syndrome by skeletal radiology is made difficult because the findings often represent the extremes of normal biological variation, particularly in Negro races. Patients are usually but not always abnormally tall. Since many have abnormal body proportions, a variety of skeletal measurements has been devised. The ratio of the upper segment to the lower one (US/LS) is considered to be one of the most reliable by McKusick (1966), who published measurements of 2,100 Baltimore children and 34 patients with the Marfan syndrome. The lower segment is from the pubic symphysis to the floor, and the upper segment is derived by subtracting this from the patient's height. McKusick found the mean value for the US/LS for whites to be just above unity at birth. As the legs grow faster than the trunk, the mid-point of the body moves upwards and the US/LS falls to about 0·93 in the adult.

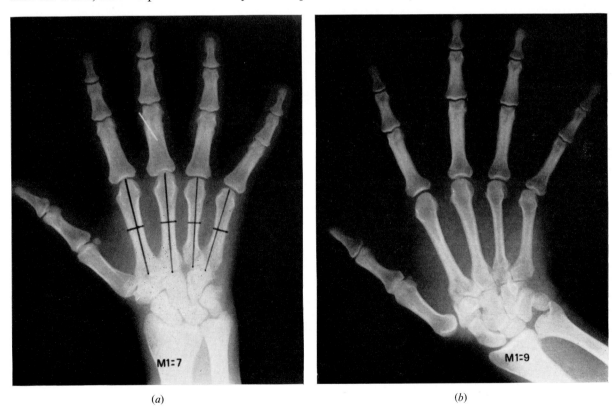

Figure 167. Metacarpal index. (a) Normal. (b) Marfan syndrome

Negroes have a slightly lower US/LS at all ages, the figure being about unity at birth and 0·87 after puberty. McKusick found no significant sex difference in either race. The ratio in Marfan is consistently lower than the mean normal; in the adult white with Marfan's syndrome it usually lies between 8 and 9, and in the Negro near or below 8.

119

Pearson and Lee (1902) measured span and height in over 2,000 normals. Unlike the US/LS ratio, they found a significant sex difference, the span being greater than the height in approximately 60 per cent of men and in only 21 per cent of women. The span was greater than the height by more than 3 inches (76 mm) in 9·3 per cent of men and in 1·8 per cent of women. Thus if Marfan's syndrome is diagnosed when the span exceeds the height by more than 3 inches, there will be at most a small false positive error in women, but the error will be greater in men. There is evidence that some patients with Marfan's syndrome have a span-to-height ratio near the mean normal (Eldridge, 1964), but according to Sinclair et al. (1960) the span has not been less than the height in any proven case.

As originally proposed by Sinclair (1958), the metacarpal index is derived from a radiograph of the right hand. The axial length of the second, third, fourth and fifth metacarpals is divided by the breadth at the exact mid-point, the average for the four being the metacarpal index (*Figure 167*). Sinclair et al. (1960) examined 100 normal people and 20 cases of Marfan's syndrome. The index in the normal group ranged from 5·4 to 7·9 and in Marfan from 8·4 to 10·4. Since this publication, it has become widely accepted that below 8 is normal while 8·4 and above is abnormal. Parish (1960) enlarged the concept of the metacarpal index by using radiographs of both hands in 26 men and 53 women. He found the metacarpal index to be higher in women and slightly higher in the left hand. The normal range for men corresponded to the figures given by Sinclair et al. (1960), but it appears from Parish's work that the upper limit of normal for women ought to be extended to 9. Parish admitted a slight overlap between the measurements of normal hands and those of the hands of patients with Marfan's syndrome, and considered the phalangeal index of the ring finger the measurement most likely to be abnormal in Marfan. This is the ratio of the length of the proximal phalanx and its minimal width (Table 8). It must be mentioned that both indices depend on breadth as well as length, so that abnormal values may be found in

TABLE 8

(a) Normal values for metacarpal index (either hand)	(b) Normal values for phalangeal index (proximal phalanx ring finger)
Men 8 or less Women 9 or less	Men 4·6 or less Women 5·6 or less

bones of normal length but unusual slenderness. Such hands were described by Achard (1902) when he coined the term arachnodactyly.

Skeletal changes which do not lend themselves to measurement are also important in the diagnosis of the Marfan syndrome. Although all the limb bones tend to be long and slender, those of the hand and foot (*Figure 167*) are most affected and the great toe often elongates out of proportion to the others. The clavicles may appear unusually long and thin. Abnormally long ribs are seen on the lateral view of the chest and may result in pectus excavatum or carinatum. Overgrowth of the skull and facial bones gives rise to dolichocephaly and high arched palate. Nelson (1958) described enlargement of the spinal canal in the lower dorsal to upper sacral region (*Figure 168*). The radiological changes are widening of the interpedicular distances, narrow pedicles, long transverse processes, posterior scalloping of the vertebral bodies and enlargement of the intervertebral foramina. Vertebral bodies may also be tall, their height being greater than their width and depth. Spinal changes are always found in the obvious Marfan and may be helpful in doubtful cases. Kypho-scoliosis due to lax ligaments and poor muscle development may become severe during active spinal growth in puberty.

Baer et al. (1943) established that the major cardiovascular abnormality of the Marfan syndrome was dilatation of the ascending aorta. The dilatation usually involves the ascending aorta, but may occasionally be seen elsewhere in the arterial system. It extends from the aortic ring to the innominate artery (*Figure 169*). On the anterior view the convex bulge of the ascending aorta is seen above the right atrial border and may be continuous with it. If the aorta bulges to the left, it may displace the pulmonary trunk or even present as a mass on the left. The lateral view confirms that the mediastinal bulge is due to the ascending aorta. Aortic regurgitation is due to ring dilatation or dissecting aneurysm and is more commonly found in the male. It may occur before aortic enlargement is visible radiologically when the dilatation is confined to the intrapericardial part of the ascending aorta (Keene *et al.*, 1971). The presence of a dissection can only be excluded on aortography. Dilatation of the pulmonary trunk is much less common than that of the aorta and may be confused with displacement of the pulmonary trunk by the aorta. Mitral regurgitation may also occur from stretching of cusps and chordae which are weakened

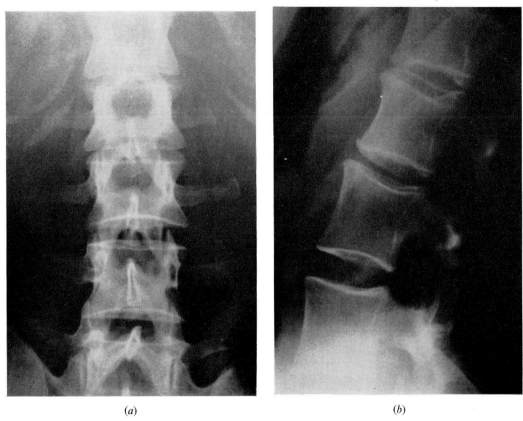

(a)   (b)

Figure 168. Marfan syndrome. Lumbar spine. (a) Anterior view. (b) Lateral view

by myxomatous degeneration (Anderson *et al.*, 1968). Cardiovascular complications are the result of abiotrophy, a term suggested by Gowers for neurological disorders in which tissues can function only for a limited time because of innate weakness. True congenital heart disease is now considered a rare association of the Marfan syndrome. For many years atrial septal defect was thought to be common, but this arose only because early authors (Salle, 1912; Boerger, 1914) included patent foramen ovale as a form of atrial septal defect. The difficulty of assessing the true incidence of congenital heart disease in the Marfan syndrome is illustrated by a case of ventricular septal defect in a 15-year-old girl reported by Ross and Gerbode (1960). At surgery the ventricular septum was found to be aneurysmal and fenestrated, suggesting abiotrophy with or without an underlying congenital lesion.

HOMOCYSTINURIA

Homocystinuria is a rare disorder due to deficiency of a specific enzyme, first described almost simultaneously by Carson and Neill (1962) and Gerritsen *et al.* (1962). The condition may resemble the Marfan syndrome clinically in that tall stature and lens dislocation occur, but there are many distinguishing features. Inheritance is recessive; mental retardation is common, although Schimke *et al.* (1965) found a normal mentality in 41 per cent of 38 affected persons. Skeletal radiology is very variable. The bones are often porotic; the long bones may be bowed and fractures may occur, the appearances somewhat resembling those of osteogenesis imperfecta tarda. Widening of epiphyseal lines in the radius and ulna, with calcifications and enlargement of epiphyses and carpal bones, are considered characteristic features (Morrels *et al.*, 1968; Dow, 1971). The skull may be small in those patients with retarded mentality.

The pattern of cardiovascular involvement is quite different from Marfan. The heart and great vessels are spared, but thrombosis is frequent in the medium-sized arteries and veins and is the commonest cause of death. Thrombosis may be precipitated by minor trauma, so that needle puncture and surgical procedures should be avoided as far as possible.

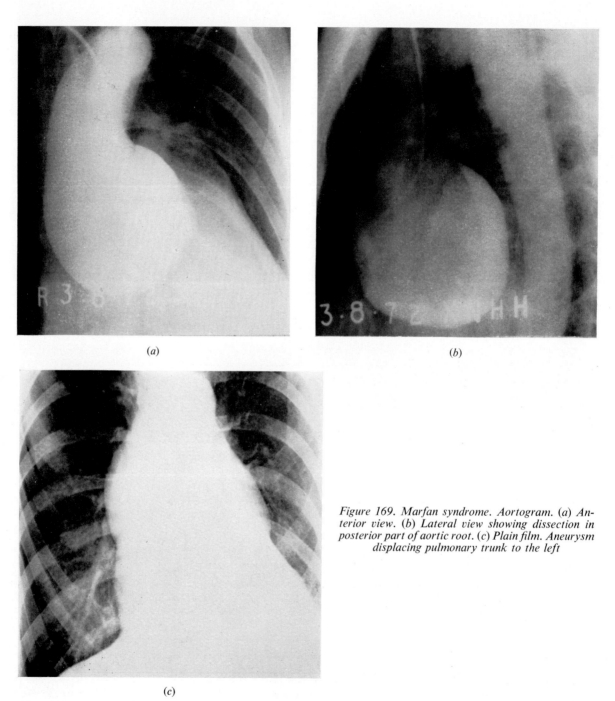

(a)

(b)

(c)

Figure 169. Marfan syndrome. Aortogram. (a) Anterior view. (b) Lateral view showing dissection in posterior part of aortic root. (c) Plain film. Aneurysm displacing pulmonary trunk to the left

HOLT–ORAM SYNDROME

Approximately 25 per cent of subjects with defects of the radial side of the forearms and hands have congenital heart disease (Birch-Jensen, 1949), whereas anomalies of the lower limb are not associated with heart disease. The reason for this may be that differentiation of the arms and the heart, particularly cardiac septation, begins during the fourth week, while the legs develop significantly later.

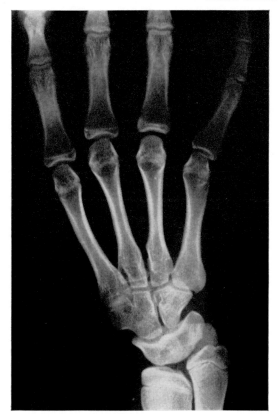

Figure 170. Holt–Oram syndrome. Absent thumb

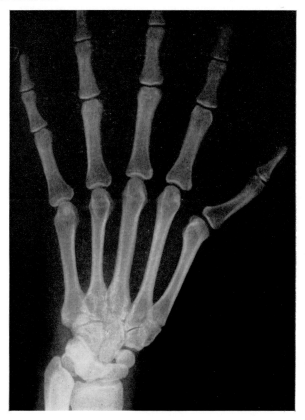

Figure 171. Holt–Oram syndrome. Hand. Finger-like thumb

Figure 172. Holt–Oram syndrome. Hand. Extra phalanx in thumb

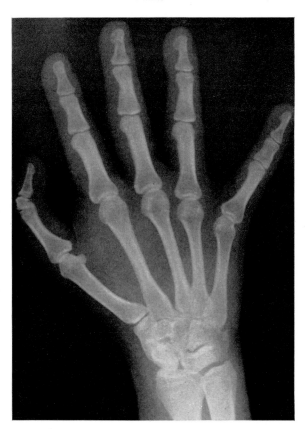

The commonest upper limb cardiovascular syndrome is that described by Holt and Oram (1960). They found the combination of atrial septal defect, upper limb deformity and dysrhythmia in four members of the same family; nine persons were thought to be affected in four generations. Many families have since been described. Although atrial septal defect is the most commonly reported lesion, ventricular septal defect is frequent. Harris and Osborne (1966) described three sporadic cases of radial

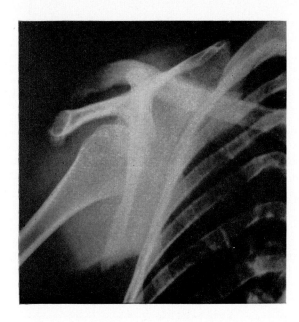

Figure 173. *Holt–Oram syndrome. Shoulder. Short clavicle with forward displacement of scapula*

dysplasia and ventricular septal defect with pulmonary hypertension, probably the result of a fresh genetic mutation. Transposition of the great arteries and other complex anomalies occasionally occur and may be responsible for early death. On the other hand, minor defects may go undetected. An anomalous right subclavian artery was reported in 3 of 11 patients fully investigated in a family of 18 affected persons by Lewis *et al.* (1965); it is interesting to note that the subclavian artery is a segmental vessel to the upper limb. Skeletal abnormality is confined to the upper limb, shoulder girdle and sternum, but Emanuel (1971) had a patient in whom one rib was shortened and constricted. Dysrhythmias are an inconstant feature and vary from a prolonged P–R interval to complex disturbances of rhythm. The cardiac and skeletal defects found in any one family are usually similar, but Holmes (1965) has reported a family with varying cardiac anomalies. The syndrome may be incomplete in that some members of a family show only skeletal changes while others have isolated heart disease (Emanuel, 1970).

Clinical examination of the musculo-skeletal system may show absent, small or finger-like thumbs, hypoplasia of the thenar muscles (Chang, 1967a), manus varus, limitation of pronation and supination of the forearms, and narrow sloping shoulders with restricted movement. Limbs may be shortened, and severe cases have phocomelia like cases of thalidomide embryopathy. Depressed sternum is common.

Radiologically a wide variety of changes is seen, the most characteristic being in the hands. The radial side of the hand and forearm is affected, the ulnar aspect often being normal; the left hand tends to be more deformed than the right (Poznanski *et al.*, 1970). The thumb with its metacarpal may be absent or hypoplastic (*Figure 170*), or the first metacarpal may be long and resemble a digital metacarpal (*Figure 171*). A small extra middle phalanx may be present in the thumb, causing ulnar deviation (*Figure 172*). The fingers are usually normal, although occasionally the fifth finger has a short middle phalanx with clinodactyly. Poznanski and his colleagues reported carpal abnormality to be more frequent than thumb deformity in 14 patients from a large family previously reported by Gall *et al.* (1966). These anomalies are radiologically but not clinically detectable. A malformed scaphoid is the commonest carpal anomaly; others include an extra ossicle, the radial central bone lying between the scaphoid and trapezium, particularly in association with severely deformed thumbs. A centrally placed extra ossicle, the os centrale, may also be present. These accessory ossicles are of phylogenetic and embryological interest. The primitive tetrapod hand contains three rows of carpal bones. The central row (the centralia) consists of two bones in primitive reptiles which correspond to the ossicles seen in the Holt–Oram syndrome. In the human embryo the os centrale is normally present at six weeks and fuses with the scaphoid. The presence of an os centrale therefore suggests that genetic damage occurs before six weeks when upper limb differentiation and cardiac septation are proceeding. Fusion of normal carpal bones may also occur, and at the wrist there may be abnormal tubulation of the radius and ulna.

Anomalies at the elbow are common and include hypoplasia and dislocation of the radial head and radio-ulnar synostosis. The humeral heads are often small and the clavicles are usually short. The scapulae are small and held abnormally far forward by the shortened clavicles (*Figure 173*). Accessory ossicles may be seen around the shoulder joint. Occasionally there is phocomelia, the whole arm being shortened with gross deficiency and fusion of bone. Usually, however, there is little or no shortening, but the bones show some abnormality of tubulation.

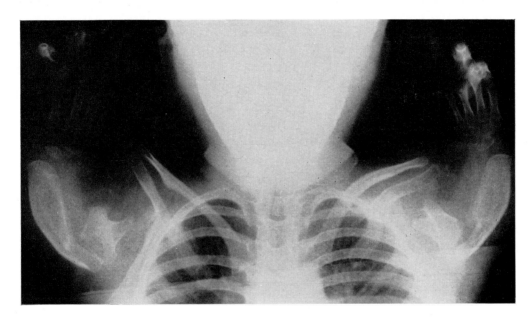

Figure 174. Thalidomide embryopathy. Shoulders and arms

One of the original cases of Holt and Oram had a depressed sternum, and this feature was recently emphasized by Antia (1971) in a description of a polygamous Nigerian family with the syndrome. Compression of the mediastinum from sternal depression may result in a very large heart shadow on the anterior view. A short bowed sternum due to deficient segmentation was noted in 3 of 14 cases by Poznanski (1970).

Radial hypoplasia with congenital heart disease is also found in Fanconi's syndrome and congenital thrombocytopenia.

THALIDOMIDE EMBRYOPATHY

Thalidomide embryopathy is discussed in this chapter because in some ways it resembles the Holt–Oram syndrome. Congenital heart disease is common, and the age period at which the foetus is at risk is the same. Congenital anomalies are, however, much more widespread and include absent gall bladder, absent appendix, bowel atresia, dysplastic ears, and haemangiomas of the face. Skeletal abnormality is more diffuse than in the Holt–Oram syndrome: all four limbs may be deformed, with underdevelopment of the scapulae and pelvis, or the upper limbs alone may be affected. The characteristic lesion is phocomelia, in which the bones between the shoulder and the hand are absent or rudimentary (*Figure 174*). The hands may be normal or may show absent thumbs, syndactyly or polydactyly; the changes in the legs are similar. In mild cases, hypoplasia or aplasia of the radial side of the arms and hands resembles that seen in the Holt–Oram syndrome. Congenital heart disease in thalidomide children does not show any specific pattern. It is the most common extraskeletal abnormality: Lenz (quoted by Taussig, 1962) found an incidence of 17 per cent in 203 children.

POLYDACTYLY AND SYNDACTYLY

Polydactyly and syndactyly are skeletal defects which may accompany congenital heart disease. Among 1,250 consecutive cases of congenital heart disease, Wood *et al.* (1958) found that there were 8 patients with polydactyly who had a ventricular septal defect and 3 patients who had syndactyly associated with Fallot's tetralogy. Polydactly and syndactyly are seen in the Ellis–Van Creveld and Laurence–Moon–Biedl–Bardet syndromes. In the latter, 69 per cent of cases coming to autopsy have cardiovascular lesions, including a variety of congenital heart disease and left ventricular hypertrophy due to systemic hypertension (McLoughlin *et al.*, 1964). Renal disease is common and is the principal cause of the hypertension. Polydactyly is also one of the many features of the trisomy 13 syndrome, in which ventricular septal defect and dextrocardia are common.

EHLERS-DANLOS SYNDROME

The syndrome is inherited as an autosomal dominant trait. The skin is hyperelastic. Bruising occurs easily and subcutaneous haematomas may calcify. Small fatty mobile nodules which form under the skin may also calcify. Joints are hyperextensible and recurrent dislocation is frequent. Diaphragmatic hernia, gastro-intestinal diverticulae, dilatation of the oesophagus, colon and trachea, perforation of the gut and spontaneous pneumothorax have been reported. Aortic dissection, intracranial aneurysm, haemorrhage from large arteries, and mitral or tricuspid regurgitation from stretching of chordae and cusps are the commonest cardiovascular complications. Isolated cases of congenital heart disease have been reported.

PSEUDOXANTHOMA ELASTICUM

The syndrome is inherited as an autosomal recessive trait. Typically the skin becomes inelastic with exaggeration of skin folds and creases, but these changes are not evident before the second decade and may be unimpressive in patients with serious ocular and vascular complications. Calcification of the dermis may occur. Angioid streaks in the fundus are characteristic, but like the skin changes they may not be seen until adult life. Retinal haemorrhage also occurs.

Cardiovascular manifestations consist of early arterial calcification, arterial occlusion and haemorrhage. The occlusions may affect the limbs, kidneys and heart, causing hypertension, angina and myocardial infarction. Aortic dilatation has been reported. Hypertension predisposes to haemorrhage, which may be fatal and may involve the gut, brain, retina, kidney or uterus.

ALKAPTONURIA

This inborn error of metabolism presents clinically with dark urine, pigmentation of cartilage and collagen, renal calculi and progressive degenerative arthritis. The arthritis is most severe in the spine, where the intervertebral discs narrow, calcify and prolapse. The hips and knees also show severe changes. Atherosclerosis and calcific aortic stenosis are common, and myocardial infarction is a frequent cause of death.

OSTEOGENESIS IMPERFECTA

This is transmitted by an autosomal dominant trait and is characterized by multiple fractures from brittle bones, deafness and blue sclera. In mild cases, blue sclera and osteoporosis may be the only manifestations, and it is in such cases (osteogenesis imperfecta tarda) that cardiovascular manifestations may become apparent. Criscitiello *et al.* (1965) reported two patients with aortic regurgitation due to a dilated aortic valve ring, and a third with abnormal aortic and pulmonary valves and an aneurysm of the anterior mitral cusp.

CHAPTER 15

General Disease and the Heart

JACCOUD'S ARTHROPATHY

Bywaters (1950) clearly separated post-rheumatic chronic polyarthropathy from rheumatoid arthritis. Jaccoud's arthropathy is a rare lesion which follows rheumatic fever and in which the small joints of the hands and feet are deformed by fibrosis of the joint capsule and the surrounding ligaments. The pathological process is similar to that seen in the valves in chronic rheumatic heart disease. The metacarpophalangeal joints are most commonly involved. The fingers show painless ulnar deviation, which is voluntarily correctable. Radiologically the deformity is not accompanied by any of the usual manifestations of rheumatoid arthritis such as osteoporosis or bone erosion. Joint cartilage is usually intact, but

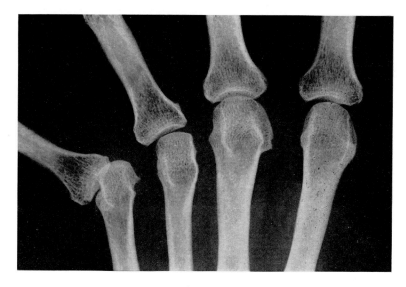

Figure 175. Jaccoud's arthropathy. Hand

may show pressure erosion as a result of subluxation or dislocation. A characteristic hook lesion was described by Bywaters (1950) resulting not from erosion but from the moulding effect of ligaments (*Figure 175*).

RHEUMATOID ARTHRITIS

Early joint changes of rheumatoid arthritis consist of subarticular decalcification progressing to articular erosions and more generalized juxta-articular osteoporosis. Joint cartilage is lost early while ulnar deviation is late (*Figure 176*). All these changes distinguish the condition from Jaccoud's arthropathy.

Rheumatoid nodules are frequently found at necropsy in epicardium, myocardium and valve tissue (Hart, 1969), but clinical manifestations of heart disease are rare. Pericardial effusion is the most frequent, but valve disease, conduction defects and congestive failure have been reported (Sokoloff, 1964). Although patients with rheumatoid heart disease are usually sero-positive with long-standing joint disease, cardiac symptoms may occasionally overshadow the arthropathy and the radiological diagnosis of rheumatoid arthritis and its differentiation from Jaccoud's arthropathy becomes important.

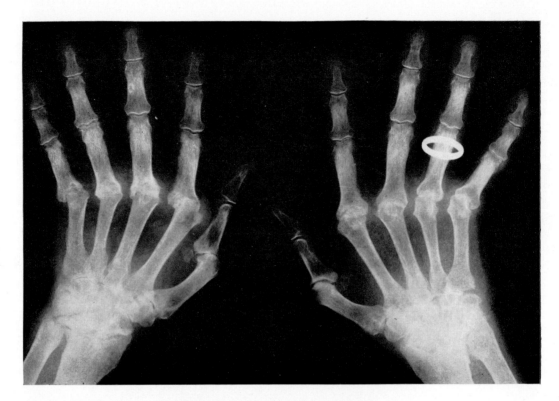

Figure 176. Rheumatoid arthritis. Hands

BONE CHANGES OF CYANOTIC CONGENITAL HEART DISEASE

Gout

Gout may complicate the polycythaemia of cyanotic congenital heart disease, but unlike primary gout it may present as an arthropathy in a patient below the age of 40 years without a family history. Somerville (1961) collected 9 cases in five years. She found that at the first attack, cyanosis had been present for at least ten years and there was severe polycythaemia with a haemoglobin of 130 per cent or more. In adults there was a correlation between haemoglobin and blood uric acid levels. The mechanism is presumably the same as in primary gout, namely precipitation of urates in the joints, but impaired renal function is an important contributory factor. The initial attack usually involves a single joint: this is most often the first metatarso-phalangeal, but the joints of the hands, ankles, knees and even elbows may be involved as well as those of the heels.

Radiological changes are similar to those seen in primary gout and do not appear until after several acute attacks. There is synovial hypertrophy, visible as eccentric soft tissue swellings or tophi. Destruction of cartilage and bone causes reduction of joint space and bone erosion. The erosions are quite unlike rheumatoid arthritis in that they are clear-cut, lie some distance from the articular surface and are unaccompanied by osteoporosis (*Figure 177*). Tophi may calcify, sometimes before bone destruction is evident (Murray and Jacobsen, 1971).

Hypertrophic osteoarthropathy

Another uncommon complication of cyanotic congenital heart disease is hypertrophic osteoarthropathy. Williams *et al.* (1963) found only 8 cases in the literature and added one of their own. The disorder occurs with long-standing cyanosis and presents with pain and swelling of the hands, wrists, ankles and knees together with clubbing. Although clinically it resembles an arthritis, the joints are unaffected

128

radiologically. Thin periosteal bone is seen at the distal ends of the radius and ulna and the tibia and fibula. The periosteal bone is usually separated from the cortex of the diaphysis by a thin radiolucent band, but fusion occurs in advanced cases (*Figure 178*). A causal relationship between cyanotic congenital heart disease and hypertrophic osteoarthropathy is strongly suggested by a case of Eisenmenger ductus arteriosus which was found to have periostitis confined to the lower limbs (Williams *et al.*, 1963).

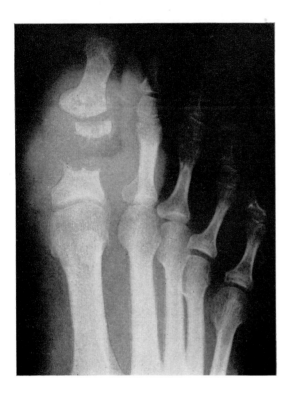

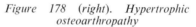

Figure 177 (left). Gout. Foot

Figure 178 (right). Hypertrophic osteoarthropathy

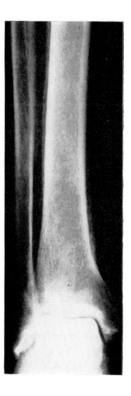

Marrow hyperplasia

The third skeletal change is marrow hyperplasia from the long-standing stimulus of hypoxia; severe polycythaemia is a constant feature. Radiologically the appearances resemble those seen in chronic haemolytic anaemia. There is enlargement of the diploic spaces in the skull. The medullary canal of long bones is widened, and bone texture in both long and short bones may be coarsened due to loss of finer trabeculae; the cortex may be thinned (Singh *et al.*, 1972). Thickening and bristling of the skull bones— 'hair on end' striations—were first described by Ascenzi and Marinozzi (1958). Nice *et al.* (1964) reported areas of sclerosis in the spine and ribs, possibly due to bone infarction.

ANKYLOSING SPONDYLITIS

Significant aortic regurgitation is found in 2 to 5 per cent of patients with ankylosing spondylitis, and 5 per cent of patients with severe aortic regurgitation have ankylosing spondylitis (Sokoloff, 1964). The incidence of aortic regurgitation increases with age and with the duration of the disease. There is evidence to suggest that cardiac involvement is more common when systemic manifestations of ankylosing spondylitis have been severe, but some patients present without a clear previous history of back pain or stiffness. Nearly all cases are male, and there is a latent period of 10–25 years between the joint symptoms and the cardiac signs.

The sacro-iliac joints show three stages during the evolution of the disease: (1) ill-defined sclerosis, more marked on the iliac than on the sacral side of the joint; (2) destruction of cartilage and subchondral bone, causing irregular widening of the joint space; (3) bony ankylosis with obliteration of the joint. The changes are bilateral and usually symmetrical (*Figure 179*). New bone formation or whiskering is seen at the attachments of certain ligaments and tendons, particularly the ischial tuberosities, the greater trochanters and the calcaneum. Squaring of the vertebral bodies is caused by an osteitis developing anteriorly at the corners of the vertebral bodies. Later, ossification of all spinal ligaments may occur. The small joints of the spine, ribs and sternum and the larger joints of the limbs may show evidence of cartilage destruction and eventual ankylosis. By the time cardiovascular involvement is detected in

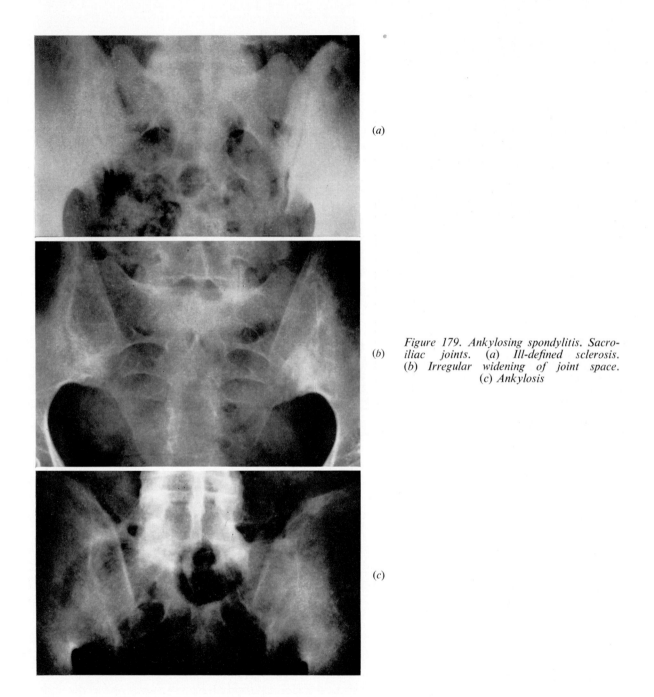

(a)

(b)

(c)

Figure 179. Ankylosing spondylitis. Sacro-iliac joints. (a) Ill-defined sclerosis. (b) Irregular widening of joint space. (c) Ankylosis

ankylosing spondylitis, the sacro-iliac joints are usually obliterated, but a joint space may be recognizable as the disease may arrest in the second stage. Spinal ligaments are usually calcified and involvement of the larger joints of the limbs is not uncommon.

The cardiovascular changes are more specific than in rheumatoid arthritis and are virtually confined to the root of the aorta, the aortic valve and the conducting tissue of the heart. Aortic regurgitation is caused by inflammation and scarring, which may lead to dilatation of the aortic sinuses and ring with cusp retraction and calcification. Heart block from conducting tissue involvement may occur with or without aortic valve disease. Pericarditis is rare.

REITER'S SYNDROME

It is now known that the cardiovascular complications of Reiter's syndrome are similar to ankylosing spondylitis both clinically and pathologically (Rodnan *et al.*, 1964). The disease is virtually confined to men and is characterized by non-bacterial urethritis and arthritis. Conjunctivitis, the third member of the triad, is inconstant, a specific dermatitis being another variable feature. The arthritis is acute or sub-acute, monarticular or polyarticular; it may be non-venereal and follow dysentery. Radiological changes

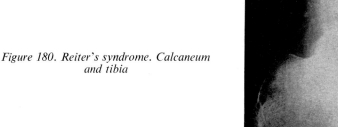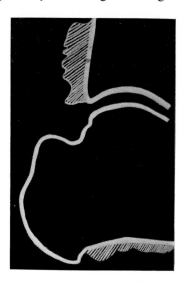

Figure 180. Reiter's syndrome. Calcaneum and tibia

may resemble those of rheumatoid arthritis or ankylosing spondylitis, but there are features which suggest the diagnosis. There is a strong predilection for the lower limbs, the ankles and knees being commonly involved. Achilles tendonitis and plantar fasciitis lead to bone erosion and periostitis on the posterior and inferior surfaces of the calcaneum (*Figure 180*). Periostitis, particularly in the bones of the feet, occurs much more frequently than in rheumatoid arthritis and is equally suggestive (Weldon and Scalettar, 1961).

The incidence of sacro-iliac joint involvement is much less than in ankylosing spondylitis. It tends to be less destructive, and bony ankylosis is less common. Articular and ligamentous changes in the spine are rarely associated with the sacro-iliitis of Reiter's syndrome.

The onset of aortic regurgitation is delayed as in ankylosing spondylitis, and heart block may be a feature. Signs of myocarditis and pericarditis—as evidenced by tachycardia, pericardial rub and electro-cardiographic abnormalities—have been reported (Neu *et al.*, 1960).

CUSHING'S SYNDROME

In this syndrome there is overproduction of adrenal cortical steroids due to hyperplasia, benign neo-plasm or rarely malignant tumour of the adrenal cortex. Hormonal effects include obesity, depression of sexual function, and hypertension which may cause cardiac enlargement. Skeletal changes consist of widespread osteoporosis with pathological fractures (*Figure 181*). Fractures are typically multiple with marked callus formation and involve the ribs and the thoracic vertebral bodies. Diminution of pain sense may render these fractures painless; it also predisposes to florid degenerative joint changes. Administration of steroids for immunosuppressive or other reasons may also produce a Cushing-like response, especially a painless avascular necrosis of the femoral head (*Figure 182*).

ACROMEGALY

Acromegaly is due to excessive growth hormone produced by an acidophil pituitary adenoma which appears after epiphyseal fusion. The tumour usually enlarges the pituitary fossa and the hormonal

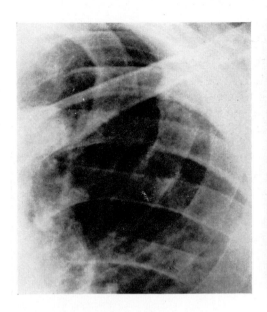

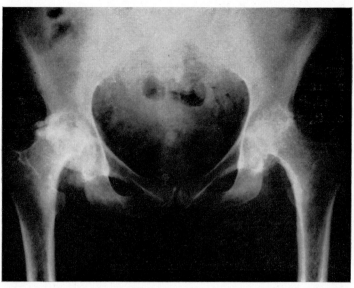

Figure 181. Cushing's syndrome. Local view of left upper ribs showing osteoporosis and fractures

Figure 182. Prolonged steroid therapy. Hips. Bilateral avascular necrosis of femoral heads

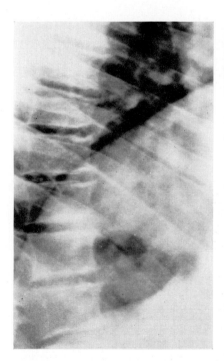

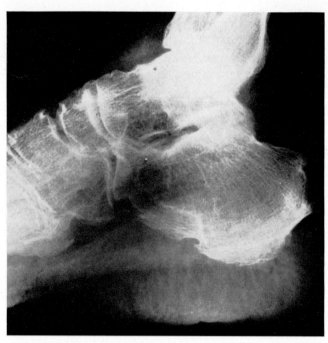

Figure 183. Acromegaly. Lateral spine

Figure 184. Acromegaly. Lateral calcaneum

effects consist of general tissue overgrowth, particularly prominent in the skeleton. The nasal sinuses and the mandible are enlarged and the skull is thick. The antero-posterior diameters of the vertebral bodies are increased (*Figure 183*) and the ribs are lengthened, causing a barrel-shaped chest. Overgrowth of bone in the extremities is seen as enlargement of the tufts of the terminal phalanges and bone ends; early degenerative arthritis is common. Hypertrophy of soft tissues can be measured posterior to the calcaneum, where it should not exceed 22 mm (*Figure 184*). There is myocardial fibrosis and an increase in the muscle bulk of the heart, causing cardiac enlargement, although hypertension, which is common, may be a factor in some cases.

CARCINOID SYNDROME

Malignant carcinoid tumours usually originate in the ileum and metastasize to the liver. A few of them secrete serotonin and other substances which cause the carcinoid syndrome. The features include cutaneous flushes, colic, diarrhoea, vomiting, bronchospasm, hypotension and valve lesions.

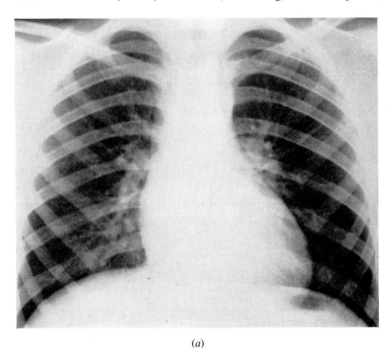

(a)

Figure 185. Rubella syndrome. (a) Anterior view showing no post-stenotic dilatation. (b) Pulmonary arteriogram. Anterior view. Multiple pulmonary stenoses. (c) Pulmonary arteriogram. Lateral view. High posterior pulmonary valve

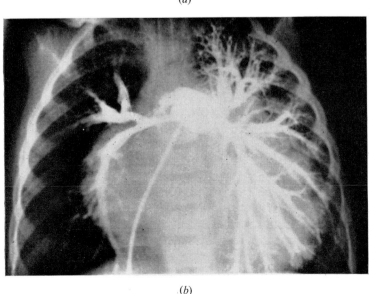

(b)

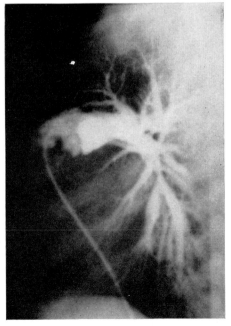

(c)

Valve lesions are caused by endocardial plaques, most often seen in relation to the pulmonary and tricuspid valves. Pulmonary stenosis and tricuspid regurgitation are usual; less often there is pulmonary regurgitation and tricuspid stenosis. The right side of the heart is dilated, but there is no post-stenotic dilatation of the pulmonary trunk. It was erroneously thought that serotonin was inactivated in the lung so that left-sided valve lesions did not occur without a right-to-left shunt or a carcinoid tumour in the lung. Mitral valve disease, similar in gross appearances to rheumatic heart disease, does however occur and is more common than aortic valve involvement. Bronchial carcinoid tumours may be associated with widespread osteoblastic skeletal metastases, flushing attacks, oedema and diarrhoea. There are left-sided valve lesions with congestive failure. Sudden death is common.

RUBELLA SYNDROME

The commonest sequelae of maternal rubella contracted in the first three months of pregnancy are deafness, cataract and congenital heart disease in the foetus. The incidence of important congenital cardiac anomalies is about 10 per cent. During epidemics, however, the heart is more often involved and widespread changes are present in other systems of the body; the condition has been termed the expanded rubella syndrome or rubella embryopathy. Affected babies usually reach full term, but their low birth weight reflects retarded growth; they may have thrombocytopenic purpura, hepato-spleno-megaly, mental retardation and microcephaly. Rudolf et al. (1965) reported bone involvement in 60 per cent of infants. The changes are most prominent in the metaphyses of long bones and are best seen in the knee. The provisional zone of calcification is poorly defined, and alternating longitudinal streaks of radiolucency and sclerosis give the metaphysis a 'celery stick' appearance which is specific to this condition. Resolution occurs within three months in clinically mild cases, but a wide dense zone of provisional calcification and abnormal trabeculation may persist. After the neonatal period, radiolucent bands and beaking at the edges of the metaphyses may remain. The skull often shows a large anterior fontanelle.

Congenital heart lesions display three patterns:

(1) Ductus arteriosus.
(2) Ductus arteriosus with pulmonary valve stenosis or pulmonary artery stenosis.
(3) Pulmonary artery stenosis alone.

Although not present in every case of post-rubella syndrome, the following appearances suggest the diagnosis (after Elliott and Amplatz, 1966) (Figure 185).

(1) No post-stenotic dilatation on the plain radiograph.
(2) A short horizontal pulmonary trunk.
(3) A high, posteriorly placed pulmonary valve with the ring lying vertically.
(4) Thickened pulmonary valve cusps.
(5) Pulmonary regurgitation.

PAGET'S DISEASE

It is rare for primary disease of bone to have important cardiovascular consequences. Paget's disease, however, is of great interest in that three different mechanisms may operate in the genesis of heart disease.

First, there is an increased incidence of arterial disease. Atherosclerosis and Monckeberg's medial sclerosis both occur with calcification (Figure 186). Sorneberger and Smedel (1952) suggested that there was an increased incidence of atheroma, but most authorities agree that occlusive vascular disease is not unduly frequent (Harrison and Lennox, 1948; Hudson, 1965) and that non-obstructive medial sclerosis is common. This is supported by the usual pattern of arterial calcification seen radiologically, which is parallel or ring-shaped and less often in separate plaques as in atheroma (Figure 186)

Secondly, there is a fivefold increase in the incidence of valve calcification compared with matched controls (Harrison and Lennox, 1948). Mitral calcification lies in the subvalvar recess between the posterior cusp and left ventricular wall (see Figures 90 and 93b); it may spread to involve the ring and posterior cusp, causing clinical valve disease or heart block. This type of calcification may occur without Paget's disease, but is then virtually confined to women. Calcification is seen less commonly in the aortic valve.

Thirdly, Paget's disease may cause a high cardiac output leading to congestive failure. Paget (1877) observed increased vascularity of bone at autopsy. Edholm *et al.* (1945) reported a 66-year-old man with

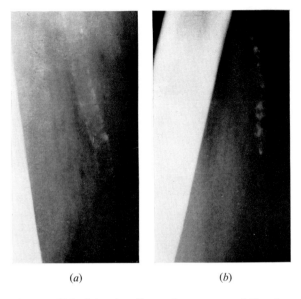

(a)   (b)

Figure 186 (above). Femoral artery calcification. (a) Monckeberg's medial sclerosis. (b) Atherosclerosis

Figure 187. Paget's disease. Femur and ischiopubic ramus. Osteolytic, mixed and sclerotic disease

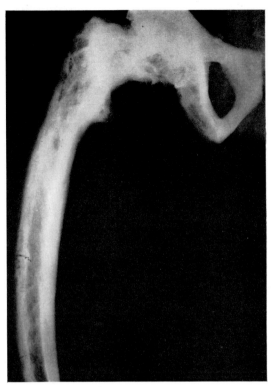

advanced Paget's disease and congestive failure who had high right atrial pressure and a cardiac output of 13·3 litres per minute. They measured blood flow through involved bone and found a tenfold to twentyfold increase. They also demonstrated that the cardiac output was normal in localized Paget's disease, although flow was increased in the affected limb. Howarth (1953) showed that a high cardiac output was not found unless at least 35 per cent of the skeleton was diseased and the alkaline phosphatase was above 45 King–Armstrong units.

Radiologically three stages of bone involvement are recognized in the natural history of Paget's disease, but all three may be seen in the same patient (*Figure 187*). In the active stage, bone destruction dominates the picture. Large osteolytic areas, characteristically seen in the skull and tibia, may be present or bone may be coarsened due to loss of the smaller trabeculae—so-called spongy Paget's disease. In the biphasic stage, sclerosis is apparent as well as destruction, and in the quiescent phase sclerosis dominates (amorphous Paget's disease). Edholm and Howarth (1953) demonstrated that blood flow through bone is increased from the very earliest radiological stage, and sometimes before radiological abnormality is apparent. The increased flow continues through the biphasic stage, but returns to normal when the disease becomes quiescent. It appears that the high output state in extensive and active Paget's disease resembles that in systemic arteriovenous fistula, although intra-osseous shunts have not been conclusively demonstrated.

PREMATURE AGEING

Premature ageing and dwarfism are seen in progeria and in Werner's syndrome. Patients with progeria usually show abnormality within 18 months of birth, with loss of hair and subcutaneous fat. Dwarfism is due to generalized skeletal hypoplasia. There is generalized osteoporosis. The long bones are short and slender; the clavicles are typically very small and may ultimately fibrose and disappear, an event not seen in any other disease. The distal phalanges may also be lost. The skull is thin, with Wormian bones and delayed closure of fontanelles. Coxa valga and joint deformities are usual. Precocious arterial calcification occurs, and premature death usually results from coronary artery disease (*Figure 188*).

Unlike progeria, the onset of Werner's syndrome is delayed until late childhood, with absence of the

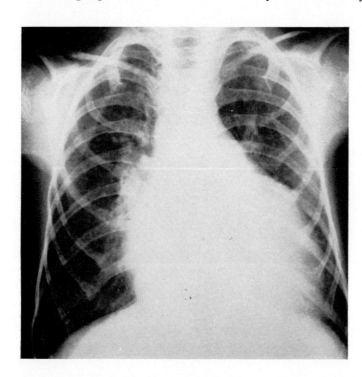

Figure 188. Progeria. Chest. Male aged 14 years. Cardiac enlargement due to severe ischaemic heart disease. Hypoplasia and osteoporosis of ribs and clavicles

adolescent growth spurt. Patients present in their twenties with dwarfism, grey hair, cataract, a thin dermis, and loss of subcutaneous fat which is replaced by thick fibrous tissue. Calcification occurs in soft tissues and in the cardiovascular system, especially the aortic valve. There is diffuse osteoporosis. Osteomyelitis, suppurative arthritis and degenerative joint disease are complications. Death from cardiovascular disease usually occurs in middle age.

PART TWO
The Clinico-radiological Approach to Heart Disease

SECTION IV
Shunts Without Cyanosis

CHAPTER 16

Atrial Shunts

This chapter deals with the group of acyanotic patients who present with a left-to-right shunt at atrial level. The clinical hallmarks are right ventricular enlargement, a pulmonary ejection systolic murmur due to increased flow, and fixed splitting of the second heart sound. The group includes:
(1) Secundum atrial septal defect.
(2) Partial anomalous pulmonary venous drainage.
(3) Primum atrial septal defect.
(4) Atrial shunts and mitral valve disease.
(5) Atrial shunts and mild pulmonary stenosis.
(6) Atrial shunts and pulmonary arterial hypertension.
Single atrium is described on page 205.

SECUNDUM ATRIAL SEPTAL DEFECT

This can be subdivided as follows.

Fossa ovalis defect is the commonest (80 per cent) and lies in the centre of the atrial septum. It may be associated with partial anomalous pulmonary venous drainage.

Inferior vena caval defect lies low in the atrial septum, is usually large, and may have no inferior or posterior border.

Sinus venosus defect lies high in the atrial septum at the superior vena cava/right atrial junction, and is always associated with partial anomalous drainage of the right pulmonary veins into the superior vena cava and sometimes into the right atrium.

There is a shunt from the left atrium to the right atrium, which produces an increase in pulmonary blood flow and imposes a volume load on the right atrium and ventricle. The right atrium, right ventricle, pulmonary arteries and pulmonary veins are dilated, but the left atrium, although also subjected to an increased flow, is usually normal in size because blood flows out of the chamber throughout the cardiac cycle. The pulmonary arterial pressure in the majority of cases is normal and the pulmonary vascular resistance is often below normal. Moderate pulmonary hypertension may occur but is rare before the age of 30 years. Extreme pulmonary hypertension with shunt reversal and cyanosis (Eisenmenger syndrome) is considered in chapter 21.

Radiology (*Figures 189* and *190*)

The heart is enlarged in 80 per cent of patients with a normal pulmonary artery pressure. The degree of enlargement varies, but bears no relation to the pulmonary flow as calculated at cardiac catheterization. There is also no correlation between the size of the defect as observed at operation and the size of the heart (*see* Appendix C).

The typical shape of right ventricular dilatation seen in the anterior view is present in 85 per cent of cases and is a useful sign in differentiating atrial septal defect from other shunts. In the lateral view right ventricular dilatation, as judged by increased contact of the heart with the sternum, is present in only 40 per cent and is therefore a less reliable sign. A useful sign, present in 56 per cent, is displacement of the heart to the left; in many cases the right border is near the edge of the spine, closely resembling sternal depression. The pulmonary trunk is enlarged in 82 per cent, in contrast to ventricular septal defect in which it is normal in 80 per cent. The enlargement is mild in 46 per cent and moderate in 36

139

per cent; marked enlargement is not seen in the absence of pulmonary hypertension. The shape of the dilated pulmonary trunk is variable, but the incidence of a long arc with a long radius is undoubtedly higher than in other causes of pulmonary trunk dilatation. The aortic arch appears small in 85 per cent and there is absence of the shadow of the ascending aorta in the right upper mediastinum, a sign not

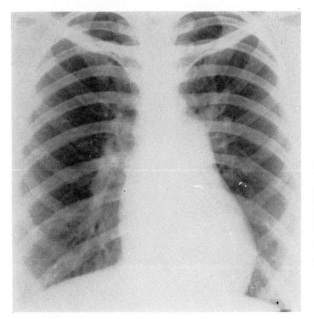

Figure 189. Typical secundum atrial septal defect

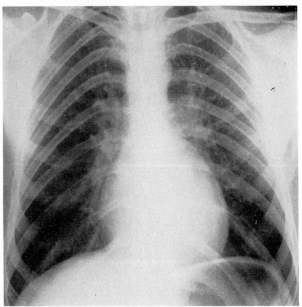

Figure 190. Atypical secundum atrial septal defect with no dilatation of pulmonary trunk

present in shunts other than at atrial level. The appearances are due to displacement of the aortic root and ascending aorta to the left as a result of dilatation of the right atrium and right ventricle; the thoracic aorta lies in the sagittal plane with little or no curving of the ascending aorta to the right or of the knuckle to the left (*Figure 191*).

Dilatation of the lowest part of the superior vena cava at the site of entry of the right upper lobe anomalous vein is occasionally seen in sinus venosus atrial septal defect and permits a diagnosis to be made (*Figure 192*). The left atrium is slightly enlarged in 10 per cent of patients without atrial fibrillation or associated mitral valve disease. The enlargement is never more than slight as judged by increased density in the mid portion of the heart or bowing of the left lower lobe bronchus, so that more obvious signs of left atrial enlargement should raise the suspicion of a complicating lesion. A left superior vena cava (present in 10 per cent) may be visible as a low density shadow in the left upper mediastinum with a vertical outer edge crossing the aortic knuckle or the pulmonary trunk and then disappearing within the heart shadow (*see Figure 13*).

The pulmonary vessels are enlarged in 100 per cent of cases. The enlargement is slight in 40 per cent and obvious or gross in 60 per cent, and the decrease in size is uniform when passing from the lobar to the segmental branches. There is no correlation between the degree of enlargement of the pulmonary trunk and the pulmonary flow, but some relationship is found between the size of the lobar and segmental vessels and the pulmonary flow. When these vessels are obviously large, the shunt is also large, but when the dilatation is unimpressive the shunt is quite unpredictable.

Atrial fibrillation does not usually occur before the age of 40 years; the heart is invariably large, the left atrium is often dilated, and basal septal lines (*see* page 87) may be visible. The shunt is large and the pulmonary artery pressure is above normal. Septal lines are occasionally found without atrial fibrillation or associated mitral valve disease. These patients also tend to be elderly with some pulmonary hypertension. The significance of the lines is not clear, but they may be related to left ventricular dysfunction. Vessels in the right lung are larger than those in the left lung in 5 per cent. There is no evidence to suggest a left pulmonary arterial stenosis and this finding, which is well documented, is not explicable.

Post-operative department films taken up to three weeks after closure of the defect usually show an increase in heart size due to pericardial and mediastinal fluid, but the plethora is less marked within a few days. Later films show a reduction of up to 13 per cent in the cardio-thoracic ratio, although the mean reduction is 4 per cent (*Figure 193*). In general, the larger the heart before closure the greater the

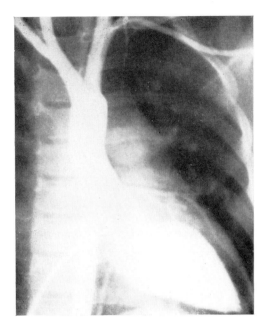

Figure 191. Position of aorta in atrial septal defect

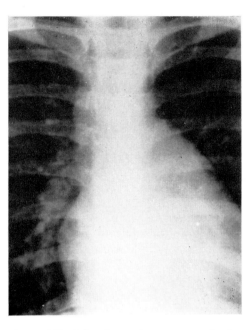

Figure 192. Dilated superior vena cava in sinus venosus atrial septal defect

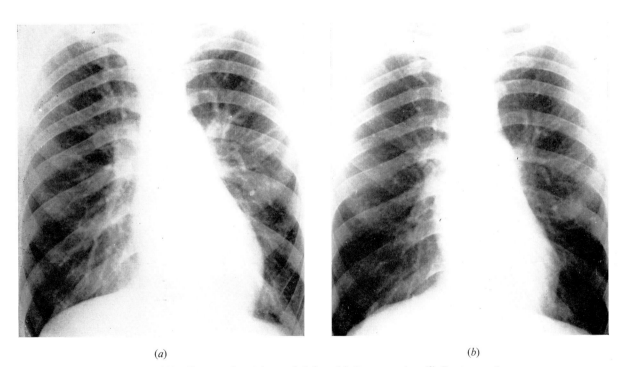

(*a*)   (*b*)

Figure 193. Closure of atrial septal defect. (a) Pre-operative. (b) Post-operative

141

diminution in size. Although the reduction in plethora is usually maximal within three weeks, a further drop is noted in later films in a few patients, suggesting that this can be a gradual process; permanent slight enlargement of proximal pulmonary vessels is usual.

PARTIAL ANOMALOUS PULMONARY VENOUS DRAINAGE

This may occur as an isolated lesion or may coexist with other forms of congenital heart disease, particularly atrial septal defect. As an isolated anomaly, the veins most commonly involved are those in the right lung, and in 50 per cent of cases these drain into the right superior vena cava. Less often they connect with the right atrium, the inferior vena cava, the azygos vein or the coronary sinus. Of particular interest to the radiologist is drainage into the inferior vena cava. Some or all of the veins in the right lung join to enter a large vessel which sweeps downward towards the right cardio-phrenic angle to join the inferior vena cava just below the diaphragm. A small volume right lung due to underdevelopment is often present, with the heart displaced to the right. The appearance of the anomalous vein has given the lesion the eponym of 'scimitar syndrome' (*see Figure 18*). Anomalous venous drainage from the left lung is rare; 85 per cent of cases of this type drain into the left superior vena cava and thence into the left innominate vein. Drainage into the left subclavian vein or coronary sinus is occasionally seen, but is rare. Anomalous venous drainage is present in 15 per cent of secundum atrial septal defects and in all cases of the sinus venosus type. In the latter the right upper pulmonary vein joins the superior vena cava just above the right atrium. The middle and lower pulmonary veins may enter the right atrium or may drain normally into the left atrium. Connection of pulmonary veins to the systemic veins or the right atrium results in a left-to-right shunt which is usually small. The pulmonary artery pressure is rarely raised. If an atrial septal defect is present as well, the proportion of the shunt carried by the anomalous veins is variable, but it may be high in the sinus venosus type and be responsible for pulmonary hypertension (Besterman, 1961).

Radiology

Recognition of anomalous pulmonary veins radiologically depends on their lying in an abnormal anatomical position in the lung. This is always the case with veins draining into the inferior vena cava, although displacement of the heart to the right may obscure the vein on the standard anterior view and it may be visible only on the penetrated film. A vein draining into the superior vena cava is difficult to identify on plain films, but easy on tomography. With veins draining into the right atrium, it is unusual to be able to recognize their anomalous position. Out of 21 patients with atrial septal defect and anomalous pulmonary veins, it was possible to identify veins in an abnormal position in 8 cases, a positive incidence of 40 per cent (*Figure 194*). Dilatation of the superior vena cava, although rare,

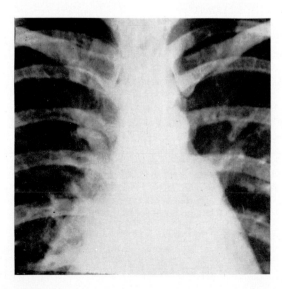

Figure 194. Partial anomalous pulmonary venous drainage. Right upper pulmonary veins are abnormally medial

suggests the diagnosis of sinus venosus atrial septal defect (*see Figure 191*). Dilatation of the left superior vena cava suggests anomalous pulmonary venous drainage from the left lung.

PRIMUM ATRIAL SEPTAL DEFECT

This defect lies low in the atrial septum below the fossa ovalis. It is associated with abnormal development of one or both atrio-ventricular valves and forms part of the spectrum of atrio-ventricular defects, the others being common atrio-ventricular canal and single atrium. It results from incomplete development of the endocardial cushions (*Figures 195* and *196*). Those patients who present clinically as cases of

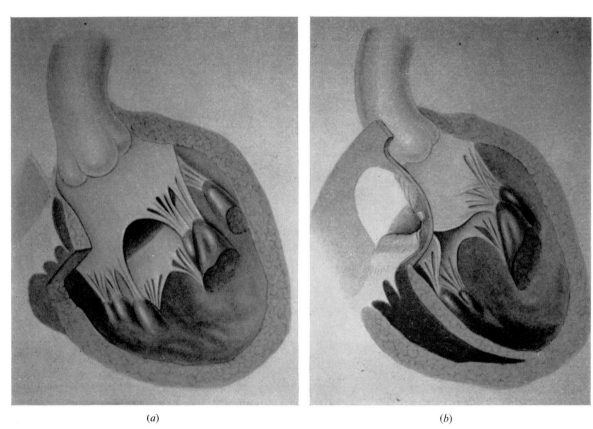

(*a*)   (*b*)

Figure 195. (a) Left ventricle. Internal anatomy, anterior view. (b) Left ventricle in atrio-ventricular defect showing mitral valve. The anterior cusp is cleft, attached to the free upper margin of the ventricular septum and displaced to form the right border of the left ventricular outflow

atrial shunt are the commonest type (70 per cent) and have an ostium primum defect in the atrial septum associated with a cleft in the anterior cusp of the mitral valve: 15 per cent have an abnormal tricuspid valve. Varying degrees of mitral regurgitation are present, but important tricuspid regurgitation is rare. The commonest associated lesions are fossa ovalis defect (17 per cent) left superior vena cava (17 per cent) and pulmonary stenosis (5 per cent) (Somerville, 1971). As the defect involves half to a third of the atrial septum, there is usually an important increase in pulmonary flow due to a shunt from the left atrium to the right atrium, and this is augmented if mitral regurgitation is present. Owing to the low position of the defect, the regurgitant blood from the left ventricle may enter the right atrium as well as the left atrium, so that in addition to the volume load on both ventricles there is a volume and pressure load on both atria.

Radiology

In children the heart is almost always enlarged (90 per cent). The shape of the left border is not specific for enlargement of either ventricle. The right atrial border is prominent in nearly all cases, but left atrial enlargement is less common (60 per cent). Dilatation of the pulmonary trunk and plethora are invariable, and vessels in the upper and lower zones are usually equal in size. Moderate or severe mitral regurgitation is associated with a larger heart, larger atria and selective upper zone vessel dilatation (*Figure 197*).

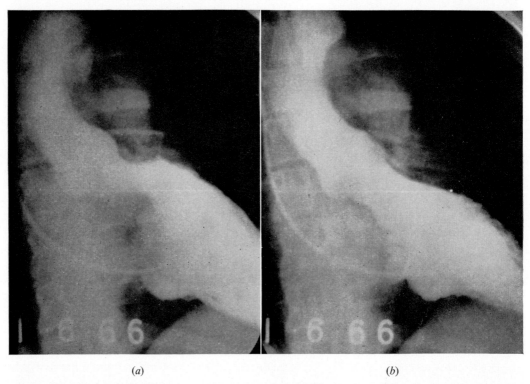

(a)   (b)

Figure 196. Ostium primum atrial septal defect. Left ventricular angiocardiogram showing abnormally placed mitral valve indenting left ventricular outflow on the right side. (a) Diastole. (b) Systole

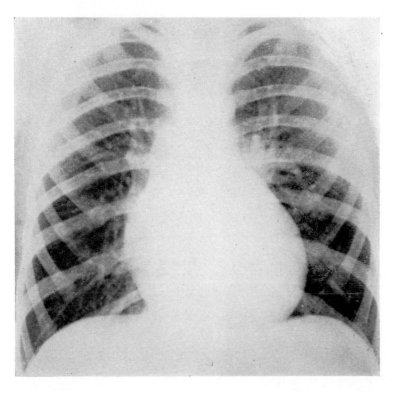

Figure 197. Ostium primum atrial septal defect in child. Plethora with upper zone vessel dilatation. Prominent right atrial border

In adults the picture is different. The heart is enlarged in only 60 per cent. As with secundum defects, the heart is frequently displaced to the left, the shape is suggestive of right ventricular dilatation and the aortic knuckle is small. Pulmonary trunk dilatation and plethora are invariably present. Left atrial enlargement is present only with moderate or severe mitral regurgitation and even then is often slight, so that the differentiation of a primum from a secundum defect on this score in an adult is difficult if not impossible (*Figure 198*). Upper zone vessel dilatation is sometimes seen with atrial fibrillation (*Figure 199*). A left superior vena cava may be visible, but does not help differentiation from other atrial shunts.

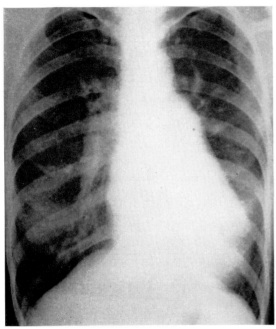
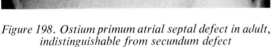
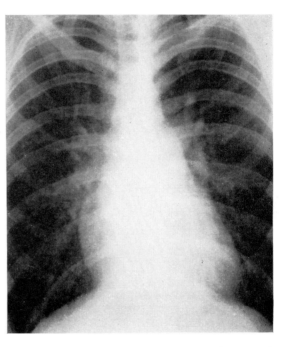

Figure 198. *Ostium primum atrial septal defect in adult, indistinguishable from secundum defect*

Figure 199. *Ostium primum atrial septal defect in adult with atrial fibrillation. Left atrial enlargement and upper zone vessel dilatation*

ATRIAL SHUNTS AND MITRAL VALVE DISEASE

Atrial shunts and mitral valve disease often cause diagnostic difficulty to the clinician, who may be helped by radiology. The clinical problem may be presentation as an atrial shunt with suspected mitral valve disease or as a mitral lesion with a suspected or unsuspected atrial shunt as well; occasionally patients may present with pulmonary hypertension of unknown cause.

The atrial shunt may be due to a septal defect or partial anomalous pulmonary venous drainage or both.

The valve lesion may be any of the following.
(1) Rheumatic mitral stenosis (Lutembacher's syndrome) with or without regurgitation.
(2) Mitral regurgitation due to:
    (*a*) Atrio-ventricular defect or an isolated congenital anomaly.
    (*b*) Cusp prolapse.
    (*c*) Rheumatic heart disease.

If the septal defect is large, a mitral lesion severe enough to cause pulmonary venous hypertension with an intact atrial septum will not do so because the left atrial pressure is immediately transmitted to the right atrium. Theoretically, therefore, pulmonary venous hypertension cannot occur without elevation of the systemic venous pressure. However, when the septal defect is small this does not apply. The effect of the mitral lesion is to increase the size of the shunt, and pulmonary hypertension is common due to a combination of high pulmonary flow and high pulmonary venous pressure.

Radiology

Signs suggestive of mitral valve disease in the presence of an atrial shunt are calcification of the mitral valve, left atrial enlargement, upper zone vessels larger than the lower ones, and interstitial oedema, particularly septal lines (*Figure 200*). One of these signs was present in 18 cases (75 per cent), two in 12 cases (50 per cent) and all three in 2 patients in a series of 24 cases of atrial septal defect and rheumatic mitral valve disease. Calcification was not seen in our series. The left atrium tends to be enlarged when there is severe mitral stenosis with a small defect in the atrial septum, but normal in cases with a large defect. The effect of an important mitral lesion is to increase pulmonary flow and pressure, with cardiac

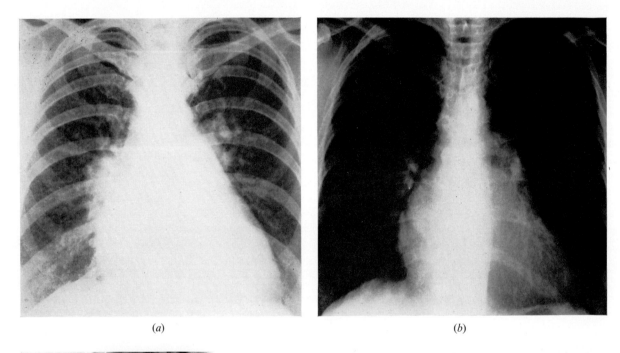

(a)   (b)

Figure 200 (above). Clinical presentation secundum atrial septal defect. (a) Upper zone vessels wider than lower. (b) Left atrial enlargement on penetrated view. Mitral valve disease correctly suspected

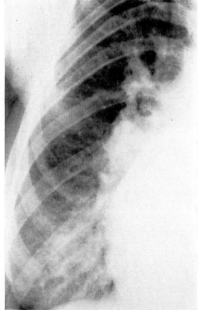

Figure 201 (left). Clinical presentation mitral valve disease. Lower lobe segmental arteries rather large, correctly suggesting a shunt

enlargement and marked plethora. The combination of plethora and relative upper zone vessel dilatation, especially with any left atrial dilatation, is suggestive of the diagnosis. This must be set against the occasional occurrence of left atrial enlargement (10 per cent) and septal lines (6 per cent) in atrial septal defect without mitral disease.

When the clinical problem is mitral disease with a possible shunt, radiology is often a help. The central vessels are often larger than those normally seen in mitral valve disease and the upper zone vessels are dilated, but so are the lower zone segmental arteries, which are always normal or small in mitral disease alone (*Figure 201*). Any suggestion that they are larger than normal or that vessel dilatation involves upper and lower zones should raise the suspicion of an associated atrial shunt, which in the authors' experience will usually prove to be correct.

ATRIAL SHUNTS AND MILD PULMONARY STENOSIS

This section deals with those patients who present clinically with a left-to-right atrial shunt but have mild pulmonary stenosis. When the stenosis is severe, patients present as cases of cyanotic congenital heart disease (*see* page 191).

Small gradients across the right ventricular outflow tract are often observed in patients with atrial septal defect, probably due to high flow. True pulmonary stenosis, documented by angiography and/or operation, is less common. The obstruction, which is at valve level, reduces the size of the shunt so that the volume load on the right ventricle is less but the pressure load greater.

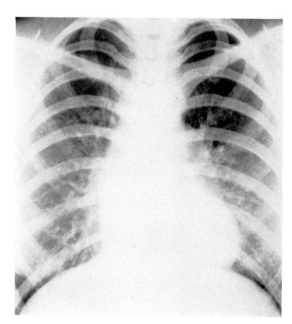

Figure 202. Atrial septal defect and mild pulmonary stenosis. Prominent left pulmonary artery due to post-stenotic dilatation

Radiology

Radiologically these patients resemble cases of atrial septal defect rather than pulmonary stenosis. The picture depends largely on the severity of the pulmonary valve stenosis, the gradients in our cases measuring from 20 to 68 mm Hg. With mild obstruction the appearances are usually indistinguishable from atrial septal defect, but features indicative of pulmonary stenosis are more likely to be present with important obstruction. There may be post-stenotic dilatation of the pulmonary trunk, which may extend into the left pulmonary artery and even into lobar and segmental arteries. The left pulmonary artery may show dilatation without any visible enlargement of the pulmonary trunk, and the commonest sign of pulmonary stenosis with atrial septal defect in our series is a larger left than right pulmonary artery (*Figure 202*). If the pulmonary stenosis is severe there may be no plethora, and its absence in a patient with clinical signs of an atrial shunt suggests the diagnosis. The heart may show only a little enlargement.

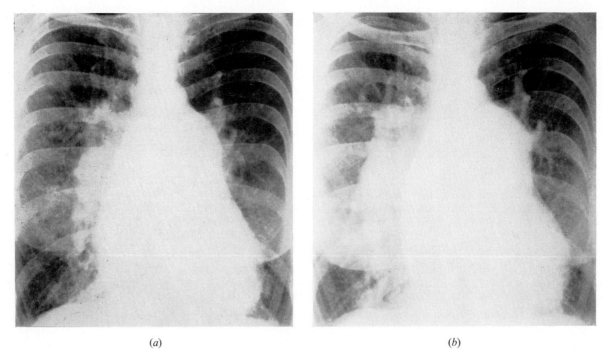

(a)   *(b)*

Figure 203. (a) Atrial septal defect and pulmonary hypertension. (b) Later film showing larger central vessels due to increasing pulmonary hypertension

ATRIAL SHUNTS AND PULMONARY ARTERIAL HYPERTENSION

A left-to-right atrial shunt may be accompanied by an increase in pulmonary arterial pressure which eventually can cause a reduction in the pulmonary blood flow. In secundum defects this is rare before the age of 30 years, but a moderate rise is frequent over 40 years of age. A very high pressure sufficient to cause shunt reversal is rare (Eisenmenger syndrome—*see* Chapter 21). In primum defects, pulmonary hypertension is more common and may be seen in children, particularly in those with significant mitral regurgitation. It is probably more frequent in sinus venosus defects when all the right pulmonary veins drain anomalously. Hypoxia of high altitude predisposes towards pulmonary hypertension.

Radiology

Cardiac enlargement is always present in hyperkinetic pulmonary hypertension and, as a general rule, increases as the pressure rises up to a point where the flow begins to fall. With the onset of the Eisenmenger situation, the heart becomes smaller and may even be normal in size.

When the pulmonary hypertension is primarily hyperkinetic, all the pulmonary vessels are enlarged, but the proximal vessels are relatively bigger than those in the periphery. This pulmonary vascular pattern is indistinguishable from that seen in other shunts with similar haemodynamics. As the pulmonary flow decreases with increase in pulmonary artery pressure, the proximal vessels become very large, with abrupt reduction in vascular calibre within the segments (*Figure 203—see also* Chapter 21).

CHAPTER 17

Ventricular Shunts

Ventricular septal defect may occur as an isolated congenital anomaly or with other lesions which may or may not dominate the picture. Associated lesions of importance include other shunts (ductus arteriosus, atrial septal defect, aortic sinus fistula), obstructive and regurgitant lesions (aortic regurgitation, coarctation, sub-aortic stenosis, mitral valve disease) and all forms of transposition. In addition to these, a ventricular septal defect is an integral part of atrio-ventricular canal, Fallot's tetralogy and related lesions, double outflow right ventricle, tricuspid atresia, and truncus arteriosus.

This chapter deals with patients whose primary clinical presentation is of a left-to-right shunt at ventricular level. The clinical hallmarks are biventricular hypertrophy and a pan-systolic murmur, although other signs may be present if there is a high pulmonary pressure and flow. The following lesions are included in this group.

    (1) Ventricular septal defect.
    (2) Atrio-ventricular canal.
    (3) Left ventricular/right atrial shunt.
    (4) Ventricular septal defect and aortic regurgitation.
    (5) Ventricular septal defect and corrected transposition.
    (6) Ventricular septal defect and ductus arteriosus.
    (7) Double outflow right ventricle.
    (8) Acyanotic Fallot's tetralogy.
    (9) Acquired ventricular septal defect.
   (10) Ventricular septal defect and pulmonary hypertension.

VENTRICULAR SEPTAL DEFECT

Isolated ventricular septal defect may be single or multiple. There are three types.

Infracristal defect (Figure 204a)
    This is the commonest type. Lying in the region of the membranous septum, it varies in size from a pinhole up to 2 cm in the adult. Above it on the right side of the septum is the crista of the right ventricle, and on the left side the right and non-coronary aortic cusps.

Muscular defects
    These lie in the muscular septum. Again variable in size and frequently multiple, they may co-exist with an infracristal defect. Acquired defects due to infarction of the ventricular septum lie in the muscular septum.

Supracristal defect (Figure 204b)
    This, the rarest, is a small defect and lies high up anteriorly in the bulbar septum, immediately below the pulmonary valve and below the right and left coronary cusps of the aortic valve.

There is a shunt from the left ventricle to the right ventricle, the size of which depends on the size of the defect and on the pulmonary vascular resistance. A small defect permits only a small shunt, so that the pulmonary flow is only slightly raised and the pulmonary artery pressure is normal. With a large defect the shunt is large if the pulmonary vascular resistance is low, and the pulmonary artery pressure may be raised because of torrential flow (hyperkinetic pulmonary hypertension). With large defects and a high resistance the shunt is either small or reversed (Eisenmenger syndrome—*see* Chapter 21). There are therefore three basic haemodynamic situations:

    (1) Low flow, normal resistance, normal pressure, acyanotic.

    (2) High flow, normal resistance, high pressure, acyanotic.

    (3) Low flow, high resistance, high pressure, acyanotic or cyanotic.

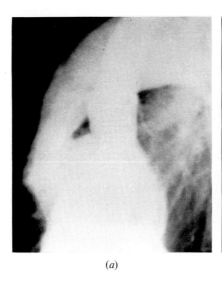 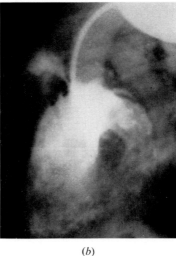

        (*a*)   (*b*)

Figure 204. Ventricular septal defect. Lateral angiograms. (a) Infracristal defect. (b) Supracristal defect

In group 1 the shunt imposes a volume load on both ventricles and on the left atrium, in group 2 there is also a pressure load on the right ventricle, and in group 3 there is primarily a pressure load on both ventricles.

Radiology (*see Figure 111b–d*)

The size of the heart correlates well with flow and pressure. With a pulmonary to systemic flow ratio of less than 2:1 and normal pressure, the heart is normal in size in 30 per cent of cases, slightly enlarged in 55 per cent, and moderately so in only 15 per cent. With a higher flow and pressure, the incidence of moderate or gross enlargement is 80 per cent.

The shape of the left border of the heart is in general non-specific for enlargement of either ventricle. Left atrial enlargement is twice as common with high flow and pressure as with low flow and normal pressure, so that it provides a good but not an absolutely reliable indicator of the pulmonary haemodynamics.

The pulmonary trunk is not enlarged in 80 per cent of those with a small shunt and normal pressure, in contrast to atrial septal defect in which dilatation is present in 82 per cent. Slight enlargement of the hilar and lower zone segmental vessels with normal upper zone vessels is the usual pattern in the lungs. The picture is distinct from that of atrial shunts, in which dilatation of the pulmonary trunk and of all the segmental vessels is seen in the majority. With a large flow, particularly when associated with hyperkinetic pulmonary hypertension, there is dilatation of the pulmonary trunk, but the correlation with the height of the pressure and the flow is not very strong. Plethora is obvious, and the dilatation involves hilar and all segmental vessels equally. Overperfusion pulmonary oedema occasionally occurs in very large shunts in children and is manifested as haziness of the hila and generalized fine mottling in the lung fields. This change is never seen with atrial shunts. The incidence of right aortic arch in isolated ventricular septal defect is 2·5 per cent (Hastreiter *et al.*, 1966).

Post-operative films show that after banding of the pulmonary artery, there is usually a reduction in heart size and always an obvious reduction in plethora. The heart is also smaller after closure of the defect by an average of about 5 per cent in the cardio-thoracic ratio, although this may not occur immediately and early films often show an increase in size. The larger the initial size of the heart, the greater the reduction. Plethora, however, is invariably less within one to three weeks, though in some cases vessels do not become normal with complete closure of the defect. Occasionally the heart and pulmonary vessels become smaller spontaneously, and this suggests natural closure of the defect or increasing pulmonary stenosis.

ATRIO-VENTRICULAR CANAL

Representing complete failure of endocardial cushion development, atrio-ventricular canal is part of the spectrum of atrio-ventricular defects, of which primum atrial septal defect is the commonest. By definition there are atrial and ventricular components to the septal defect, and clefts are also present in the tricuspid septal cusp and the mitral anterior cusp, causing varying degrees of regurgitation (*Figure 205*). Atrio-ventricular canal is commonly found in Down's syndrome. The most frequent associated anomalies are fossa ovalis defect (53 per cent), left superior vena cava (50 per cent) and pulmonary stenosis (14 per cent) (Somerville, 1971).

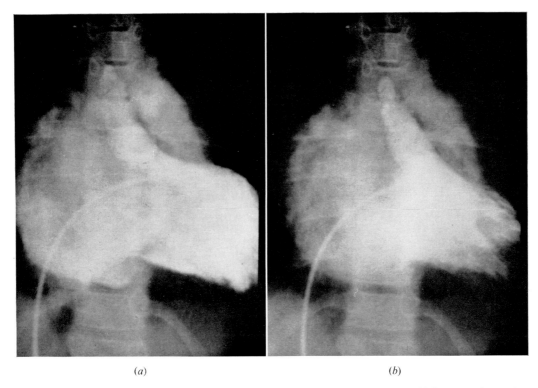

(a)   (b)

Figure 205. Atrio-ventricular canal. Anterior angiogram. Indentation of right side of left ventricular outflow from abnormally placed mitral valve. Shunt from left ventricle into pulmonary trunk and right atrium.
(a) Diastole. (b) Systole

The shunt is complex, but is predominantly from the left-sided chambers into the right. Some degree of mixing may occur in atrio-ventricular canal, giving slight arterial desaturation. Obvious cyanosis occurs with high pulmonary vascular resistance or severe pulmonary stenosis (*see* Chapters 19 and 21).

Radiology

The heart is always enlarged, but most obviously so with pulmonary hypertension. The shape is typically globular due to large ventricles combined with a prominent right atrial border (*Figure 206*). Absence of this shape suggests a small shunt and mild mitral regurgitation. The shape of the left border may resemble the right ventricular dilatation of secundum atrial septal defect, but is usually nonspecific for enlargement of either ventricle. The left atrium is enlarged unless the shunt is small and mitral regurgitation slight. A large pulmonary trunk and plethora are the rule and are most obvious with hyperkinetic pulmonary hypertension. When the Eisenmenger situation is present, the heart may

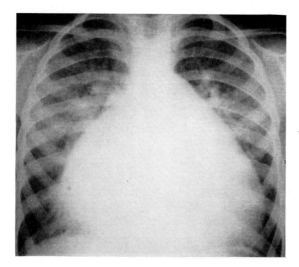

Figure 206. Atrio-ventricular canal. Large globular heart with plethora

not be very large and there may be only slight proximal vessel dilatation resembling Eisenmenger ventricular septal defect. A left superior vena cava may be visible.

LEFT VENTRICULAR/RIGHT ATRIAL SHUNT

This is known as the Gerbode defect (Gerbode *et al.*, 1958) (*Figure 207*).

There are two types of communication between the left ventricle and the right atrium. In the direct type there is a defect in the atrio-ventricular septum just above the tricuspid ring. In the indirect type, a defect in the membranous ventricular septum opens into the right ventricle behind the septal cusp of the tricuspid valve, which is often abnormal, and thence into the right atrium through a second defect inside the tricuspid ring. Shunting may occur into right ventricle and right atrium, but if the cusps of the tricuspid valve are adherent to the ventricular defect, right atrial shunting alone occurs. The indirect form is the more common. There is an unusually high incidence of bacterial endocarditis.

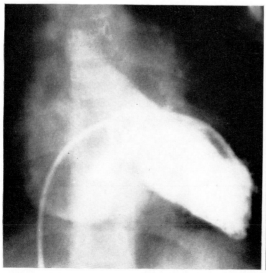

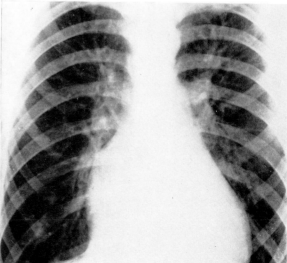

Figure 207. Left ventricular/right atrial shunt. Angiocardiogram

Figure 208. Left ventricular/right atrial shunt. Prominent right atrial border

As the defect is usually small, pulmonary hypertension is rare. There is a volume load on all four chambers.

Radiology

The appearances closely resemble those of ventricular septal defect. The only clue which may be helpful is disproportionate enlargement of the right atrium (*Figure 208*). On plain films it is not possible to differentiate the Gerbode defect from ostium primum atrial septal defect or from complete canal—in fact, all these lesions result from defective development of the endocardial cushions. Rupture of an aortic sinus aneurysm into the right atrium and ventricular septal defect with tricuspid regurgitation produce similar features.

VENTRICULAR SEPTAL DEFECT AND AORTIC REGURGITATION

Aortic regurgitation occurs in about 5 per cent of ventricular septal defects. The defect may be infra-cristal or supracristal. The lesion is basically a maldevelopment of the aortic root consisting of a defect in the membranous or bulbar septum, a defective support for the aortic valve ring, and sometimes anomalies of the cusps such as commissural fusion. In some cases there is displacement of the parietal band of the crista causing infundibular pulmonary stenosis. The regurgitation is usually due to prolapse of the right coronary cusp and sometimes of the non-coronary cusp as well (*Figure 209*). Rarely all three cusps prolapse. If the right coronary cusp prolapses through the defect, it may obstruct the right ventricular outflow tract. Right ventricular obstruction is rarely severe enough to cause cyanosis.

Aortic regurgitation usually appears after the age of two years. The shunt is from left ventricle to right ventricle in systole, but in diastole part of the regurgitating blood from the aorta enters the right ventricle. There is a volume load on both ventricles, but mainly on the left because of increased diastolic inflow from the left atrium as well as the aortic regurgitation.

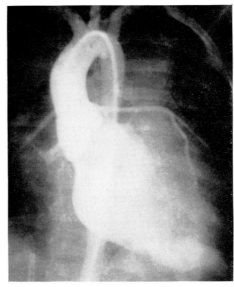

Figure 209. Ventricular septal defect and aortic regurgitation. Aortogram showing cusp prolapse

Radiology (*Figure 210*)

Heart size is dependent more on the degree of aortic regurgitation than on the size of the shunt or the defect. There is always cardiac enlargement, which is typically more conspicuous than the degree of plethora. Slight enlargement is unusual and occurs only with mild regurgitation. The shape of the left border is always suggestive of left ventricular dilatation. Aortic dilatation is usually absent, and when present is only exceptionally seen in patients under 20 years of age. Pulmonary trunk dilatation is also usually absent, particularly when there is infundibular stenosis. Plethora is slight or moderate but not gross. It may decrease with time due to progressive obstruction of the ventricular septal defect by a prolapsing right coronary cusp. Lack of plethora may also be caused by right ventricular outflow obstruction. Left atrial enlargement is common, but upper zone vessel dilatation is seen less often. Infundibular stenosis may show as an infundibular chamber or bay in the middle of the left cardiac border.

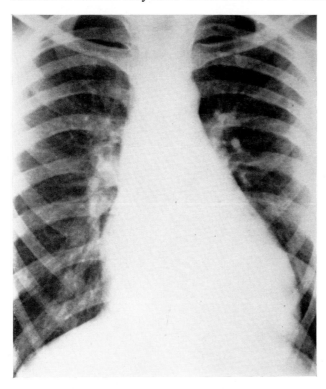

Figure 210. Ventricular septal defect and aortic regurgitation. Gross cardiac enlargement out of proportion to degree of plethora. Some aortic dilatation

VENTRICULAR SEPTAL DEFECT AND CORRECTED TRANSPOSITION

The importance of this lesion lies in its recognition before surgery, as closure of the defect carries a high risk of heart block and is usually contra-indicated. The ventricles are inverted. The aorta lies to the left and in front of the pulmonary trunk, so that it forms the left border of the cardiovascular shadow above the ventricles. Malposition of the heart is often present.

As the transposition is corrected, the circulation within the heart is basically normal and there is a shunt from the left-sided to the right-sided ventricle.

Radiology

The important sign which distinguishes this lesion from uncomplicated ventricular septal defect is alteration of the upper left border of the cardiovascular shadow, which is formed by the ascending aorta. The appearances are obvious in about half the patients and suggestive in a further quarter. Five important features may be seen (*Figure 211*).

(1) The border may be concave, straight or convex, but it is always long, which distinguishes it from the pulmonary trunk.

(2) The border is continuous above with the aortic knuckle.

(3) Below the border formed by the ascending aorta, there is a bulge which is formed by the right ventricular outflow and the aortic sinuses.

(4) There is a high positioning of the right and left pulmonary arteries, which may lie at the same level (*Figure 262*).

(5) The pulmonary arteries in the right upper zone may be wider than on the left (*see Figure 134*).

The theoretical background to transposition is discussed in Chapter 5.

VENTRICULAR SEPTAL DEFECT AND DUCTUS ARTERIOSUS

Approximately 10 per cent of patients presenting with a ventricular shunt have an associated ductus.

Most of them present in infancy. If the ventricular shunt is large with hyperkinetic pulmonary hypertension, the pressures on either side of the ductus will be roughly equal, so that there may be no shunt across it and therefore no duct murmur. However, recognition is important before corrective surgery as the ductus must be ligated before cardio-pulmonary by-pass is set up.

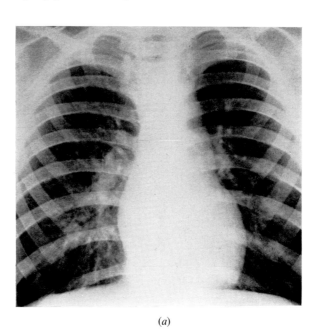

Figure 211. Corrected transposition. Left upper cardiac border formed by ascending aorta. Bulge below formed by 'right' ventricular outflow and aortic sinuses. (a) Convex aorta. (b) Flat aorta. (c) Concave aorta

(a)

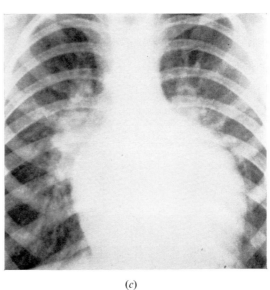

(b)

(c)

Radiology

As with other ventricular shunts, the radiology of the heart and lungs is dependent on the balance of the pressure and flow. A ductus may be suspected if an aortic infundibulum can be identified (*see* pages 36 and 163). This cannot be done in infants, but in older patients the infundibulum may be seen on the penetrated film.

DOUBLE OUTFLOW RIGHT VENTRICLE

There are basically two types of double outflow right ventricle (Neufeld *et al.*, 1962b), depending on the position of the ventricular septal defect (*see Figure 288*). In type 1, which is considered in this

155

section, the defect lies below the crista and is anatomically and functionally sub-aortic (*Figure 212*). In type 2 the defect lies above the crista and is sub-pulmonary; this type includes the Taussig–Bing anomaly (*see* page 207). Double outflow right ventricle may also be associated with pulmonary stenosis (*see* page 186).

Type 1 may present as the Eisenmenger syndrome (*see* Chapter 21), but if the vascular resistance is low, left ventricular blood is directed through the defect predominantly into the aorta. The clinical presentation is of a left-to-right shunt at ventricular level without cyanosis but usually with pulmonary hypertension.

Radiology

Although the aorta arises anteriorly from the right ventricle, the great vessels are normally related in the anterior view. The lesion is therefore indistinguishable on the plain film from ventricular septal defect.

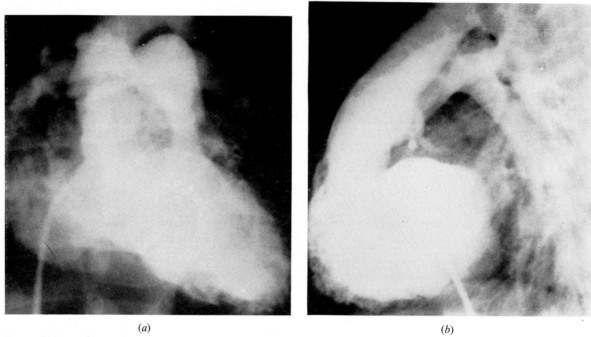

(a)   (b)

Figure 212. Double outflow right ventricle; left ventricular angiogram. (a) Anterior view. (b) Lateral view: the great vessels lie side by side

ACYANOTIC FALLOT'S TETRALOGY

This somewhat controversial term is used synonymously with ventricular septal defect and right ventricular outflow tract obstruction, but with a left-to-right shunt. The defect may be infracristal or supracristal, but the former is much more common. The stenosis is almost always at infundibular level.

Angiocardiography shows an abnormality of the crista and its bands similar to ordinary Fallot's tetralogy (Varghese *et al.*, 1970) but less marked (*Figure 213*). A similar deformity may be found in ventricular septal defect without any outflow gradient but with the probability of obstruction developing later. There is a left-to-right shunt at ventricular level, the size of which is determined by the degree of outflow obstruction. The shunt rarely exceeds 2:1, and systolic gradients up to 100 mm Hg may be encountered. Endocardial thickening usually results in increasing obstruction which eventually causes shunt reversal and a late onset of cyanosis. The right ventricle has a volume and pressure load, and there is also a small volume load on the left ventricle.

Radiology

The heart is enlarged only when the left-to-right shunt is important. Typically the heart decreases in size and the plethora disappears with the onset of cyanosis (*Figure 214*). The shape of the left border

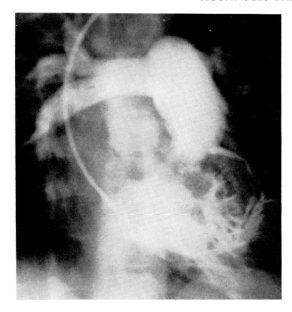

Figure 213. Acyanotic Fallot's tetralogy; angiogram. Infundibular stenosis, normal-sized pulmonary valve ring

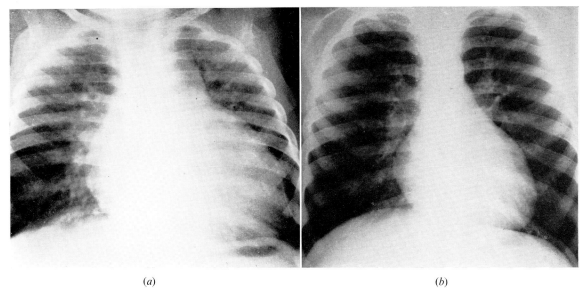

(a)   (b)

Figure 214. Acyanotic Fallot's tetralogy. (a) Plethora and large heart. (b) Reduction of plethora and heart size due to increasing right ventricular outflow obstruction. The patient developed cyanosis

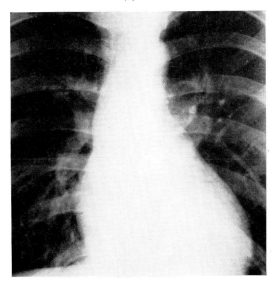

Figure 215. Acyanotic Fallot's tetralogy. Localized bulge on left heart border formed by outflow above infundibular stenosis

157

may suggest right ventricular hypertrophy, but the classical *coeur en sabot* is not seen. There may be a definite localized bulge above the ventricular border, which on right ventricular angiocardiograms is shown to be formed by the infundibulum above the stenosis and the sinus portion of the pulmonary trunk (*Figure 215*). In other patients there may be pulmonary trunk dilatation without an infundibular chamber below, a normal pulmonary trunk above an infundibular chamber, or a bay resembling Fallot's tetralogy. A right arch in a child increases the chance of a ventricular septal defect being acyanotic Fallot's tetralogy (Nadas, 1963). No case of right arch was encountered by the authors, but their patients were older (mean age 17 years).

ACQUIRED VENTRICULAR SEPTAL DEFECT

The ventricular septum may rupture for the following reasons.

(1) Myocardial infarction.
(2) Trauma:
    (*a*) Penetrating (Leaver *et al.*, 1970).
    (*b*) Non-penetrating (Gahagen and Green, 1965).

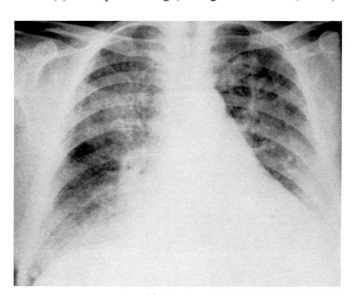

Figure 216. Acquired ventricular septal defect. (a) Interstitial oedema. (b) Plethora. (c) Return to normal after closure

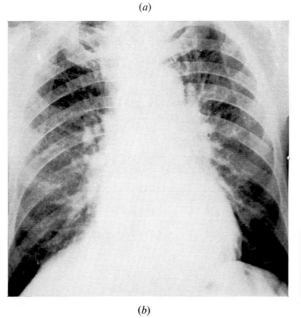

(*a*)

(*b*)

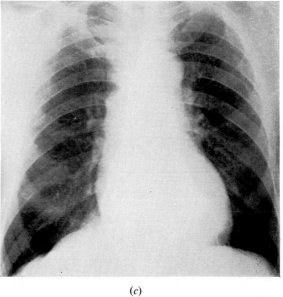

(*c*)

The rupture is almost always in the muscular septum and there may be multiple defects (*see Figure 343*).

If the patient survives, there is a shunt from left to right. The sudden increase in volume load on both ventricles results in left-sided and right-sided failure. In myocardial infarction, left ventricular dysfunction is an important factor in the production of pulmonary venous hypertension. There may also be a low cardiac output from cardiogenic shock following infarction or from pericardial tamponade with penetrating wounds. If the circulation recovers, the left-to-right shunt persists, often with pulmonary hypertension.

Radiology

Ward films taken in the acute phase show varying degrees of cardiac enlargement, left atrial enlargement, pulmonary oedema and pleural effusion. The presence or absence of plethora is difficult to evaluate in the early stages because of pulmonary oedema, and it is usually impossible to differentiate ventricular septal defect from the clinically similar condition of acute mitral regurgitation due to papillary muscle infarction. It should always be borne in mind, however, that these conditions may coexist. Department films taken after recovery from the acute phase show plethora, so that it may be possible to confirm the diagnosis at this stage (*Figure 216*).

VENTRICULAR SEPTAL DEFECT AND PULMONARY HYPERTENSION

Ventricular septal defect is the commonest cause of hyperkinetic pulmonary hypertension. In contrast to cases with normal pressures, the pulmonary trunk is invariably large and plethora is marked, with the proximal vessels appearing a little larger than the more distal ones. In children particularly, it is difficult to predict the onset of a rise in pulmonary vascular resistance because the radiology changes very little until shunt reversal occurs. Then the heart and pulmonary vessels all become smaller and may approach normality (*see Figure 257*); there is no abrupt reduction in calibre along the segmental arteries, unlike atrial septal defect but like ductus arteriosus (*see* page 195).

CHAPTER 18

Aorto-pulmonary Shunts

This chapter deals with left-to-right shunts originating distal to the aortic valve. The clinical hallmark is a continuous murmur. The lesions to be considered are:

(1) Ductus arteriosus.
(2) Aorto-pulmonary septal defect.
(3) Aortic sinus fistula.
(4) Coronary artery fistula.
(5) Surgical systemic/pulmonary anastomoses.

Continuous murmurs due to an arteriovenous shunt may also arise from systemic/pulmonary collaterals in pulmonary atresia (*see* page 182), from arteriovenous fistulae in the lung (*see* page 210), and from vascular malformations of the chest wall such as intercostal fistula. Other causes of continuous murmurs are vessel narrowing (atheroma, peripheral pulmonary stenosis, venous hum, total anomalous pulmonary venous drainage with stricture), increased flow (coarctation, tumour, mammary souffle) and intracardiac shunts (ventricular septal defect and aortic regurgitation).

Venous hum is an important differential diagnosis of ductus arteriosus, although the murmur disappears in the supine position. The murmur of aorto-pulmonary septal defect is usually systolic because pulmonary hypertension is common. The continuous murmur of aorto-pulmonary shunts, which occurs throughout the cardiac cycle, typically shows a late systolic crescendo before the second heart sound and differs from other continous murmurs such as those heard in ventricular septal defect and aortic regurgitation.

DUCTUS ARTERIOSUS

A ductus may occur as an isolated anomaly or be associated with other congenital anomalies such as ventricular septal defect, Fallot's tetralogy, pulmonary atresia and transposition. Isolated ductus is considered in this section. The ductus is an arterial communication between the distal part of the aortic arch and the left pulmonary artery. In foetal life it carries blood ejected by the right ventricle into the descending thoracic aorta and thence into the lower part of the body and the placenta. It normally closes functionally within 24 hours of birth and ultimately forms the ligamentum arteriosum. The typical small ductus is conical in shape with a wide aortic end and a narrower pulmonary end. A large ductus may have a lumen as wide as that of the aorta. The aorta at the origin of the ductus has a local dilatation termed the infundibulum.

The ductus is developed from the distal end of the left sixth aortic arch, connecting the proximal sixth arch (the left pulmonary artery) to the dorsal aorta. The right distal sixth arch disappears early along with the right dorsal aorta. If the aortic arch is right-sided, the right dorsal aorta persists and the ductus is usually on the right. Persistence of the distal sixth arch on the opposite side to the aortic arch is occasionally seen, but rarely as an isolated anomaly; usually the arch is right-sided, the left pulmonary artery is connected via the ductus to the innominate or subclavian artery, and there may be a vascular ring.

The shunt is from left to right, resulting in increased pulmonary flow. There is a volume load on the left atrium and left ventricle. If the ductus is large and carries a large shunt, there may be hyperkinetic pulmonary hypertension. Extreme pulmonary hypertension with shunt reversal (Eisenmenger syndrome) can also occur (*see* Chapter 21).

Radiology

In a ductus with a normal pulmonary artery pressure, it is unusual for cardiac enlargement to be more than slight and a normal-sized heart is encountered in a third of the cases. The shape of the left border usually suggests left ventricular dilatation, and the left atrium is slightly enlarged in about 25 per cent. Pulmonary trunk dilatation is the rule but is nearly always slight (*Figure 217*): gross dilatation does not occur under the age of 50 years without pulmonary hypertension. Plethora is variable and may be

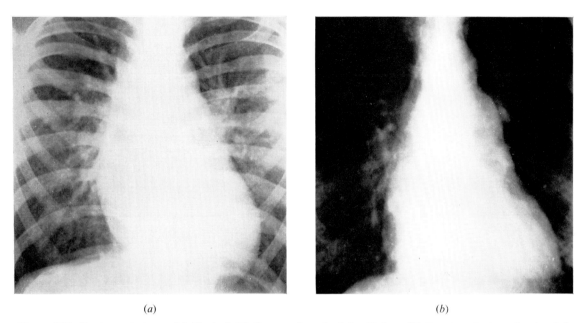

(a)   (b)

Figure 217. Ductus arteriosus. (a) Typical. Plethora and aortic infundibulum. (b) Penetrated view showing left atrial enlargement

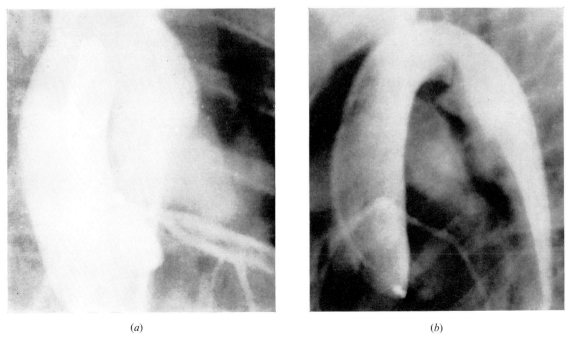

(a)   (b)

Figure 218. Ductus arteriosus. Aortogram. (a) Anterior view showing infundibulum. (b) Lateral view showing funnel-shaped ductus

absent, but is usually present and not gross. The degree of plethora corresponds to the cardiac enlargement, and patients without plethora tend to have a normal-sized heart. Measurements of pulmonary flow are done so infrequently in patients with a ductus that observations on the relationship of flow to radiological signs are not possible. However, a strong correlation exists between the size of the ductus as assessed at surgery and the size of the heart (*see* Appendix C).

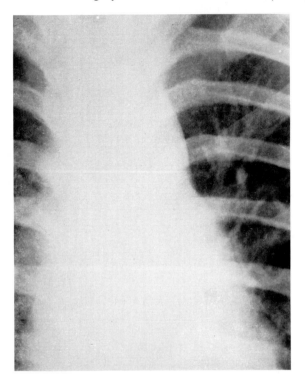

Figure 219. Ductus arteriosus. Large knuckle

With pulmonary hypertension (excluding Eisenmenger) the ductus and the shunt are large. The heart, left atrium and pulmonary trunk are correspondingly large and plethora is obvious. In the elderly patient occasionally encountered who has not developed irreversible pulmonary hypertension, central vessel dilatation may be gross and of similar proportion to that seen in pulmonary hypertension with atrial septal defect.

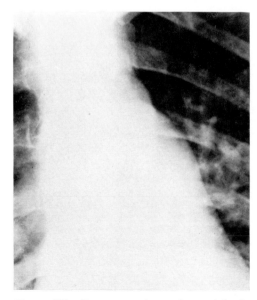

Figure 220. Ductus arteriosus. Large infundibulum

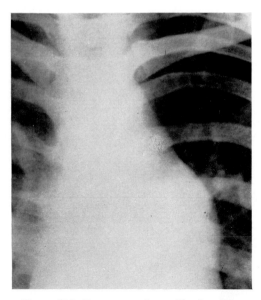

Figure 221. Ductus arteriosus. Flat knuckle

Radiologically the cardinal feature of a ductus is the infundibulum, a localized dilatation of the aorta around the ductus orifice (*Figure 218*) which may be apparent on the anterior view as:

(1) A larger than normal knuckle (50 per cent) (*Figure 219*).

(2) An aortic bulge to the left below the knuckle seen through the pulmonary trunk (60 per cent) (*Figure 220*).

(3) A flat knuckle (15 per cent) (*Figure 221*).

(4) Filling in of the angle between the knuckle and the pulmonary trunk (5 per cent) (*Figure 222*).

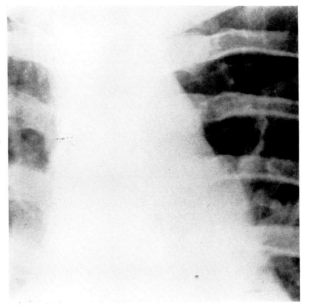

Figure 222. Ductus arteriosus. Filling in between aortic knuckle and pulmonary trunk

On the standard view the size of the knuckle and the presence of a bulge below it may be difficult to appreciate, and they may be seen only on the penetrated view. However, it is exceptional for one or more signs of an infundibulum not to be present on close scrutiny except in infants and children. Calcification

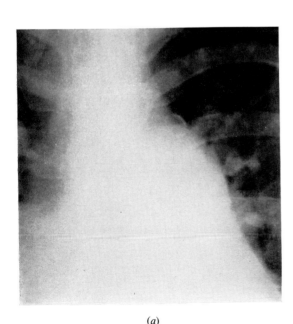

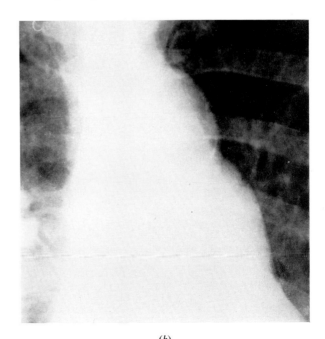

(a)   (b)

Figure 223. Ductus arteriosus. (a) Calcium in ductus. (b) Calcium in infundibulum

163

of the ductus is found in middle-aged patients with pulmonary hypertension (*Figure 223a*). Calcification also occurs in the aorta around the ductus (*Figure 223b*) and in the pulmonary artery as atheroma with pulmonary hypertension and right-to-left shunt.

Post-operative films taken after closure of the ductus show early disappearance of the plethora. The heart returns to normal if the enlargement was initially only slight, but with larger hearts, and particularly with pulmonary hypertension, reduction in heart size may be slower and is occasionally incomplete after several months. Disappearance of left atrial enlargement is unusual. Reduction in pulmonary trunk dilatation from moderate to slight but not to normal is common, but in patients who initially had only slight enlargement there is rarely any change and it is unusual for the pulmonary trunk to return to normal. The aortic infundibulum does not alter.

AORTO-PULMONARY SEPTAL DEFECT (AORTO-PULMONARY WINDOW)

Although this lesion physiologically resembles a ductus, a continuous murmur is found in only a minority (Neufeld *et al.*, 1962a) owing to the frequency of severe pulmonary hypertension. The defect lies above the aortic sinuses and connects the ascending aorta to the pulmonary trunk. It varies from a defect a few millimetres wide to an absence of much of the truncal septum. Both semilunar valves are present, and this is the important feature which distinguishes the condition from truncus arteriosus (*Figure 224*). Associated lesions have been reported including ductus arteriosus (Coleman *et al.*, 1967), coarctation, sub-aortic stenosis, bicuspid aortic valve and right aortic arch (Somerville, 1959).

If the defect is small, the shunt is small and from left to right. Larger defects are much commoner and are associated with hyperkinetic pulmonary hypertension or with a high vascular resistance and a bidirectional shunt (*see* Chapter 21).

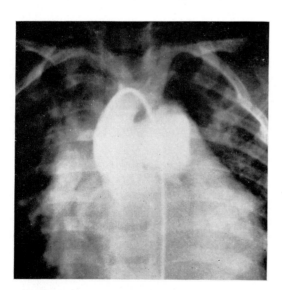

Figure 224. Aorto-pulmonary septal defect. Aortogram

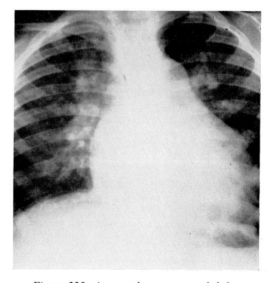

Figure 225. Aorto-pulmonary septal defect. Plain film

Radiology

The appearances are dependent on the size of the shunt and the state of the pulmonary circulation. In general they are indistinguishable from those of a ventricular septal defect or a ductus arteriosus (*Figure 225*) except that a normal or small aortic knuckle with a continuous murmur suggests that the shunt is not through a ductus.

AORTIC SINUS FISTULA

Rupture of an aortic sinus aneurysm into a chamber in the right heart results in an aortic sinus fistula. The aneurysm may be congenital or due to bacterial endocarditis, but the exact aetiology is often difficult if not impossible to establish with certainty (Hudson, 1965). The right and non-coronary sinuses are involved with roughly equal frequency, aneurysms of the right sinus usually rupturing into the right ventricle and those of the non-coronary sinus into the right atrium (*Figure 226*). Aneurysms of the left sinus are rare; rupture may occur into the left atrium (Magidson and Kay, 1963) but more often occurs into the pericardium causing sudden death. (Aneurysms which rupture into the left atrium or left ventricle do not, of course, produce an aorto-pulmonary shunt but an overload on the left heart). Aneurysms are occasionally multiple and may be associated with ventricular septal defect. Sinus aneurysms in the Marfan syndrome do not rupture into the right heart.

The shunt is from the aorta into the right heart, causing a volume load on the right heart, left atrium and left ventricle. The continuous murmur is heard lower than the typical ductus murmur and may be transmitted to the right of the sternum.

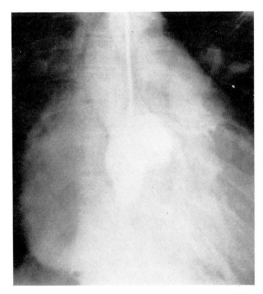

Figure 226. Aortic sinus fistula. Aortogram. Communication between right coronary sinus and right atrium

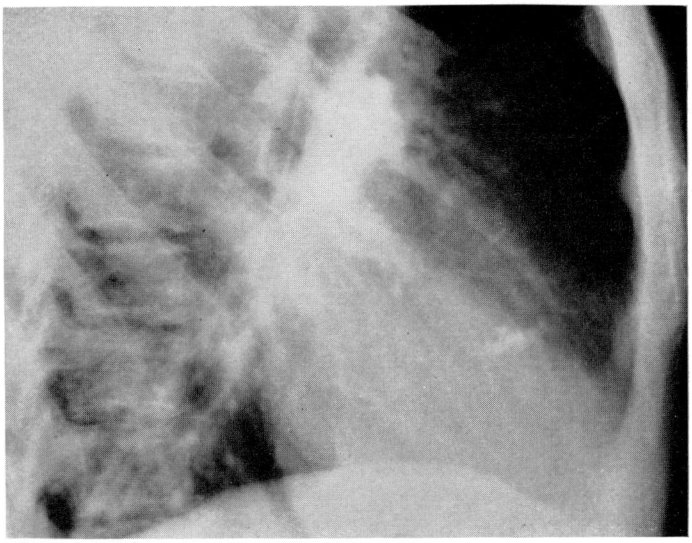

Figure 227. Aortic sinus fistula. Calcification

Radiology

Sinus aneurysms are rarely large enough to be seen as an increased density within the cardiovascular shadow. Exceptionally they may appear as an unusual bulge on either side, which on the left may be mistaken for the left atrial appendix. The onset of the shunt is often abrupt and, in the early stages, there may be pulmonary oedema due to left ventricular failure. Cardiac enlargement and plethora are dependent on the size of the shunt and are usually slight to moderate. The aorta is unremarkable, and prominence of the right border of the heart due to right-sided dilatation is not significant enough to be a sign of diagnostic value. Eggshell calcification may occur in the wall of the aneurysm, but amorphous clumps may also be seen and be difficult to distinguish from the aortic valve (*Figure 227*).

CORONARY ARTERY FISTULA

Coronary artery fistula is a congenital communication between a coronary artery and a chamber of the heart or the pulmonary trunk. There are two forms:
   (1) Origin of a coronary artery from the pulmonary trunk.
   (2) Coronary arteriovenous fistula.

ORIGIN OF LEFT CORONARY ARTERY FROM PULMONARY TRUNK

Death usually occurs in infancy from severe ischaemia of the left ventricle, but infants may also present with severe mitral regurgitation due to papillary muscle dysfunction or dilatation of the mitral valve ring. Patients may survive beyond infancy and into adult life if a good collateral circulation develops. There is a left-to-right shunt from the aorta through the right and the left coronary arteries into the pulmonary trunk; the myocardium may be ischaemic, since much of the arterial blood entering the coronary circulation is shunted past the capillaries. The right coronary artery is dilated and tortuous and many collaterals, particularly through the ventricular septum, fill the left coronary (*Figure 228*). Adult patients may be asymptomatic and present with a continuous murmur in the left second interspace so that a diagnosis of ductus is made. However, premature angina, cardiac enlargement, left ventricular aneurysm (Kafkas and Miller, 1971) and sudden death all occur.

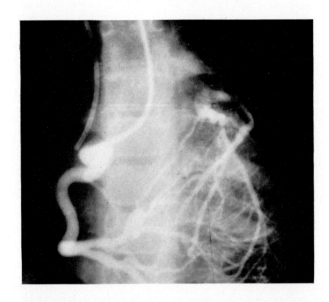

Figure 228. Origin of left coronary artery from pulmonary trunk. Angiogram, anterior view

Radiology

In infancy the picture is that of left ventricular failure or mitral regurgitation. There is a progressive reduction of heart size in surviving patients. In adult life the left ventricle may be only slightly enlarged (*Figure 229*), and left atrial dilatation is absent unless there is mitral regurgitation. Fluoroscopy may show an area of antero-lateral akinesis and there may be a bulge suggesting an aneurysm. Plethora is

Figure 229. Origin of left coronary artery from pulmonary trunk. Plain film

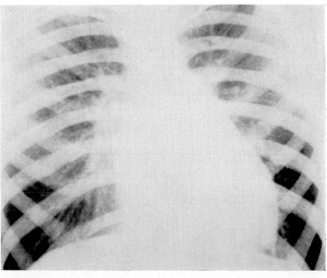

usually not obvious as the shunt is rarely large. The differential diagnosis includes endocardial fibro-elastosis and cardiomyopathy in infancy, other causes of mitral regurgitation, ductus arteriosus and other lesions which give rise to a continuous murmur.

ORIGIN OF RIGHT CORONARY ARTERY FROM PULMONARY TRUNK

Origin of the right coronary artery from the pulmonary trunk causes no symptoms, physical signs or radiological abnormality. It has been reported in a patient aged 90 years (Cronk *et al.*, 1951).

Origin of both coronary arteries from the pulmonary trunk is rare and incompatible with life for more than a few weeks.

CORONARY ARTERIOVENOUS FISTULA

This is a malformation in which a main coronary artery or one of its branches communicates directly with a vein which may enter any of the cardiac chambers, the pulmonary trunk or the coronary sinus. The affected artery is dilated and usually tortuous; the fistula may enter the heart directly or, before doing so, end in an aneurysm or a complex of vessels. The right coronary artery is most often involved and the fistula terminates in the right atrium, right ventricle (*Figure 230*), pulmonary trunk, left atrium or left ventricle in that order of frequency (Neufeld *et al.*, 1961). A fistula to the right atrium may involve the coronary sinus, which is dilated often to aneurysmal proportions (Harris *et al.*, 1969) (*Figure 231*).

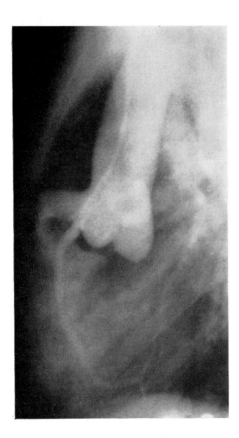

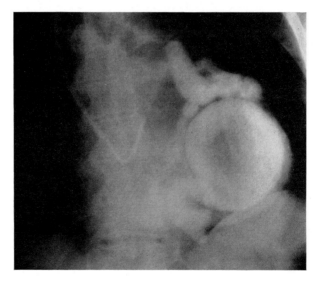

Figure 230 (left). Coronary artery fistula. Conus branch of right coronary artery enters right ventricular outflow. Angiogram

Figure 231 (below). Coronary artery fistula. Circumflex branch of left coronary enters coronary sinus, which is grossly dilated. Angiogram

With large communications, congestive failure may occur in early life. Most commonly, however, the shunt is small and produces no symptoms, so that patients present with a continuous murmur. The site of the murmur is related to the entry point of the fistula into the heart, and if this is the right ventricular outflow (*see Figure 230*) or the pulmonary trunk, the position of the murmur is similar to that of a ductus. Rarely the fistula enters the left ventricle, and then only a diastolic murmur may be audible. Other modes of presentation are congestive failure in later life, bacterial endocarditis, an abnormal heart shape on the chest radiograph and, rarely, angina or rupture. A few coronary arteriovenous fistulae have been reported in association with other congenital heart diseases such as persistent ductus, Fallot's tetralogy (de Nef *et al.*, 1971) and atrial septal defect (Bestermann, 1972). In pulmonary atresia with intact septum and a competent tricuspid valve, right ventricular sinusoids may be dilated and communicate with the coronary arteries with right-to-left shunting as a result of the high right ventricular systolic pressure: in effect, a coronary veno-arterial fistula.

Radiology

As the left-to-right shunt is usually small, the heart is rarely enlarged and pulmonary plethora is often absent. The chamber or pulmonary artery receiving the fistula, however, may be dilated. In the rare cases in which the fistula enters the left atrium, this chamber may be enlarged and the lungs normal; if the left ventricle is involved, the picture may resemble aortic regurgitation. The aneurysm itself may cause an abnormal cardiac shape, which is most often seen with dilatation of the circumflex branch of

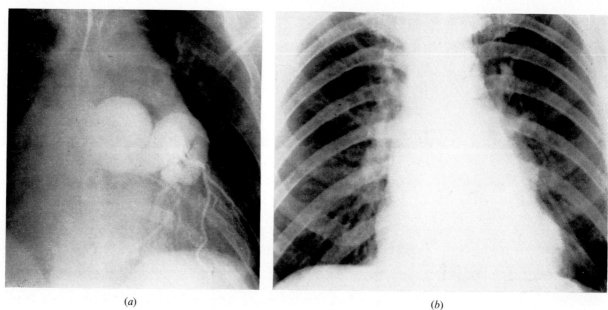

(a)   *(b)*

Figure 232. Coronary artery fistula. Left atrial circumflex branch enters right atrium. (a) Angiogram. (b) Plain film showing bulge on left heart border due to dilated circumflex branch

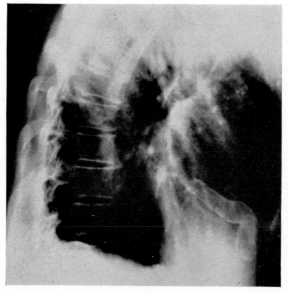

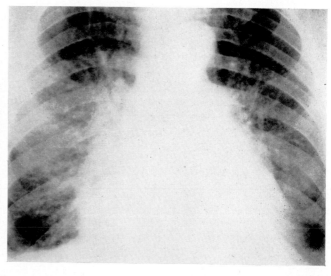

Figure 233. Calcified coronary artery fistula

Figure 234. Coronary artery fistula (left coronary artery to coronary sinus) causing congestive failure

the left coronary artery, producing a localized bulge easily mistaken for the left atrial appendix (*Figure 232*). Usually the bulge is small, but the aneurysm can be big enough to cause bizarre cardiac enlargement (Meyer *et al.*, 1967). Calcification of the fistula occurs but is rare (*Figure 233*). Dilatation of the ascending aorta has been reported by Gasul *et al.* (1960), but has not been encountered by the authors. In older patients who present with congestive failure, there is cardiac enlargement with signs of pulmonary venous hypertension (*Figure 234*). If a coronary artery fistula is associated with another congenital heart disease, the latter usually dictates the radiological picture. Congenital aneurysms of the coronary arteries without fistulous communications may also cause abnormal cardiac bulges and show calcification.

SURGICAL SYSTEMIC/PULMONARY ANASTOMOSES

Continuous murmurs may be produced by surgical shunts created to increase the pulmonary blood flow in certain types of cyanotic congenital heart disease. They include:

    (1) Blalock (subclavian/pulmonary) (Blalock and Taussig, 1945).
    (2) Potts (descending aorta/pulmonary) (Potts *et al.*, 1946).
    (3) Waterston (ascending aorta/pulmonary) (Waterston, 1962).
    (4) Glenn (superior vena cava/pulmonary) (Glenn and Patino, 1954).

Other arteries have occasionally been used, such as the left aortic infundibulum or the innominate artery (Rees and Somerville, 1969).

The size of the resulting shunt depends on the size of the anastomosis and on the pulmonary vascular resistance. In practice a Blalock shunt rarely if ever causes pulmonary hypertension, but a Waterston or Potts shunt may do so. Angiography shows that blood passing through the shunt may predominantly or entirely enter one lung, especially after the Waterston operation. The shunt imposes a volume load on the left ventricle.

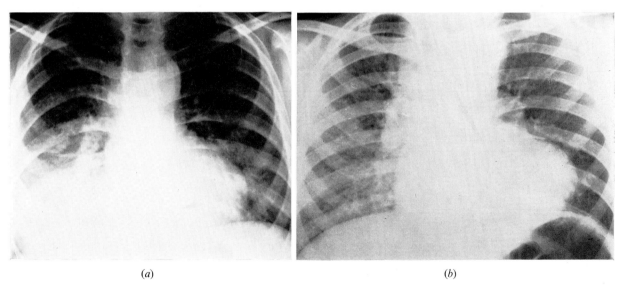

(*a*)   (*b*)

Figure 235. Right Waterston operation. (a) Overperfusion oedema at right base. (b) Unilateral plethora

Radiology

In the early post-operative period, particularly after a Potts or Waterston shunt, there may be obvious unilateral pulmonary plethora and sometimes overperfusion oedema (*Figure 235a*). This settles with medical treatment, but the vessels on the affected side remain large (*Figure 235b*). Pulmonary hypertension is suggested by tortuosity of the segmental arteries. Unequal vascularity is less obvious after a Blalock shunt but may be seen with a Glenn, particularly if the vessels on the opposite side are small. Notching of the upper three or four ribs may occur after a Blalock shunt due to dilatation and tortuosity of the intercostal arteries (*see* page 105 and *Figure 146*). An upper thoracic scoliosis, concave to the side of the shunt, has also been noticed to develop with some frequency.

SECTION V
Shunts With Cyanosis

CHAPTER 19

Fallot's Tetralogy

INTRODUCTION

Historically the tetralogy of Fallot consists of pulmonary stenosis, ventricular septal defect, overriding aorta and hypertrophy of the right ventricle (Fallot, 1888). Haemodynamically only obstruction to right ventricular ejection and the ventricular septal defect are of importance.

The embryological fault in Fallot's tetralogy is displacement of the trunco-conal septum towards the right ventricle and pulmonary trunk, with the result that the outflow tract of the right ventricle is compromised and the aorta is larger than normal. As the displaced conal septum fails to fuse with endocardial cushion tissue, a defect in the ventricular septum results. Obstruction to right ventricular outflow may be caused by one or more of the following: infundibular stenosis, pulmonary valve stenosis, a small valve ring, a small pulmonary trunk, and pulmonary artery or branch stenosis (*Figure 236*). Infundibular stenosis results from upward displacement and hypertrophy of the parietal and often of the septal band, forming a constricting collar around the right ventricular outflow; another result of band displacement is hypoplasia of the outflow tract, which contrasts with the hypertrophy of the inflow or body of the right ventricle. The infundibulum may be uniformly narrow, or the constriction may be localized at the junction of the inflow and outflow portions of the right ventricle or lie higher up just below the valve. With a low stenosis there may be post-stenotic dilatation of the infundibulum, improperly called the third ventricle. Endocardial thickening often contributes to the right ventricular obstruction. Angiocardiographic and surgical findings indicate that infundibular stenosis is the commonest form of obstruction and is present in 90 per cent of cases; valve stenosis occurs in about two-thirds. Infundibular stenosis alone (20 per cent) is commoner than valve stenosis alone (10 per cent). Rarely the pulmonary valve cusps are absent or rudimentary and pulmonary regurgitation occurs, usually with a mildly stenotic infundibulum (Macartney and Miller, 1970) (*see Figure 239*).

If distortion of the right ventricular outflow by the abnormal bands is minimal, no obstruction may be present for years and the patient will present as a left-to-right shunt at ventricular level (acyanotic Fallot); increasing obstruction by band hypertrophy and endocardial thickening occurs later, causing reversal of the shunt and a late onset of cyanosis. Fallot's tetralogy may be associated with an absent left pulmonary artery (*see Figure 133*), the left lung filling via collaterals from systemic arteries. Alternatively, the left pulmonary artery may be hypoplastic and disconnected from the pulmonary trunk, in which case it will fill from a ductus or from systemic collaterals. Ductus arteriosus is uncommon in uncomplicated Fallot, but the bronchial arteries tend to be larger than normal.

The ventricular septal defect is large and approximates to the size of the aortic root. It is nearly always infracristal in position below the right coronary cusp. In the presence of a markedly distorted right ventricular outflow, the aorta is displaced forward and to the right to override the ventricular septum (dextroposition of the aorta). The fourth component of the tetralogy, right ventricular hypertrophy, results from right ventricular ejection against systemic pressure.

The combination of a large ventricular septal defect and severe obstruction to right ventricular outflow in classical Fallot's tetralogy means that the right and left ventricular pressures are identical during systole. The heart is not subjected to a volume overload, but the right ventricle acts against a pressure overload. Right ventricular hypertrophy without much dilatation occurs but is rarely severe enough to cause more than slight cardiac enlargement. In pulmonary stenosis with an intact ventricular septum, the right ventricle is able to raise its systolic pressure so as to maintain a normal cardiac output, whereas in Fallot's tetralogy the right ventricular systolic pressure is limited to the systemic pressure.

173

As resistance to flow across the obstructed outflow is greater than the systemic vascular resistance, pulmonary blood flow is reduced and a right-to-left shunt occurs across the ventricular septal defect. Unoxygenated blood is ejected into the aorta, with the production of cyanosis. Reduction in pulmonary

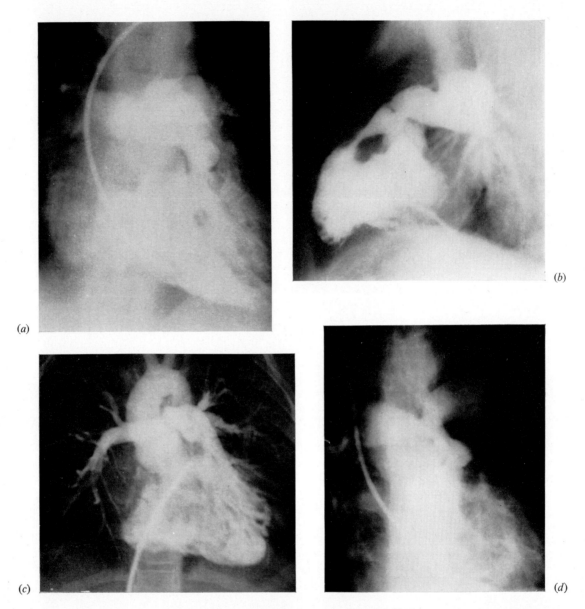

Figure 236. Fallot's tetralogy. Right ventricular angiograms. (a) Infundibular stenosis. Anterior view. (b) Valve stenosis with cristal hypertrophy. Lateral view. (c) Small ring. Anterior view. (d) Pulmonary trunk stenosis. Anterior view

blood flow limits oxygen uptake in the lungs and results in hypoxia. The body reacts anatomically by hypertrophy of the bronchial arteries and physiologically by polycythaemia.

RADIOLOGY

The heart is rarely more than slightly enlarged and is normal in about half the cases. Cardiac enlargement bears no relationship to clinical severity. Anaemia, pulmonary regurgitation and surgical shunts are causes of an unusually large heart in Fallot's tetralogy. The right atrium is very rarely enlarged, and marked right atrial dilatation should suggest an alternative diagnosis. The left atrium is invisible.

The classical ventricular contour on the frontal view is a high or upturned apex, described as the *cœur en sabot* shape; nevertheless this is seen in only 10 per cent of patients. The most common ventricular shape is that of ordinary right ventricular enlargement (*see* page 22) with the apex not far above the diaphragm.

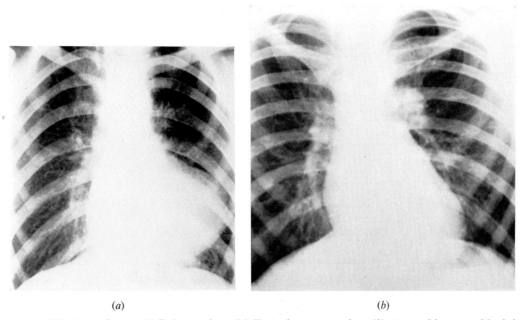

(a)   (b)

Figure 237. Heart shape in Fallot's tetralogy. (a) Typical coeur en sabot. *(b) Atypical low apex-like left ventricular enlargement*

Often the contour is normal; less commonly it may be evenly rounded with the apex roughly in the middle of the ventricular border, and rarely the shape suggests left ventricular enlargement.

The incidence of these various shapes is as follows.

Apex low (classical right ventricle—*see Figure 38*)	45 per cent
Normal shape	25 per cent
Apex middle (rounded—*see Figure 37*)	15 per cent
Apex high (*cœur en sabot—Figure 237a*)	10 per cent
Apex at or below diaphragm (classical left ventricle—*Figure 237b*)	5 per cent

Whatever the contour on the frontal view, the left ventricle is displaced upwards, outwards and backwards by the enlarged right ventricle. It may form all the ventricular border, only its upper part, or none of it if the right ventricle is particularly large and the left ventricle is small (*see* page 22 for detailed discussion of right ventricular enlargement).

A concavity or bay in the middle segment of the left cardiac border due to right ventricular outflow hypoplasia is one of the most important features of Fallot's tetralogy and is seen in at least two-thirds of cases (*Figure 238a*). When this segment is straight or convex (*Figure 238b* and *d*) it usually means a large infundibular chamber and/or muscular hypertrophy (thickening of bands). Sometimes an infundibular chamber or muscle hypertrophy may show as a small convexity within the bay (*Figure 238c*). The pulmonary trunk is invisible in 80 per cent of cases, but it may be normal or enlarged (*Figure 238e*) if there is lone or dominant obstruction at valve level; occasionally it is prominent with dominant infundibular stenosis. Post-stenotic dilatation of the left pulmonary artery, not extending into its branches, is seen in about 20 per cent, again associated with valve stenosis. Gross dilatation of the pulmonary trunk and of the right and left pulmonary arteries, in combination with small intrapulmonary vessels, is characteristic of absence of the pulmonary valve with pulmonary regurgitation (*Figure 239*). Normal-sized hilar arteries with small intrapulmonary vessels are very suggestive of obstruction at valve level or at the pulmonary trunk bifurcation with or without infundibular stenosis. Normal hilar vessels

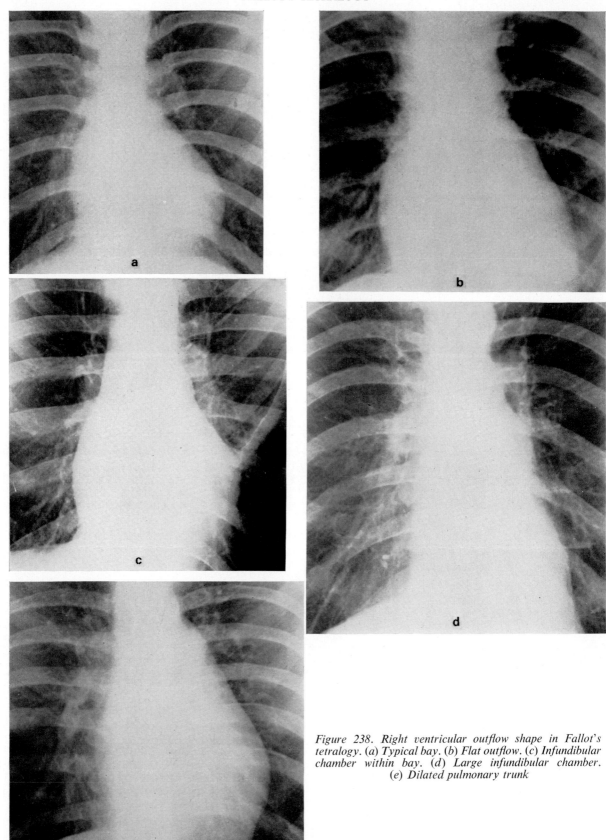

Figure 238. Right ventricular outflow shape in Fallot's tetralogy. (a) Typical bay. (b) Flat outflow. (c) Infundibular chamber within bay. (d) Large infundibular chamber. (e) Dilated pulmonary trunk

probably reflect the presence of central post-stenotic dilatation; they are not related to the severity of cyanosis or, as a corollary, to the degree of obstruction to right ventricular outflow. The left pulmonary artery is occasionally abnormally high in relation to the right (*Figure 240*); this is seen when the right

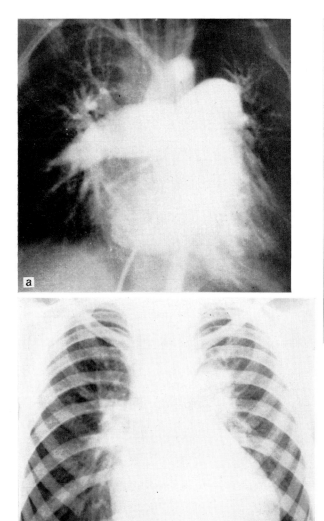

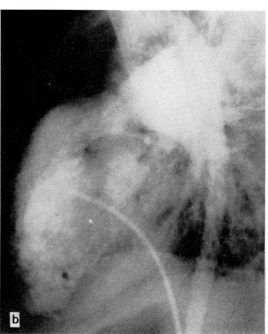

Figure 239. Fallot with absent pulmonary valve. (a) Angiogram, anterior view. (b) Angiogram, lateral view. (c) Anterior view

ventricular outflow is tilted to the right so that the left pulmonary artery has to form a long arc over the left main bronchus. Either pulmonary artery may be elevated following Blalock's operation.

Intrapulmonary arteries and veins are usually smaller than normal and reflect a reduction in pulmonary blood flow. The incidence of oligaemia is related to the clinical severity. Ninety per cent of patients with severe Fallot's tetralogy and 70 per cent of mild cases show oligaemia—an incidence much higher than in lone pulmonary stenosis, in which right ventricular hypertension usually maintains a normal output into the lungs. In Fallot the right ventricular systolic pressure cannot exceed the systemic level because of the large ventricular septal defect. Usually the normal difference in size between the smaller upper zone vessels and the larger lower zone vessels is retained, but severe cases show a more uniform reduction throughout all zones. Unilateral asymmetry of intrapulmonary vessels is seen in Fallot's tetralogy, and the right lung vessels are more often enlarged than the left (Wilson and Amplatz, 1967).

The causes are as follows.

Right pulmonary vessels larger than left
    Right ventricular outflow tilt to right.
    Hypoplastic left pulmonary artery (*Figure 241*).
    Absent left pulmonary artery (*see Figure 133*).
    Right-sided surgical shunt (*see Figure 235*).

Left pulmonary vessels larger than right
    Right ventricular outflow tilt to left, often with pulmonary valve stenosis.
    Compression of right pulmonary artery by a right aortic arch.
    Left surgical shunt.

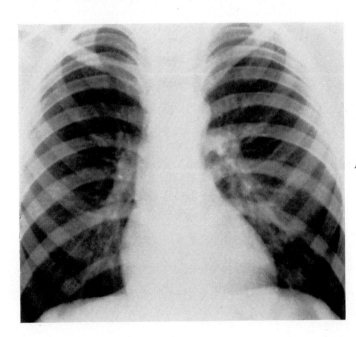

Figure 240. Fallot's tetralogy with high left pulmonary artery

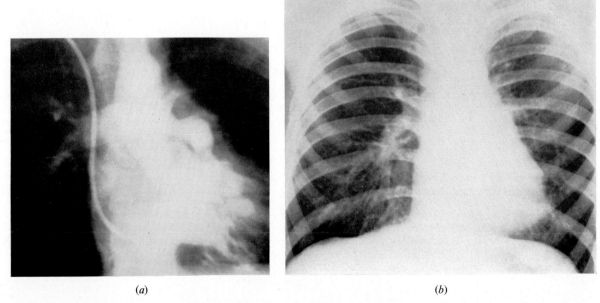

(a)   (b)

Figure 241. Vessel asymmetry in Fallot's tetralogy due to small left pulmonary artery. (a) Angiogram. (b) Anterior view

178

The right ventricular outflow tends to point towards the right pulmonary artery when there is marked band distortion with severe obstruction; selective ejection into the right lung results, and there is increased flow with enlarged vessels on this side. Abnormally small left lung vessels, with a compensatory increase in size of those in the right lung, may be due to hypoplasia or absence of the left pulmonary artery. A persistent ductus or systemic vessels fill a hypoplastic left pulmonary artery which is not connected to the pulmonary trunk: systemic vessels form the only vascular supply to the left lung when the pulmonary artery is absent. In both cases the lung is often reduced in size and, as the left pulmonary artery is usually invisible on the plain film, angiography is necessary to differentiate hypoplasia from absence. In Fallot's tetralogy the right ventricular outflow is occasionally directed to the left, and may

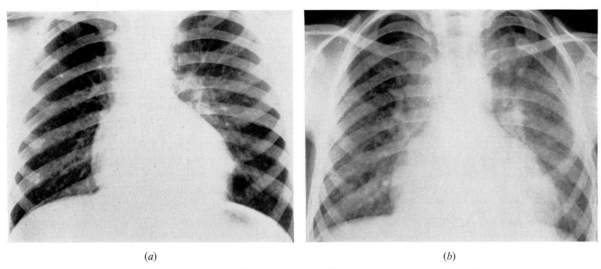

(a)   (b)

Figure 242. Blalock's anastomosis. (a) Pre-operative. (b) Post-operative showing plethora

Figure 243. Left pulmonary artery aneurysm following Blalock's operation

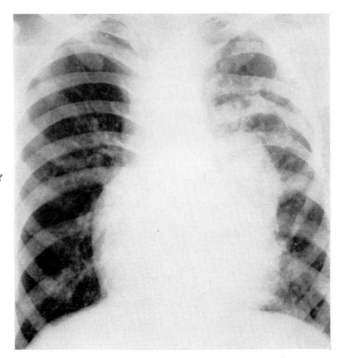

be so when pulmonary valve stenosis is the sole or dominant obstruction; the left pulmonary vessels then appear larger than the right. Compression of the right pulmonary artery by the ascending aorta as a cause of diminished right pulmonary vessels has been reported with a right aortic arch by Porstmann *et al.* (1967). In some severe cases of Fallot's tetralogy, bronchial arteries may be visible on the plain film, showing as an increase in the number of fine vessels in the hilar regions.

The ascending aorta and the aortic arch are usually wider than normal. Dilatation of the ascending aorta may not be visible on the plain film, particularly in children when it is hidden by the thymus or the superior vena cava; an indirect sign of dilatation may be lateral displacement of the superior vena cava. A large aortic arch is commoner in severe than in mild Fallot, but it may also be seen in acyanotic cases. This would suggest that deviation of the trunco-conal septum towards the pulmonary artery side of the truncus is more important as a cause of aortic enlargement than increased aortic flow (not present in acyanotic cases).

The arch is right-sided in 25 per cent of cases (*see Figure 61a*). When a right arch is both enlarged and high in position, pulmonary atresia rather than Fallot's tetralogy should be suspected.

Emanuel and Pattinson (1956) reported a 60 per cent incidence of right aortic arch with absence of the left pulmonary artery in Fallot's tetralogy. Other congenital heart lesions associated with right aortic arch are truncus arteriosus (50 per cent), pulmonary atresia (25 per cent) and uncomplicated ventricular septal defect (2·6 per cent). The descending aorta is normal in size. When a right arch is present, the descending aorta usually travels downwards to the right of the spine to reach the midline above the diaphragm. It presents as a right paraspinous shadow on the penetrated anterior view.

SURGERY IN FALLOT'S TETRALOGY

Blalock's operation (subclavian/pulmonary artery anastomosis) usually produces an increase in pulmonary vessel size (*Figure 242*). Vessels in both lungs often enlarge, but the change may be evident only on the ipsilateral side. Aneurysmal dilatation of the pulmonary artery is occasionally seen (*Figure 243*).

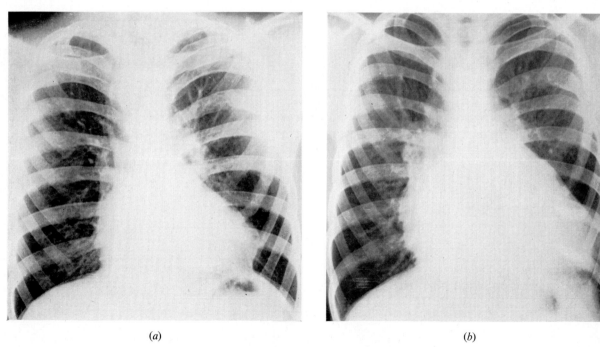

(a)   (b)

Figure 244. Open ventricular septal defect following total correction. (a) Pre-operative. (b) Post-operative showing enlarged heart, dilated right ventricular outflow and plethora

Occasionally the upper lobe vessels are obstructed during the anastomotic procedure and localized upper lobe oligaemia is evident. Rib notching may slowly develop on the side of the anastomosis (*see Figure 146*). Heart size is often unchanged. After the Waterston operation (ascending aorta/pulmonary artery anastomosis—*see Figure 235*), increase in vessel size is usually greater than following the Blalock procedure and is often confined to the side of the shunt because kinking of the proximal part of the pulmonary artery prevents flow into the other lung. Unilateral pulmonary oedema is common, but subsides provided the shunt is not too large. It presumably reflects acute overperfusion of the lung. Pulmonary hypertension is suggested by tortuous segmental vessels and is particularly liable to occur after the Potts operation (descending aorta/pulmonary artery anastomosis). A successful Brock procedure (dilatation of the right ventricular outflow) causes a slight increase in vessel and heart size.

Total correction of Fallot's tetralogy consists of closure of the ventricular septal defect and relief of right ventricular obstruction. The latter is achieved by infundibular resection and pulmonary valvotomy. If obstruction is severe, insertion of a gusset or an aortic homograft may be necessary. After successful operation the most striking change is disappearance of the bay in the middle of the left cardiac border. The concavity may be replaced by a convexity and the pulmonary trunk may become visible. A prominent bulge indicates an aneurysm of the right ventricular outflow (*Figure 244*) and raises the possibility of continuing right ventricular hypertension, persisting ventricular septal defect or important pulmonary regurgitation (Anderson *et al.*, 1965). Calcification is seen in about 80 per cent of stored homografts three to six months after insertion into the right ventricular outflow; it tends to lie in the wall and not in the cusps and does not obstruct the right ventricle (*see Figure 95*). The heart is enlarged for some weeks after correction. Ultimately the overall heart size is often slightly increased, but it may decrease if a surgical shunt was closed at the time of operation, or it may show no real change apart from filling in of the right ventricular outflow. If much enlargement occurs, one of the complications mentioned above should be suspected. In those cases in which no pre-operative surgical shunt was present, hilar and pulmonary vessels usually enlarge after total correction, but obvious plethora will suggest persistence of the ventricular shunt (*Figure 244*).

CHAPTER 20

Differential Diagnosis of Fallot's Tetralogy

Lesions in this group have in common a similar physiological state to Fallot's tetralogy, namely obstruction somewhere in the right heart limiting pulmonary blood flow and causing shunt reversal. They include:

(1) Pulmonary atresia.
(2) Pulmonary stenosis and double outflow right ventricle.
(3) Pulmonary stenosis, ventricular septal defect and corrected transposition.
(4) Pulmonary stenosis and complete transposition.
(5) Pulmonary stenosis and single ventricle.
(6) Two-chambered right ventricle and ventricular septal defect.
(7) Pulmonary stenosis and atrial septal defect or atrio-ventricular defect.
(8) Hypoplastic right ventricle.
(9) Tricuspid atresia (*see* Chapter 23, page 220).

PULMONARY ATRESIA

In pulmonary atresia there is complete obstruction between the ventricular portion of the heart and the pulmonary arteries. The pulmonary valve cusps are rudimentary and fused and the infundibulum is hypoplastic (*Figure 245*). When the ventricular septum is intact, the pulmonary trunk and pulmonary arteries are present and are supplied by a persistent ductus. Right-to-left shunting usually occurs through a patent foramen ovale or atrial septal defect. Greenwold *et al.* (1956) and Cole *et al.* (1968) described two types of ventricle: a normal or large right ventricle associated with tricuspid regurgitation, and a small or minute right ventricle with a competent tricuspid valve. In the latter type the right ventricle generates a high pressure, venous sinusoids may dilate and communicate with the coronary arteries, and a systolic right ventricular/aortic shunt develops (*Figure 246*). Patients present as neonates with severe cyanotic heart disease.

Much more commonly, pulmonary atresia is combined with a right-to-left shunt through a ventricular septal defect. The degree of pulmonary artery development is variable, and the vascular supply to the lungs is derived from a persistent ductus arteriosus or from systemic arteries which vary in size, number, origin and course (Jefferson *et al.*, 1972). When a ductus persists, it fills a full set of pulmonary arteries—usually to both lungs, but sometimes only the ipsilateral pulmonary artery and the pulmonary vessels are present (*Figure 247*). When the pulmonary blood supply is via systemic collaterals, they may be multiple, small and tortuous, with a widespread origin from the aorta and its branches; they connect with the hilar arteries, and central pulmonary arterial development is complete, sometimes with the exception of the pulmonary trunk (*Figure 248*). A different pattern is seen with large systemic arteries. These mostly originate from the descending thoracic aorta; they may be up to 2 cm in diameter and are not more than five in number. They enter the hilum and become continuous with the hilar arteries. The pulmonary trunk and the right and left pulmonary arteries are absent, but the intrapulmonary vessels are present. Stenoses are common at the junction of systemic and hilar vessels (*Figure 249*). If there is no stenosis, the systemic artery from the descending aorta can join directly with the right or left pulmonary artery, which may or may not be connected with its fellow across the midline. The arteries in the lungs are large,

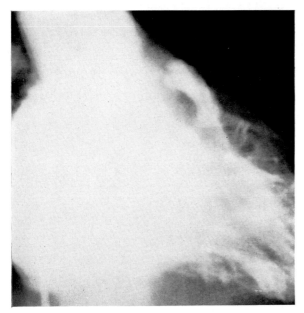

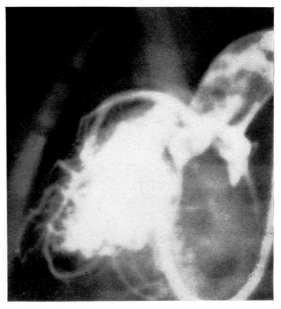

Figure 245. Pulmonary atresia. Right ventricular angiogram, anterior view

Figure 246. Pulmonary atresia with intact septum and competent tricuspid valve. Right ventricular angiogram. Lateral view shows filling of venous sinusoids, coronary arteries and aorta from right ventricle

tortuous and at systemic pressure (*Figure 250*). Combinations of persistent ductus and small and large systemic arteries occur (Jefferson *et al.*, 1972).

Continuous murmurs are frequently present in pulmonary atresia; they were heard in 27 of 32 patients studied by Zutter and Somerville (1971). They are related to flow in the systemic/pulmonary collaterals. A murmur may be heard whether the collaterals are large or small, but may not be audible if the lungs

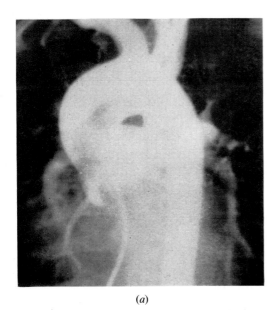

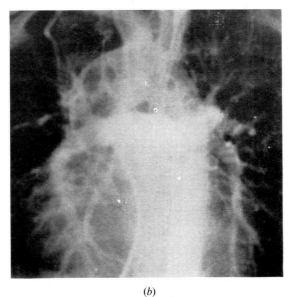

(a)

(b)

Figure 247. Pulmonary atresia. Aortogram. Anterior view. (a) Early phase. (b) Late phase. Ductus filling a complete pulmonary artery tree

are perfused by large vessels at systemic pressure with decreased flow. Sometimes the murmur is absent with multiple very fine vessels. When heard only beneath the left clavicle, it is good evidence of a ductus (Zutter and Somerville, 1971).

Radiology

It may not be possible to differentiate pulmonary atresia from Fallot's tetralogy on the plain film. There are, however, a few features which suggest the former condition. Large hearts are more frequent in pulmonary atresia than in Fallot's tetralogy (*Figure 251*), and the classical *cœur en sabot* is more common (*Figure 252*). Progressive enlargement is seen in the neonatal period in cases with an intact ventricular septum and tricuspid regurgitation. There is a marked concavity in the middle segment of the left

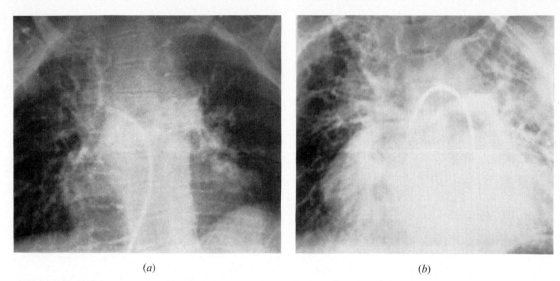

(a)   (b)

Figure 248. Pulmonary atresia. Aortogram. Anterior view. (a) Filling of multiple small collaterals. (b) Later, filling of right and left pulmonary arteries and intrapulmonary vessels

cardiac border, but without any central convexity because of the extreme hypoplasia of the infundibulum (*Figure 252*). The combination of an unusually high and dilated aortic arch makes pulmonary atresia much more likely than Fallot's tetralogy; this is particularly striking with a right arch (*Figure*

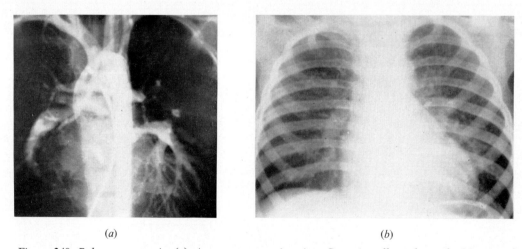

(a)   (b)

Figure 249. Pulmonary atresia. (a) Aortogram, anterior view. Stenotic collateral vessels. No central pulmonary arteries. (b) Plain film. Normal hilar vessels

251). Of 30 fully investigated patients with pulmonary atresia, 8 (25 per cent) had a right arch, 21 had a left arch and one had a double arch (Jefferson *et al.*, 1972). A right arch was most commonly present with large systemic arteries to the lung (6 out of 15 patients, or 40 per cent).

Hilar and pulmonary vessels are small except when large systemic arteries connect directly with the right or left pulmonary arteries or continue into hilar arteries without any stenosis. Large vessels are then seen either locally or generally; in the latter situation, the radiological appearances resemble the Eisenmenger syndrome (*Figure 253*). Uneven pulmonary perfusion due to hilar stenoses and a variable

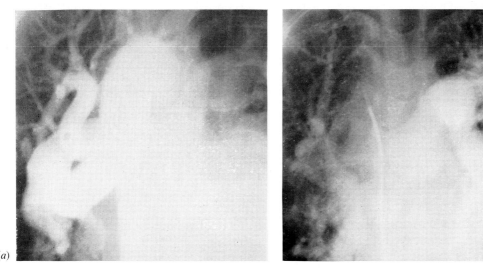

(a)   (b)

Figure 250. Pulmonary atresia. Aortogram. (a) Early phase. (b) Late phase. A large systemic artery from descending aorta continuing into right and then left pulmonary artery

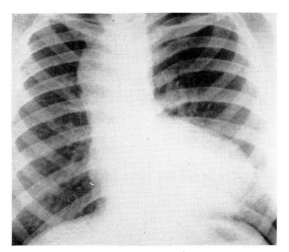

Figure 251. Pulmonary atresia. Large heart with high dilated and right-sided aortic arch

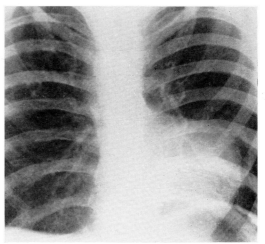

Figure 252. Pulmonary atresia. Cœur en sabot

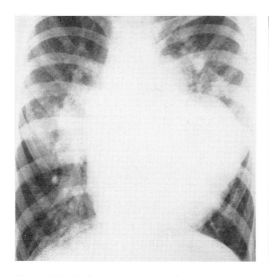

Figure 253. Pulmonary atresia. Severe pulmonary hypertension

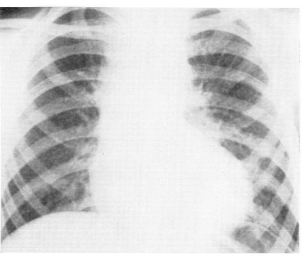

Figure 254. Pulmonary atresia. Uneven pulmonary vessels

185

systemic supply is a valuable differentiating feature from Fallot's tetralogy (*Figures 254* and *256b*). The intrapulmonary vessels show the normal branching pattern, and only rarely is a systemic artery seen in an anomalous position in the lung. The multiple small type of systemic vessels may sometimes be

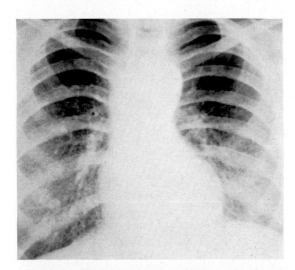

Figure 255 (left). Pulmonary atresia. Reticular pattern in both hilar regions

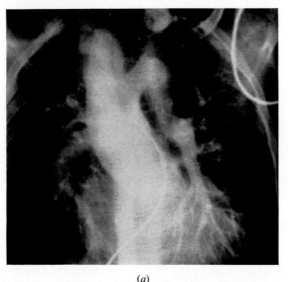

(a)

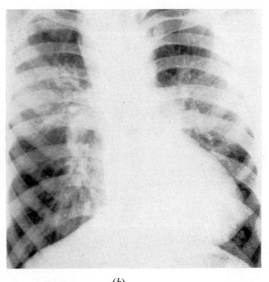

(b)

Figure 256. Pulmonary atresia. (a) Aortogram. Large systemic vessels. No central pulmonary arteries. (b) Plain film. Normal hilar vessels. Uneven pulmonary vascularity

identified as a reticular pattern in the hilum (*Figure 255*). They indicate that the central pulmonary arteries are present and that the case is surgically correctable (*see Figure 248*). Identification of the hilar vessels themselves does not necessarily mean that the right and left pulmonary arteries are present, because the large systemic vessels may continue as the hilar arteries with complete absence of the central pulmonary arteries (*see Figures 249* and *256*). A large systemic artery may sometimes cause an unusual mediastinal bulge. Rarely rib notching is seen when intercostal arteries form part of the collateral supply to the lung (*see* page 105 and *Figure 147*).

PULMONARY STENOSIS AND DOUBLE OUTFLOW RIGHT VENTRICLE

In double outflow right ventricle, both the aorta and the pulmonary trunk arise entirely from the right ventricle. Both outflow tracts lie side by side and, as they contain bulbar muscle, the aortic and pulmonary valve rings lie at about the same height above the right ventricle (*Figures 257* and *258*). As there is discontinuity between the aortic and mitral valve rings, the anomaly should be classed as a transposition. The only outlet from the left ventricle is through a ventricular septal defect, and so a left-to-right shunt occurs through the ventricular septal defect with veno-arterial mixing in the right

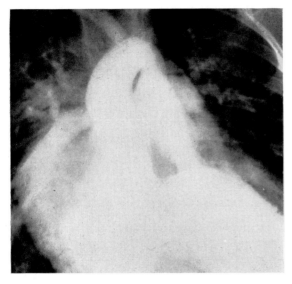

Figure 257. Pulmonary stenosis and double outflow right ventricle. Infundibular stenosis. Right ventricular angiogram, anterior view

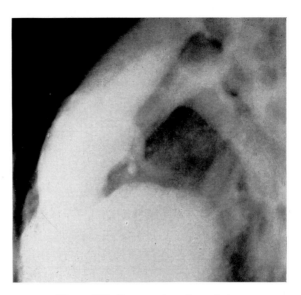

Figure 258. Same patient, lateral view

ventricle. The right ventricular obstruction is infundibular, with or without valve stenosis, and the ventricular septal defect is infracristal (Dayem *et al.*, 1967). Double outflow right ventricle may also occur without pulmonary stenosis (*see* pages 155 and 207).

Radiology

The plain x-ray appearances are indistinguishable from those of Fallot's tetralogy (*Figure 259*).

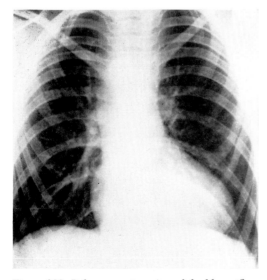

Figure 259. Pulmonary stenosis and double outflow right ventricle resembling Fallot's tetralogy

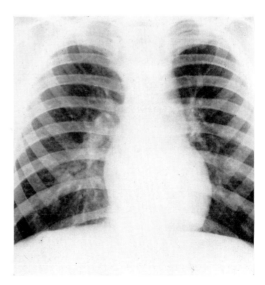

Figure 260. Pulmonary stenosis, corrected transposition and ventricular septal defect. Convex ascending aorta

PULMONARY STENOSIS, VENTRICULAR SEPTAL DEFECT AND CORRECTED TRANSPOSITION

In corrected transposition the ventricles are inverted (right ventricle to the left of the left ventricle) and the great vessels are parallel (*see* page 44 and *Figure 71*). The two abnormalities are physiologically self-correcting, and the circulation is normal unless associated defects are present. Pulmonary stenosis and ventricular septal defect are together the commonest associated lesions, and the haemodynamics are similar to those of Fallot's tetralogy. The stenosis may be at or below valve level (Levy *et al.*, 1963). Malposition of the heart, particularly dextroversion, may be associated.

Radiology

On the anterior view the left cardiac contour is formed below by the right ventricle and above by the ascending aorta. The pulmonary trunk takes no part as it lies centrally and posteriorly. The ascending aorta usually presents as a long straight, concave or convex left upper border leading towards a normally placed aortic knuckle, and in many cases provides the clue to the diagnosis (*Figure 260—see also* page 154). The ascending aorta may turn quite sharply inwards towards the midline to produce a bay so that the appearances resemble those of Fallot's tetralogy (*Figure 261*). The aortic root may be prominent and cause what appears to be a high bulge and a rounded contour to the ventricular border (*Figure 261*). Other features differing from Fallot are a high and sometimes level position of the hilar arteries, a larger right than left pulmonary artery, and wider vessels in the right upper zone than in the left (*Figure 262*).

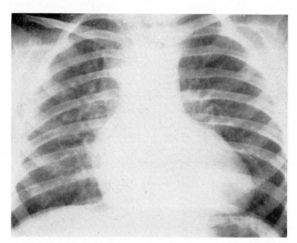

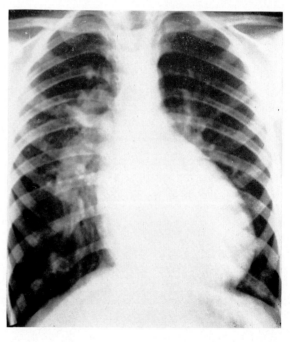

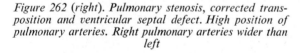

Figure 261 (above). Pulmonary stenosis, corrected transposition and ventricular septal defect. Concave left border like Fallot's tetralogy

Figure 262 (right). Pulmonary stenosis, corrected transposition and ventricular septal defect. High position of pulmonary arteries. Right pulmonary arteries wider than left

PULMONARY STENOSIS AND COMPLETE TRANSPOSITION

When pulmonary stenosis is present with complete transposition (*see* page 44 and *Figure 69*), there is usually a ventricular septal defect as well. Pulmonary blood flow depends on the severity of the pulmonary stenosis and the size of the ventricular septal defect; if these two factors are nicely balanced, the prognosis may be good and some patients will reach adult life. The stenosis may be at or below the pulmonary valve (Shaher *et al.*, 1967).

Radiology

The radiological picture is similar to that of Fallot's tetralogy (*Figure 263*). The heart is not large and does not often show an 'egg on side' appearance as in transposition without pulmonary stenosis.

There may be a concavity on the left cardiac border due to the central position of the pulmonary trunk. Unlike Fallot's tetralogy, however, the ascending aorta and arch may appear small because they lie

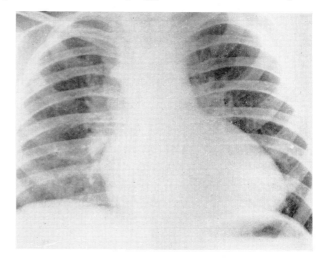

Figure 263. Pulmonary stenosis and complete transposition

centrally in the sagittal plane. The antero-posterior relationship of aorta and pulmonary trunk, together with absence of the thymic shadow, may cause a narrow vascular pedicle. The lungs are usually oligaemic; the right pulmonary artery may be wider than the left as in corrected transposition and pulmonary stenosis.

PULMONARY STENOSIS AND SINGLE VENTRICLE

A single or common ventricle denotes one ventricular chamber into which the tricuspid and mitral valves, or a common atrio-ventricular valve, open. Two types are distinguished by their gross anatomical appearance.

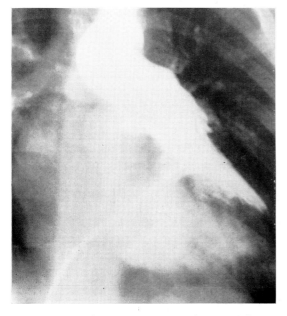

Figure 264. Pulmonary stenosis and single ventricle, with outflow chamber

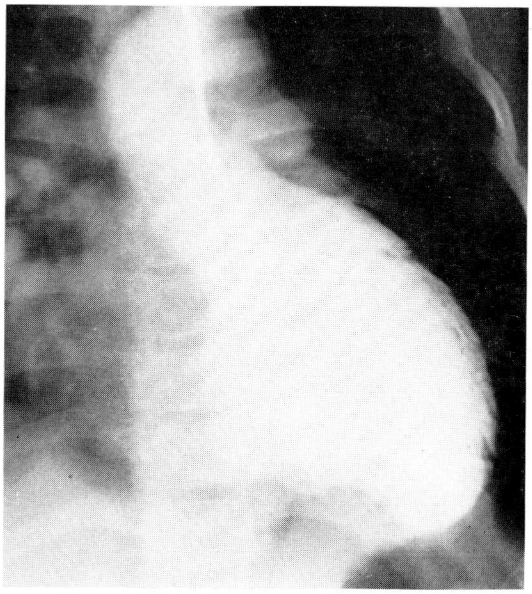

Figure 265. Pulmonary stenosis and single ventricle. No outflow chamber. Ventricular angiogram

Absence of right ventricular inflow (sinus)

The single ventricle represents the anatomical left ventricle, which communicates via the bulboventricular foramen with an outlet chamber representing the right ventricular infundibulum (distal part of bulbus cordis—*Figure 264*). This type comprised 78 per cent of a series of 60 cases reported by Van Praagh *et al.* (1964).

Absence of ventricular septum

The free walls and outflow tracts of both ventricles develop normally and no outflow chamber is present (*Figure 265*). Variants are absence of the left ventricular sinus and absence of both sinuses. This heterogeneous group without an outlet chamber comprised 22 per cent of the 60 cases of Van Praagh *et al.* (1964).

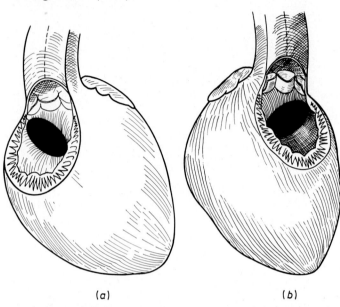

Figure 266. *Single ventricle and transposition with* (a) d-*loop and* (b) l-*loop*

(a)   (b)

Any type of single ventricle may be associated with normally related great vessels or with transposition. If a *d*-loop with *d*-transposition is present, the right ventricular part of the common ventricle lies to the right of and anterior to the left ventricle and is continuous with the anterior aorta. If an *l*-loop is present, the inverted (left-sided) outlet chamber or right ventricular part of the common ventricle is continuous with the anterior aorta on the left (*Figure 266*). Transposition was present in 84 per cent in the series of Van Praagh *et al.* (1964), with an almost equal number of *d*-loops and *l*-loops. The following convenient clinico-pathological classification of single ventricle is suggested.

With outlet chamber (single left ventricle)
  Normally related great vessels⎫
  D-transposition (complete) ⎬ Plus or minus pulmonary stenosis
  L-transposition (corrected) ⎭

With no outlet chamber (absent ventricular septum)
  Normally related great vessels⎫
  D-transposition (complete) ⎬ Plus or minus pulmonary stenosis
  L-transposition (corrected) ⎭

The terms *d*-transposition and *l*-transposition should be used in preference to complete and corrected transposition as the latter are patently inappropriate in single ventricle. Pulmonary stenosis (or atresia) occurs in approximately 50 per cent of all cases (Fontana and Edwards, 1962; Elliott *et al.*, 1964). With normally related great vessels, obstruction to pulmonary blood flow may be caused by the outlet chamber (small bulbo-ventricular foramen) or by valve stenosis. With transposition and an outlet chamber, a small bulbo-ventricular foramen may result in aortic outflow obstruction.

Radiology

The appearances depend on the presence or absence of transposition. With normally related great vessels they resemble Fallot's tetralogy. Single ventricle with absent right ventricular sinus may be suggested by a notch on the left heart border between the right ventricular outflow chamber and the body of the left ventricle (Hallermann *et al.*, 1966). With transposed great vessels, the radiological features are similar to those of ordinary complete or corrected transposition.

TWO-CHAMBERED RIGHT VENTRICLE AND VENTRICULAR SEPTAL DEFECT

The inflow portion of the right ventricle may be obstructed by aberrant muscle bands dividing the chamber into two portions. The narrowing is in the region of the moderator band and is more proximal than that in Fallot's tetralogy. The infundibulum is normal (*Figure 267*). Ventricular septal defect is the commonest associated abnormality. If it lies distal to the right ventricular obstruction, the features are those of an ordinary ventricular septal defect; if the defect is in the proximal high pressure chamber, a right-to-left shunt occurs and haemodynamically the condition is indistinguishable from Fallot's tetralogy (Gale *et al.*, 1969; Barnes *et al.*, 1971; Perloff *et al.*, 1965).

Radiology

In the cyanotic type, there is no bay in the middle of the left cardiac border as the infundibulum is not hypoplastic (*Figure 268*). The heart is normal or only slightly enlarged, and the pulmonary trunk and hilar and pulmonary vessels tend to be small as in Fallot's tetralogy. The acyanotic type is indistinguishable from a ventricular septal defect.

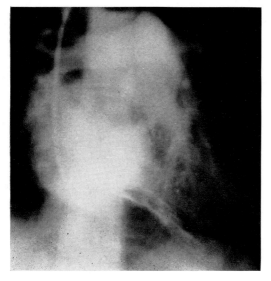

Figure 267. *Two-chambered right ventricle. Right ventricular angiogram*

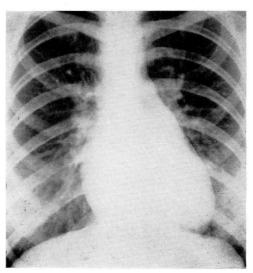

Figure 268. *Two-chambered right ventricle*

PULMONARY STENOSIS AND ATRIAL SEPTAL DEFECT OR ATRIO-VENTRICULAR DEFECT

In severe pulmonary stenosis, the pressure in the right atrium exceeds that in the left and a right-to-left shunt may then occur across the atrial septum. This may be through a patent foramen ovale, a fossa ovalis defect or an atrio-ventricular defect. Cyanosis may be present from birth or appear later, commonly in adolescence. With an atrial shunt the stenosis is at valve level, but with an atrio-ventricular defect the obstruction may be valvar or infundibular. With atrio-ventricular canal, the shunt is at ventricular as well as atrial level.

Radiology

Patients present radiologically as cases of pulmonary stenosis and not of atrial septal defect. The main difference from pulmonary valve stenosis with intact atrial septum is that the pulmonary vessels are

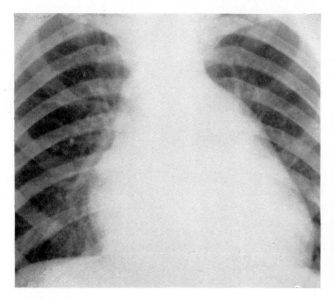

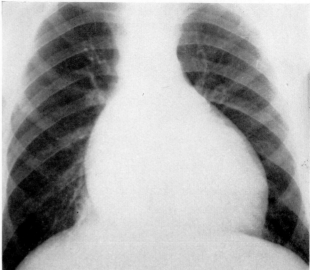

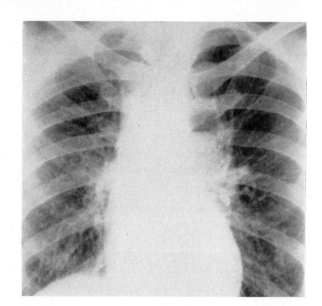

Figure 269 (above). Pulmonary stenosis and atrial septal defect showing oligaemia

Figure 270 (above right). Pulmonary stenosis and atrial septal defect. Congestive failure. Large heart with right atrial and right ventricular dilatation and extreme oligaemia

Figure 271 (right). Pulmonary stenosis and complete canal. Obstruction at infundibular and valve levels. Post-stenotic dilatation of left pulmonary artery. Bay in left heart like Fallot's tetralogy

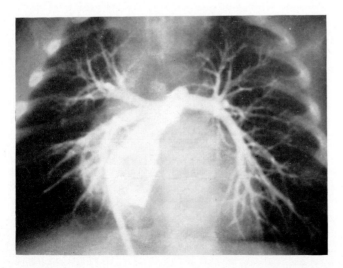

Figure 272. Hypoplastic right ventricle. Right ventricular angiogram. Small ventricular cavity. No outflow obstruction

consistently smaller than normal (*Figure 269*). The heart tends to be a little larger than in pure pulmonary stenosis, probably reflecting the severity of the right ventricular and right atrial hypertension associated with reversed atrial shunt. Congestive cardiac failure causes cardiac enlargement, which may reach extreme limits and be mistaken for pericardial effusion or Ebstein's anomaly. Whatever the size of the heart, contour changes usually indicate right ventricular and right atrial enlargement (*Figure 270*). The pulmonary trunk is dilated in virtually all cases, and the dilatation extends into its left branch in about half.

Pulmonary stenosis with complete canal may resemble Fallot's tetralogy if the obstruction is at infundibular level and pulmonary stenosis if it is at valve level (*Figure 271*).

HYPOPLASTIC RIGHT VENTRICLE

In this condition there is isolated hypoplasia of the right ventricle without obstruction at the tricuspid or pulmonary valves (*Figure 272*). The basic defect is resistance to inflow by the small right ventricle and a right-to-left shunt across the atrial septum when the right atrial pressure exceeds the left. The anomaly tends to be familial (Okin *et al.*, 1969).

Radiologically there is usually only slight cardiac enlargement because the right ventricle is small. The pulmonary trunk is small and the lungs show oligaemia.

CHAPTER 21

The Eisenmenger Syndrome

INTRODUCTION

In 1897 Eisenmenger described the case of a man aged 32 years with a history of cyanosis since infancy. He developed heart failure and died following a massive haemoptysis. Necropsy revealed a large defect in the membranous ventricular septum, right ventricular hypertrophy and normal semilunar valves. The lungs showed extensive infarction. Eisenmenger's interpretation was partly correct. He concluded that pulmonary hypertension was present, but thought it was terminal due to pulmonary arterial thrombosis. Unlike many others later, he felt that the overriding aorta was unimportant and suggested that the cyanosis was peripheral due to a poor systemic circulation. The combination of cyanosis and ventricular septal defect has since been called the Eisenmenger complex, but it is now known that severe pulmonary hypertension is always present and is responsible for the reversed shunt, so producing central cyanosis. Wood (1958) put the disease on a firm physiological basis and suggested that the term Eisenmenger syndrome should be used to describe all cases of pulmonary hypertension with reversed shunt, irrespective of the site of the defect. He pointed out that the bedside diagnosis of the essential physiological situation was usually easy but localization of the shunt level could be difficult, although Sutton *et al.* (1968) have subsequently shown that auscultation may provide a useful clue from the behaviour of the second heart sound. Important and often diagnostic clues can also be obtained from radiology (Rees and Jefferson, 1967).

All systemic/pulmonary communications may be complicated by a right-to-left shunt and cyanosis due to extreme pulmonary hypertension. However, in the more complex lesions, veno-arterial mixing is due to many factors, of which pulmonary hypertension is but one, and these are considered separately in Chapter 22. In the present section the Eisenmenger syndrome will be discussed in relation to:

(1) Atrial septal defect.
(2) Ventricular septal defect.
(3) Atrio-ventricular canal.
(4) Double outflow right ventricle.
(5) Ductus arteriosus.
(6) Aorto-pulmonary septal defect.

The pulmonary vascular resistance is very high. With ventricular and aorto-pulmonary shunts it equals the systemic resistance, but with atrial shunts it may not be identical. By definition there is a right-to-left shunt, but in practice the shunt is nearly always bidirectional. The effect of the altered pressure and flow on the heart is variable, but a pressure load on the right ventricle is common to all cases.

There appears to be general agreement that the natural history of shunts at atrial level complicated by pulmonary hypertension is different from that of shunts at other levels (Wood, 1958). In atrial septal defect there is very little shunting at birth, as the ventricular compliances and filling resistances are equal and this results in equal atrial pressures. Normal involution occurs with reduction in right ventricular thickness; at the same time there is fragmentation of elastic tissue with muscle loss in the pulmonary artery media, indicating a transition from the foetal to the adult type of pulmonary artery. A left-to-right shunt is established in early childhood and in the majority of patients the pulmonary vascular bed remains dilated throughout adult life. Pulmonary hypertension is uncommon and is rare before the third decade. The vasoconstrictive and occlusive changes initially involve the small arteries, but gradually move centrally. The large arteries dilate progressively and the extreme proximal dilatation contrasts

194

with the distal narrowing, resulting in an abrupt point of change in vessel calibre. The whole process is progressive over many years, and clinical cyanosis does not appear until the vessel changes are far advanced.

With a large ventricular septal defect, atrio-ventricular canal, ductus arteriosus or aorto-pulmonary septal defect, the slight drop in right ventricular pressure which occurs after birth results in an immediate left-to-right shunt. If the pulmonary vascular resistance fails to drop to normal, the pulmonary artery pressure remains high and a vicious circle of hypertension and vascular narrowing is established. The pulmonary blood flow is initially increased, but progressively falls. Shunt reversal with clinical cyanosis is often present in childhood and occasionally in infancy, rarely appearing after the third decade. Histologically the large pulmonary arteries retain their foetal structure with persistence of orderly elastic tissue and smooth muscle in the media.

RADIOLOGY

In secundum atrial septal defect the heart is enlarged in 80 per cent and grossly enlarged in 25 per cent; this contrasts with ventricular and aorto-pulmonary shunts, in which the heart is of normal size in 50 per cent of cases and gross cardiac enlargement is rare. In all groups, older patients tend to have larger hearts.

In atrial septal defect, displacement of the heart to the left is very common; however, this may some-times be accounted for by scoliosis, which occurs more frequently than with other lesions. Left atrial enlargement is rare with atrial septal defect but is common with ventricular and aorto-pulmonary shunts, particularly in childhood.

The aortic knuckle is small or invisible in atrial septal defect, normal or slightly small in ventricular septal defect, and enlarged in ductus arteriosus. The shape of the knuckle and its relationship to the pulmonary trunk are important in the diagnosis of ductus arteriosus. The most common sign is filling in of the angle between the aortic knuckle and the pulmonary trunk; this is most obvious in the presence of considerable enlargement of both vessels, but is also apparent without great enlargement of either. The arc formed by the knuckle may be elongated and the descending aorta just distal to the ductus may show a distinct bulge to the left (the infundibulum), best seen on the penetrated film (*see Figures 218–222*). Calcification in the ductus occurs in about 25 per cent (*see Figure 223*).

Each type of lesion appears to have a typical vessel pattern in the lungs, and in the majority of cases a diagnosis can be made on this alone (*Figures 273–275*). The differences between the groups are well illustrated by the degree of arterial enlargement at each level in the lung, graded out of three and averaged in the groups as a whole (Table 9). The peripheral arteries are not included as they are always the most difficult to assess; most patients show a reduction in size and number, most obvious in atrial shunts and least so with ventricular shunts.

TABLE 9

Pulmonary Arterial Patterns (Rees and Jefferson, 1967)

	A.S.D. (26 cases)	V.S.D. (30 cases)	Ductus (25 cases)
Pulmonary trunk	+2·3	+1·0	+2·2
Lobar arteries	+2·2	+0·9	+0·8
Proximal segmental arteries	+1·4	+0·8	+0·6
Distal segmental arteries	+0·2	+0·4	0

In atrial septal defect, the pulmonary trunk and lobar arteries are always moderately or grossly enlarged and may contain calcified atheromatous plaques (*see Figures 104 and 115*). Reduction in size occurs at proximal, mid or distal segmental artery level and is usually abrupt (*Figure 273*). With ventri-cular shunts, enlargement of the pulmonary trunk is seldom more than slight and there is little or no abrupt reduction in size of the segmental arteries, these vessels appearing either slightly enlarged or normal. The striking difference from atrial septal defect is that the central arteries are never very big and in 40 per cent, mostly children, the whole radiograph can be passed as normal or showing only minor vessel dilatation (*Figure 274*). This is particularly so with atrio-ventricular canal, in which it may be impossible to differentiate shunt reversal due to pulmonary hypertension or pulmonary stenosis.

The pattern in some patients with a ductus arteriosus closely resembles ventricular septal defect, but the majority have moderate or gross enlargement of the pulmonary trunk and this, together with

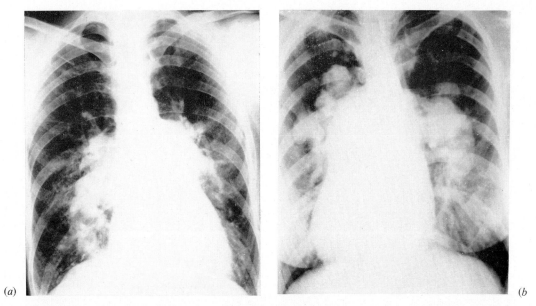

(a)   (b)

Figure 273. Typical Eisenmenger atrial septal defect. (a) Very large pulmonary trunk and central vessels, small aorta. (b) Enormous hilar pulmonary arteries (dextrocardia)

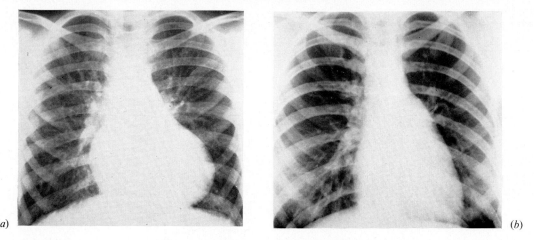

(a)   (b)

Figure 274. Typical Eisenmenger ventricular septal defect. (a) Child. Pulmonary vessels virtually normal. (b) Adolescent. Dilatation of pulmonary trunk only

slightly enlarged or normal lobar and segmental arteries, seems to represent the typical pattern (*Figure 275*). Calcified atheroma is occasionally seen in ductus, but is rare with ventricular septal defect. Aorto-pulmonary septal defects are indistinguishable from ventricular shunts.

Study of serial radiographs shows that there is usually a reduction in heart size before or with the appearance of cyanosis. With atrial shunts there is a tendency for the proximal arteries to enlarge slightly and for the peripheral vessels to become smaller (*Figure 276*), but it may not always be possible in the individual case to differentiate radiologically moderate pulmonary hypertension without cyanosis from severe pulmonary hypertension with cyanosis. With other shunts the onset of the Eisenmenger reaction is nearly always accompanied by an increase in the size of the pulmonary trunk, but the other arteries, including those in the hilum, tend to become smaller (*Figures 277* and *278*).

Anterior bowing of the sternum is commonly seen in ventricular and aorto-pulmonary shunts, implying that hyperkinetic pulmonary hypertension preceded the Eisenmenger situation (Davies, 1959; Davies *et al.*, 1962) (*see Figure 112*). Correlation with the vessel pattern shows that the central arteries are significantly larger in patients with sternal bowing, which suggests that those without bowing have

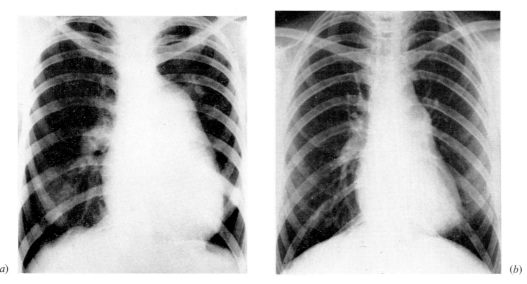

(a)   (b)

Figure 275. Eisenmenger ductus arteriosus. (a) Typical dilatation of pulmonary trunk disproportionate to hilar pulmonary arteries. (b) Atypical with proportionate dilatation of pulmonary trunk and hilar arteries. Size and shape of aortic knuckle would suggest the diagnosis

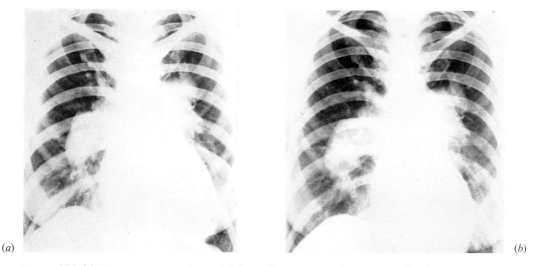

(a)   (b)

Figure 276. (a) Eisenmenger atrial septal defect. (b) Four years later. Central pulmonary arteries larger, heart smaller

never had a high pulmonary flow and the Eisenmenger situation has been present from early infancy (Rees, 1968).

The differences in vessel patterns are probably related to the different natural history of atrial from other shunts. The late onset of pulmonary hypertension in atrial septal defect means that the elastic arteries are fully involuted. They are more distensible than foetal type pulmonary arteries and dilate from a long-standing left-to-right shunt: an increase in pressure serves to produce more dilatation, which often becomes gross.

This must be contrasted with shunts at ventricular or aorto-pulmonary levels, which show modest or even absent proximal vessel dilatation. They differ from atrial shunts in the following ways.

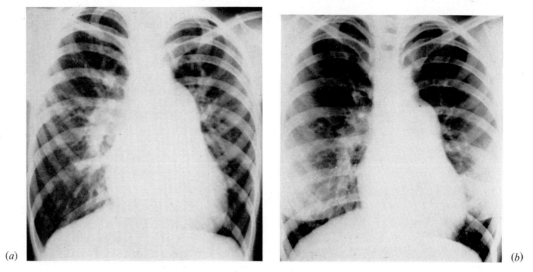

Figure 277. (a) Ventricular septal defect and hyperkinetic pulmonary hypertension. (b) Three years later. Cyanosed. Heart and pulmonary vessels smaller

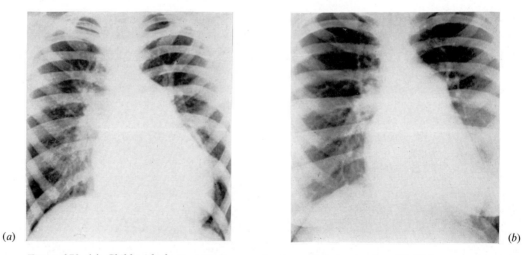

Figure 278. (a) Child with ductus arteriosus and pulmonary hypertension. (b) Eight years later. Differential cyanosis. Hilar vessels and heart smaller

(1) Retention of the foetal structure in the arteries so that they are thicker-walled and less distensible than normal (Harris et al., 1965).

(2) A pulmonary blood flow which may never have been high, suggested by the absence of sternal bowing.

Those patients in whom the pulmonary vascular resistance fails to show a significant drop after birth have little or no increase in pulmonary blood flow and radiologically normal or minimally enlarged proximal pulmonary arteries (with no sternal bowing). More commonly the pulmonary vascular resistance drops sufficiently for a left-to-right shunt to operate for months or years. These patients show partial involution of pulmonary artery media and radiologically up to moderate but never gross dilatation of proximal pulmonary arteries (often with some sternal bowing).

Most patients with a ductus arteriosus present a major radiological difference from all other shunts in the disproportionate dilatation of the pulmonary trunk compared with the pulmonary arteries. Contributory factors probably include transmission of the aortic diastolic pressure and retrograde diastolic flow into the pulmonary trunk, often with ensuing pulmonary regurgitation, which itself causes further dilatation (Rees, 1968).

The point at which pulmonary hypertension becomes irreversible is of great practical importance in deciding whether or not to recommend surgical treatment. It is the authors' impression that radiology lags behind the haemodynamic changes. It is therefore easier to diagnose irreversibility than to predict when it is about to occur. With atrial shunts, it is largely age which dictates the interpretation of the changes, since obvious central vessel dilatation in a patient aged under 30 years is more likely to herald the Eisenmenger reaction than in a patient over this age. With hyperkinetic pulmonary hypertension in other shunts, the earliest sign of impending irreversibility—and it may not always be early—is obvious tapering of the segmental vessels. By the time the hilar arteries or the heart begin to get smaller, it is too late.

CHAPTER 22

Veno-arterial Mixing Lesions

Included under this heading are lesions in which cyanosis is due to mixing of venous and arterial blood for reasons other than obstruction in the right heart or extreme pulmonary hypertension and a reversed shunt. If veno-arterial mixing occurs proximal to the lungs, cyanosis will be accompanied by radiological evidence of increased flow and usually increased pressure. Mixing in the lungs is caused by arteriovenous fistulae, which are usually visible but rarely cause cardiac enlargement. If mixing occurs distal to the lungs, cyanosis will be present with normal lungs and heart unless there is some other congenital cardiovascular anomaly. The lesions to be considered are as follows.

Mixing proximal to the lungs
    (1) Complete transposition.
    (2) Total anomalous pulmonary venous drainage.
    (3) Single atrium.
    (4) Single ventricle.
    (5) Double outflow right ventricle without pulmonary stenosis.
    (6) Truncus arteriosus.

Mixing in the lungs
    (7) Pulmonary arteriovenous fistula.

Mixing distal to the lungs
    (8) Superior or inferior vena cava draining into left atrium.

MIXING PROXIMAL TO THE LUNGS

COMPLETE TRANSPOSITION

The anatomical and embryological background to transposition is discussed in Chapter 5 (*see* page 41). The following discussion applies only to viscero-atrial situs solitus (normal position of viscera and atria) with *d*-transposition (*see Figures 68* and *69*). The essential features are as follows.

(1) All four cardiac chambers are normal in position (non-inversion of the ventricles; atrioventricular concordance; viscero-atrial concordance).

(2) The great vessels are parallel; the aorta arises from the right ventricle and the pulmonary artery from the left ventricle.

(3) The aortic valve lies anterior to and often just to the right of the pulmonary valve, and is higher in position. There is discontinuity between the aortic and mitral valve rings due to the presence of bulbar muscle beneath the aortic valve.

(4) The ascending aorta, the arch and the descending aorta all lie approximately in the sagittal plane. The pulmonary trunk lies posterior to and often just to the left of the ascending aorta and underneath the aortic arch.

(5) There is a variable incidence of associated abnormalities including patent foramen ovale, atrial septal defect, ventricular septal defect, persistent ductus and pulmonary stenosis. Coarctation is particularly lethal. More complicated congenital heart disease is common including tricuspid atresia, single ventricle and single atrium.

The foetus with complete transposition develops normally because oxygenated blood from the placenta reaches the systemic circulation by two pathways: (1) right atrium, right ventricle, ascending aorta, upper part of body; (2) right atrium, left atrium, left ventricle, pulmonary trunk, ductus, descending aorta, lower part of body.

After birth the systemic circulation loses its oxygenated blood from the placenta because oxygenation of blood is transferred to the lungs and useless recirculation of saturated blood occurs through the pulmonary circuit. No oxygenated blood reaches the ascending aorta unless there is shunting from the pulmonary into the systemic circulation through a central communication. If there is no mixing between the two circulations, they remain independent and death occurs immediately after birth. Conversely, the greater the mixing between the two circuits, the less the cyanosis. In the majority of cases, mixing is

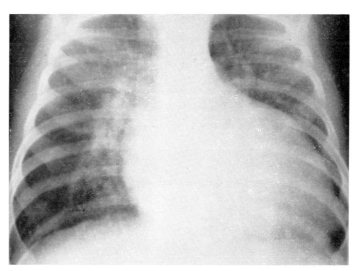

Figure 279. Complete transposition. Narrow vascular pedicle

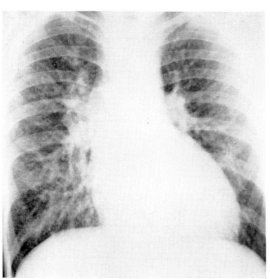

Figure 280. Complete transposition. Ascending aorta to the right

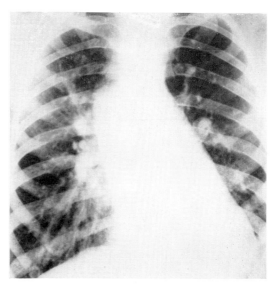

Figure 281. Complete transposition. Pulmonary hypertension. Dilated pulmonary trunk (presenting to the right) and proximal pulmonary arteries

inadequate and 90 per cent of patients die from anoxia or congestive cardiac failure in the first year of life (Grainger, 1970) unless palliative surgery is performed. In surviving patients, especially those with a ventricular septal defect, pulmonary vascular disease is usually established by the age of one year. The best tolerated situation is a large atrial septal defect with bidirectional shunt and little or no pulmonary hypertension; moderate pulmonary stenosis is also favourable as it protects the lungs from excessive pressure and flow, and in either of these situations the patient may reach adult life.

Radiology

Typically the heart is normal in size at birth but begins to enlarge during the first two weeks of life, reaching a maximum at 2–3 months. In the majority of cases, all four chambers of the heart enlarge to produce a characteristic shape—the 'egg-on-side' appearance. The blunt end of the egg is represented by the dilated right atrium and the sharp end by the apex, the axis of the heart being oblique (*Figure 279*). The left border of the heart is usually long and convex. A prominent bulge may be seen in its upper part, due to a dilated atrial appendix. When complete transposition is associated with left juxtaposition of the atrial appendices, the bulge is even greater and the cardiac configuration is characteristic. The apex is usually above the diaphragm and pointed, suggesting right ventricular enlargement. As the pulmonary trunk lies centrally within the heart, it is invisible unless extremely dilated. The pulmonary artery segment is replaced by the continuation of the left heart border upwards to the vascular pedicle. This contour is slightly convex or concave and may reach a high position level with the aortic knuckle in big hearts.

If the aorta lies in the sagittal plane with the pulmonary trunk immediately behind the ascending part, the vascular pedicle is narrow; hypoplasia of the thymus may contribute to this appearance (*Figure 279*). The pedicle is broader in the left anterior oblique and in the lateral projection. More often the ascending aorta lies slightly to the right of the pulmonary trunk, so that the vascular pedicle will appear normal (*Figure 280*). The aortic arch is nearly always left-sided. The tracheal bifurcation may lie in an abnormally posterior position due to interposition of the aorta and the pulmonary trunk between the sternum and the trachea.

Because of the central position of the pulmonary trunk, the right and left pulmonary arteries may not be seen in the hila. This causes a characteristic discrepancy between unimpressive hilar vessels and prominent intrapulmonary vessels (Grainger, 1970). Pulmonary plethora is difficult to assess in the first two weeks of life, but becomes definite after that. It appears to be due to an increase in the number of visible vessels as well as in their size. Marked plethora is seen with a large ventricular septal defect, but the pulmonary vascular pattern may change with elevation of pulmonary vascular resistance and show proximal vessel dilatation and peripheral vessel narrowing (*Figure 281*). Vessels may appear larger in the right upper zone, as is sometimes seen in corrected transposition and uncomplicated shunts. The pulmonary trunk may become very large and bulge to the right or left of the midline (*Figure 281*). A large pulmonary trunk may also be due to post-stenotic dilatation with pulmonary stenosis; the vessels in the lungs may then be large, normal or small, depending on the degree of obstruction. Complete transposition and pulmonary stenosis is discussed further on page 188.

Total Anomalous Pulmonary Venous Drainage

In total anomalous pulmonary venous drainage, all the pulmonary veins connect anomalously to the right atrium or one of its tributaries. Both systemic and pulmonary venous blood returns to the right atrium, which acts as a common mixing chamber. A patent foramen ovale or atrial septal defect is essential to life. The mixed venous blood passes to the lungs in the normal way through the tricuspid valve into the right ventricle and also into the systemic circulation across the atrial septum through the left heart. The oxygen saturation is therefore identical in all four chambers as well as in the systemic and pulmonary arteries. As all the pulmonary venous blood enters the right atrium and some of it recirculates in the lungs, there is increased pulmonary flow. The size of the atrial septal defect and the relative resistances of the pulmonary and systemic circulations determine the pulmonary flow, which is usually 3–5 times the systemic. Pulmonary arterial hypertension is often initially mild, but may be high in those patients reaching late childhood and beyond. In obstructed total anomalous pulmonary venous drainage there is pulmonary venous hypertension, pulmonary oedema and increased pulmonary vascular resistance. As mixed venous and arterial blood crosses the atrial septum to enter the systemic circulation, moderate cyanosis is present.

Radiology

It is logical from the radiological (not the embryological) point of view to classify total anomalous pulmonary venous drainage into four types as certain common radiological features may be found in each.

Supracardiac (Figure 282)

Connection to left superior vena cava, right superior vena cava or azygos vein. The cardiovascular shadow may have a characteristic shape.

Cardiac

Connection to right atrium or coronary sinus. There are no characteristic features in the heart or lungs.

Infracardiac (Figure 283)

Connection to portal vein, ductus venosus, inferior vena cava or hepatic vein. The pulmonary veins are obstructed, causing pulmonary oedema.

Mixed

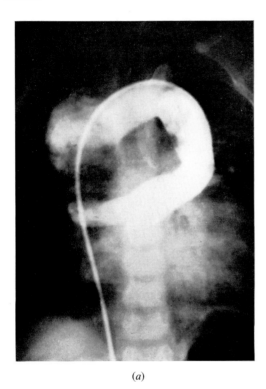

(a)

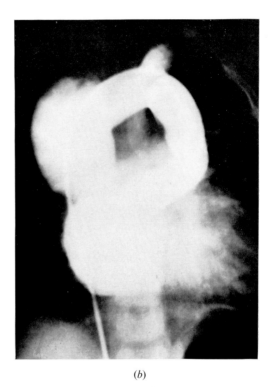

(b)

Figure 282 (above). Total anomalous pulmonary venous drainage. Angiograms, supracardiac type. (a) Injection into common pulmonary vein. Early phase. (b) Late phase. Filling of both superior venae cavae and right atrium

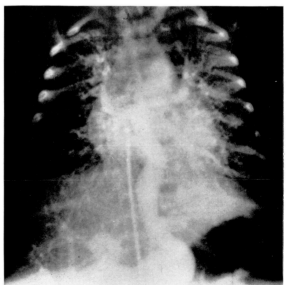

Figure 283 (right). Total anomalous pulmonary venous drainage. Angiogram. Pulmonary venous phase after right atrial injection showing common pulmonary vein draining into portal vein

All types show the combination of cyanosis and plethora. Two-thirds of patients have total anomalous pulmonary venous drainage as an isolated lesion, and one-third have another major anomaly. Total anomalous pulmonary venous drainage is one of the anomalies that may be present in asplenia.

The commonest type of total anomalous pulmonary venous drainage is connection of the pulmonary veins to the left superior vena cava. All the veins join a common chamber, situated behind but unconnected with the left atrium. A vertical vein, usually referred to as the left superior vena cava, arises from the left side of the confluence and joins the left innominate vein, from whence blood flows into the right superior vena cava and right atrium (*see Figure 282*). There is usually no obstruction, but occasionally the vertical vein is stenosed or compressed between the pulmonary artery and bronchus in the left hilum (normally it courses in front of both structures). The characteristic radiological appearance is caused by dilatation of both superior venae cavae producing the 'figure of eight', 'cottage loaf' or 'snowman'

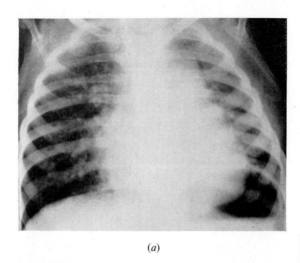

(*a*)

Figure 284. Total anomalous pulmonary venous drainage, supracardiac type. (a) Neonate. Dilated left superior vena cava. (b) Adult. Both venae cavae dilated

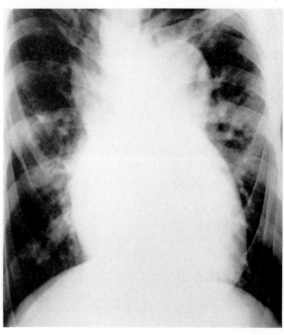

(*b*)

shape, but this may not be evident during the first few months of life (Owen, 1962; Bonham Carter *et al.*, 1969) (*Figure 284*). The right superior vena cava may appear larger than the left as it carries the systemic venous return from the head and arms in addition to all the pulmonary venous blood. The heart is enlarged due to dilatation of the right atrium and right ventricle. The pulmonary trunk is dilated but hidden by the left superior vena cava. There is pulmonary plethora and the appearances may suggest hyperkinetic pulmonary hypertension. In the rare obstructed cases the lungs show pulmonary oedema. Much less frequently the confluence of pulmonary veins joins the right superior vena cava or the azygos vein, and these structures are then dilated.

In the cardiac type of total anomalous pulmonary venous drainage, the pulmonary veins join the right atrium or coronary sinus. As the venous connections are invisible radiologically, the plain radiograph merely shows non-specific enlargement of the right heart and pulmonary trunk with evidence of increased pulmonary flow and/or pulmonary hypertension.

In the infracardiac type, the pulmonary veins join to form a single long vessel which descends behind the heart to penetrate the diaphragm through the oesophageal hiatus (*see Figure 283*). Most commonly it joins the portal vein at the junction of the splenic and superior mesenteric veins. Less often it enters the ductus venosus, a hepatic vein or even the inferior vena cava. Pulmonary venous obstruction is the rule where the drainage is below the diaphragm except when connection is to the inferior vena cava. The main cause is an increased resistance to flow across the hepatic sinusoids, but the width and length of the descending vein, narrowing within the oesophageal hiatus and stricture formation may contribute. The pulmonary venous pressure is high and the pulmonary arterial pressure is usually at systemic level.

Patients present with cyanosis and congestive failure at or soon after birth. The heart is normal or only slightly enlarged. The lungs show generalized mottling, most marked in the hilar areas, indicative of pulmonary oedema (*Figure 285*). Septal lines are not often identified, and upper zone vessel dilatation is not evident. The radiological appearances may suggest diffuse lung disease rather than a congenital heart anomaly and the diagnosis may be missed.

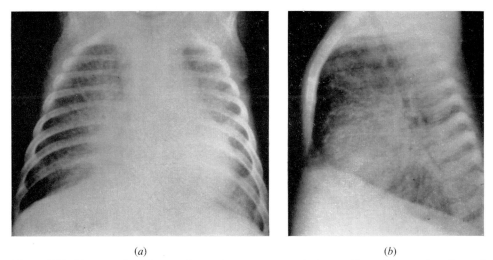

(a)   (b)

Figure 285. Obstructed total anomalous pulmonary venous drainage. Normal heart size. Generalized mottling due to pulmonary oedema

SINGLE ATRIUM

In single or common atrium, the atrial septum is absent and the atrio-ventricular valves are nearly always abnormal (*Figure 286*). When the inferior border of the defect is formed by the atrio-ventricular valves, the anterior cusp of the mitral valve is cleft and the condition is comparable to a large ostium primum defect, but with the atria forming a common mixing chamber. When the inferior border of the defect is formed by the ventricular septum, both atrio-ventricular valves are deformed and the condition

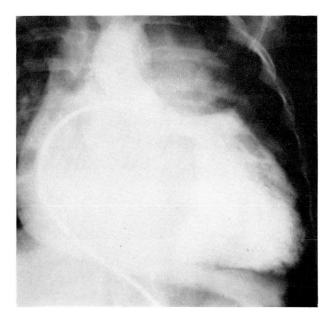

Figure 286. Single atrium. Left ventricular angiogram. Deformity of left ventricular outflow indicating an atrio-ventricular defect (ostium primum—see Figure 195). Single atrial cavity

is comparable to a complete canal, but with a common atrio-ventricular mixing chamber. Patients with a single atrium, a competent mitral valve and no ventricular component to the defect have little or no

205

incapacity or cyanosis and show increased pulmonary flow with normal pulmonary pressures. Patients with atrio-ventricular regurgitation and a functioning ventricular septal defect behave like those with a complete canal. They present in early life with congestive failure and, if they survive, develop the Eisenmenger reaction. A left superior vena cava is present in 60–70 per cent of cases of single atrium (Somerville, 1972) and may connect with the coronary sinus or occasionally with the left atrium just medial to its appendix. A single atrium is present in about 60 per cent of patients with the Ellis–Van Creveld syndrome (*see* page 118).

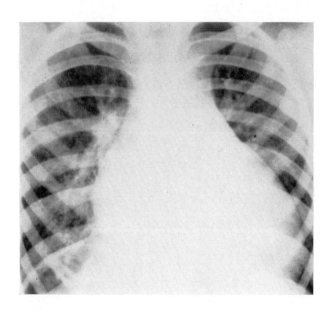

Figure 287. Single atrium showing large heart due to dilatation of single atrium and right ventricle

Radiology

The radiological appearances resemble those of secundum atrial septal defect when the mitral valve is competent and the ventricular septum intact. Munoz-Armas *et al.* (1968) reported four cases in which the atrio-ventricular valves were normal: the radiological appearances were those of a large atrial septal defect except that the right atrium was only mildly enlarged. Their explanation was that the single atrium shares the atrial blood, whereas in atrial septal defect active shunting occurs into the distensible right atrium, which contains a greater proportion of atrial blood than the left atrium. With important mitral and tricuspid regurgitation, the heart may be very large due to dilatation of the common atrium and right ventricle (*Figure 287*). The right atrial border is prominent; the dilated pulmonary trunk and marked plethora reflect the greatly increased pulmonary flow. Pulmonary hypertension due to increased pulmonary vascular resistance, especially likely in the presence of a ventricular septal defect, is indicated by proximal vessel enlargement. A left superior vena cava may be seen as a vertical shadow of low density in the left upper mediastinum.

SINGLE VENTRICLE

The anatomical types of single ventricle are discussed on page 189 under the heading of pulmonary stenosis and single ventricle. About 50 per cent of patients have an unobstructed outflow to the lungs. A variable amount of veno-arterial mixing occurs in the common ventricular chamber, and ejection into the lungs takes place at systemic pressure. When the great vessels are normally related, streaming is such that most of the venous blood flows into the pulmonary artery and the arterial blood into the aorta. Cyanosis may be mild or even absent, and patients present as cases of ventricular septal defect with high flow and pressure; eventually the Eisenmenger reaction develops with obvious cyanosis. Similar flow pathways are seen in patients with *l*-transposition, and the clinical features are similar. However, when *d*-transposition is present, venous blood from the right atrium shows preferential flow into the aorta and cyanosis is usual.

Radiology

With normally related great vessels the radiological features are similar to those of ventricular septal defect with high flow and high pressure or to a ventricular septal defect with reversed shunt (Eisenmenger syndrome). With *d*-transposition the picture resembles ordinary complete transposition. With an *l*-loop the features may be indistinguishable from corrected transposition and ventricular septal defect. A notch is occasionally seen on the left heart border corresponding to the junction between the hypoplastic right ventricle and the left ventricle (Hallermann *et al.*, 1966).

DOUBLE OUTFLOW RIGHT VENTRICLE WITHOUT PULMONARY STENOSIS

Veno-arterial mixing occurs in the right ventricle, venous blood entering through the tricuspid valve from the right atrium, and oxygenated blood through the ventricular septal defect from the left ventricle. Although mixing takes place, considerable streaming of venous and arterial blood may occur, its pattern depending on the position of the ventricular septal defect. Ejection into the lungs is at systemic pressure.

There are two types without pulmonary stenosis (Neufeld *et al.* 1962b).

Type 1 (Figure 288a)

The ventricular septal defect is infracristal in position and as it lies close to and below the aortic valve, oxygenated blood from the left ventricle is directed predominantly through the aortic valve. The right ventricular stream crosses the left and is directed towards the pulmonary valve. Patients present as a ventricular septal defect with pulmonary hypertension but without cyanosis.

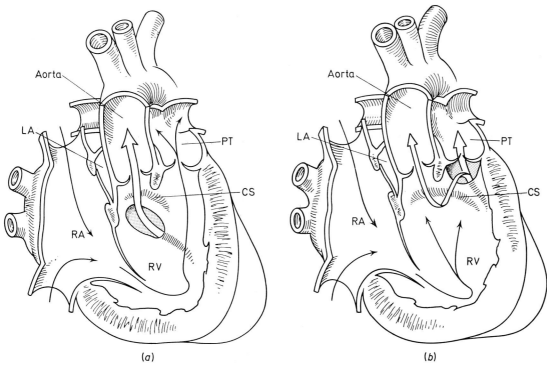

Figure 288. Double outflow right ventricle without pulmonary stenosis: (a) Type 1; (b) Type 2. LA = left atrium; RA = right atrium; RV = right ventricle; PT = pulmonary trunk; CS = crista supraventricularis. (Neufeld et al., 1962b)

Type 2 (Figure 288b)

The ventricular septal defect is supracristal in position and lies immediately below the pulmonary valve. Left ventricular blood shows preferential streaming into the pulmonary trunk, and right ventricular blood into the aorta. The result is that these patients present as a ventricular septal defect with pulmonary hypertension and cyanosis. The Taussig–Bing anomaly (Taussig and Bing, 1949) is a variant (Van Praagh, 1968).

Radiology

Radiologically the two types are similar and cannot be distinguished from ventricular septal defect with plethora and pulmonary hypertension, although plethora is usually more obvious in the second type (Carey and Edwards, 1965). The heart is enlarged and the left atrium may appear dilated. The pulmonary trunk and proximal pulmonary arteries are large, with some reduction in size in the periphery. Appearances resembling the Eisenmenger syndrome occur (*see* Chapter 21) when the pulmonary vascular resistance is high.

TRUNCUS ARTERIOSUS

In truncus arteriosus, a single vessel representing the embryological truncus emerges from the ventricles above a ventricular septal defect and gives origin to systemic, coronary and pulmonary arteries. Collett and Edwards (1949) classified the anomaly into four types (*Figure 289*).

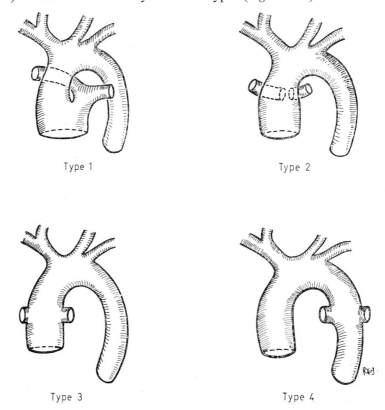

Figure 289. The four types of truncus arteriosus (Collett and Edwards, 1949)

Type 1

The aorta and the pulmonary trunk are largely separate and arise from a short common trunk just above the truncal valve (*Figure 290*).

Type 2

The right and left pulmonary arteries arise close together from the dorsal aspect of the truncus arteriosus.

Type 3

One or both pulmonary arteries arise independently from the lateral aspect of the truncus.

Type 4

The vascular supply to the lung is derived from the descending aorta. In the authors' view this condition should not be regarded as a type of truncus arteriosus as the pulmonary arteries do not arise from the embryological truncus and thus the anomaly does not satisfy the definition of truncus arteriosus. Furthermore, the pulmonary arteries may or may not be present (Jefferson *et al.*, 1972).

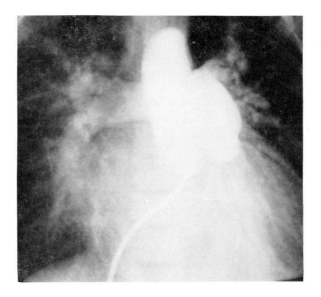

Figure 290. Truncus arteriosus. Aortogram. Type 1 with the pulmonary trunk present

The term pseudotruncus has also been applied to this condition. Both terms should be abandoned and the anomaly be called what it is, pulmonary atresia (*see* page 182).

Another classification of truncus (Van Praagh and Van Praagh, 1965) includes hemitruncus, associated hypoplasia of the aortic isthmus and rare cases with an intact ventricular septum.

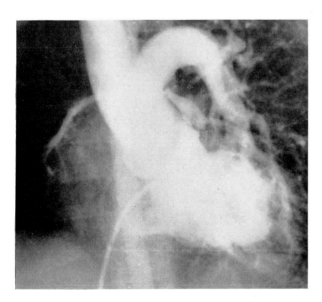

Figure 291. Hemitruncus. Right ventricular angiogram. The left lung is supplied by the hemitruncus and the right lung through a stenotic right ventricular outflow

The truncal valve usually has three cusps as it is embryologically the aortic valve, but there may be two or even four cusps. It may be regurgitant but is rarely stenotic. The aortic arch is on the right in 50 per cent of cases. The ventricular septal defect is large and lies immediately below the truncal valve. The right and left pulmonary arteries are almost always wide.

Hemitruncus is a condition in which one lung is supplied by a vessel arising from the ascending aorta and the other from the right ventricle. The right ventricular outflow may be normal, stenotic as in Fallot's tetralogy or atretic, the lung in the last case being supplied by a ductus or systemic vessels from the aorta (*Figure 291*).

Aorto-pulmonary septal defect is closely related embryologically to truncus arteriosus in that there is partial failure of truncal septation. The distinguishing feature is that the lower part of the trunco-conal septum has developed normally to separate the aortic and pulmonary valves from the sinus portions of the aorta and pulmonary trunk (*see* page 164).

Both ventricles act as a common pumping chamber and eject blood at systemic pressure into the truncus, where venous and arterial mixing occurs. Initially the pulmonary blood flow is increased and cyanosis may be slight. Later the pulmonary vascular resistance rises, the pulmonary blood flow falls and cyanosis becomes marked.

Radiology

In patients with increased pulmonary flow, there is quite marked cardiac enlargement involving all four chambers. With an increased pulmonary vascular resistance, the pulmonary flow may be similar to or less than the systemic; the heart is then slightly or moderately enlarged and the picture of plethora

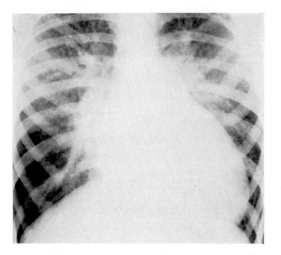

Figure 292. Truncus, type 1. Pulmonary trunk visible. Dilatation of pulmonary trunk and proximal pulmonary vessels

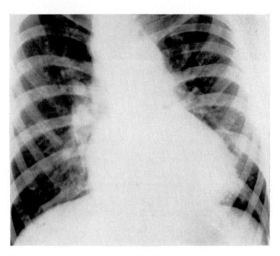

Figure 293. Truncus, type 2. A concavity in the middle of the left cardiac border

changes to one indicating pulmonary arterial hypertension, namely proximal vessel dilatation with narrowing at segmental level. In type 1 of Collett and Edwards (1949), the pulmonary trunk is present and, as it is usually large, produces a convexity on the left cardiac border (*Figure 292*). In types 2 and 3, which are much less common, there is a concavity as the pulmonary trunk is absent (*Figure 293*). The right and left pulmonary arteries may be higher than normal (*see Figure 292*); in type 1 the left pulmonary artery may arch out into the lung, sometimes reaching the level of the aortic knuckle (Keith *et al.*, 1967). The aortic arch is right-sided in about half the cases, and is frequently high in position whichever its side (*Figure 293*).

MIXING IN THE LUNGS

PULMONARY ARTERIOVENOUS FISTULA

Pulmonary arteriovenous fistulae are direct communications between pulmonary arteries and veins, usually through dilated thin-walled channels which by-pass the pulmonary capillaries. The result is a mixing of desaturated blood from the pulmonary arteries with oxygenated blood in the pulmonary veins.

The amount of systemic arterial desaturation and cyanosis depends on the size of the right-to-left shunt.

Single lesions do occur, but the fistulae are usually multiple and are more common in the lower lobes. They may occupy a whole segment or lobe, and rarely are diffusely distributed throughout both lungs. Pulmonary arteriovenous shunting is seen in some types of liver disease with cirrhosis (Karlish *et al.*, 1967). Complications include cerebral thrombosis (with polycythaemia), paradoxical embolus, brain abscesses, rupture and infection. Sixty per cent of patients with pulmonary arteriovenous fistulae have hereditary telangiectasia (Osler–Weber–Rendu disease). Such patients have cutaneous, mucosal and visceral vascular lesions from which bleeding may occur. The pulmonary fistulae are multiple and more prone to complications (Gomes and Bernatz, 1970).

Radiology

A fistula presents as a round or oval opacity, most often in the lower lobe (*Figure 294*). Visible feeding and draining vessels, best shown on tomography, enable the diagnosis to be made with confidence. Sometimes these vessels are visible but not the malformation itself: the vessels are dilated and often

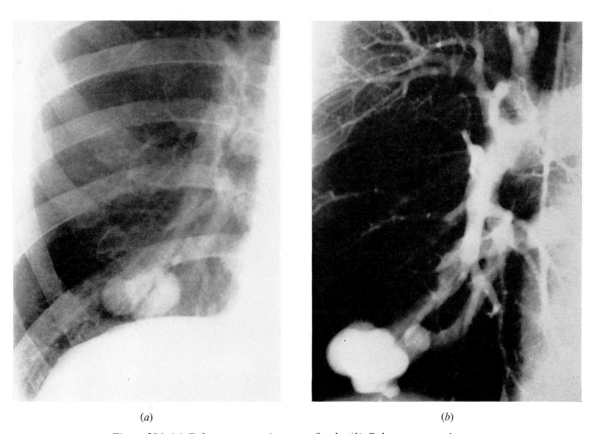

(a)   (b)

Figure 294. (a) Pulmonary arteriovenous fistula. (b) Pulmonary arteriogram

tortuous, and do not taper normally as they are traced to the periphery. Occasionally a complex arteriovenous malformation occupies a segment or a lobe and may be mistaken for such lesions as pulmonary tuberculosis (*Figures 295–297*); if extensive enough, the fistulae may steal blood from the rest of the lung, which will appear oligaemic. Very rarely the fistulae are small and multiple, producing no visible changes in the lungs except diffuse punctate shadowing. Calcification in a fistula is very rare. Fistulae may be observed to become smaller during the Valsalva manoeuvre and larger during the Müller procedure. Tomography clearly demonstrates the lesions and may also show up others that were not previously detected; for this reason both lungs should be examined even if only a single lesion is visible on plain radiography. Cardiac enlargement is rare except when there are systemic as well as pulmonary arteriovenous fistulae as part of the Osler–Weber–Rendu syndrome.

A fistula must be distinguished from a pulmonary varix, which is a localized enlargement of a pulmonary vein, the pulmonary arteries and capillaries being normal (Bartram and Strickland, 1971). The dilated vein usually drains into the left atrium, but may have anomalous connections.

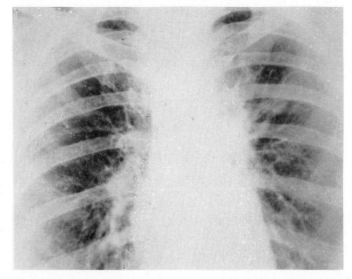

Figure 295. Pulmonary arteriovenous fistula. Lesion above left hilum

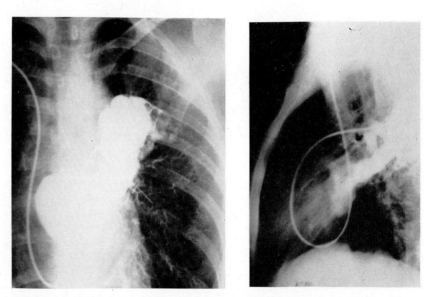

Figure 296 (left). Pulmonary arteriogram in same case. Anterior view

Figure 297 (right). Pulmonary arteriogram in same case. Lateral view. Fistula in apical segment of left lower lobe

MIXING DISTAL TO THE LUNGS

ANOMALOUS SYSTEMIC VENOUS DRAINAGE TO LEFT ATRIUM

The superior or the inferior vena cava may terminate in the left instead of the right atrium. If there are no other congenital cardiac anomalies, the patient may present with central cyanosis and normal radiological appearances of the heart and lungs. Sometimes, however, the abnormal systemic venous return is in the pathway of a left-to-right shunt from the left to the right atrium and there may be no arterial desaturation (Meadows and Sharp, 1965). It is more common for the left than the right superior vena

212

cava to enter the left atrium. The left superior vena cava joins the roof of the left atrium, the coronary sinus is absent, and associated cardiovascular anomalies are nearly always present and complex (*Figure 298*). Defects of the atrial septum are common including single atrium, ostium primum atrial septal defect and a particular type of postero-inferior defect (Raghib *et al.*, 1965). Complex heart disease with asplenia is frequent. Radiological features may suggest a left superior vena cava and the associated congenital heart disease.

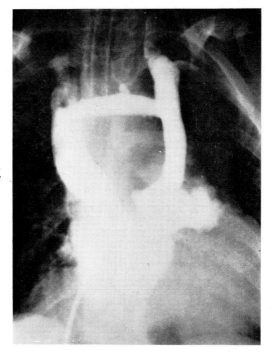

Figure 298. Left superior vena cava entering roof of left atrium. Injection into right superior vena cava with flow across innominate vein into left superior vena cava and thence to left atrium

The inferior vena cava may drain into the left atrium in association with an intact atrial septum, in which case the patient will be cyanosed with a normal chest x-ray; as an alternative pathway for the caval blood is through the azygos vein, it would be expected that the greater the azygos venous return, the less would be the cyanosis. The inferior vena cava may straddle an atrial septal defect or may enter the right atrium with some streaming of venous blood into the left atrium by an enlarged Eustachian valve (inferior vena caval type of defect). In each case the radiological picture is that of atrial septal defect.

SECTION VI
Obstruction and Regurgitation

CHAPTER 23

Tricuspid Obstruction and Regurgitation

INTRODUCTION

The following lesions are described.
(1) Tricuspid stenosis.
(2) Tricuspid regurgitation.
(3) Ebstein's anomaly of the tricuspid valve.
(4) Tricuspid atresia.

Radiological signs which may occur are:
(1) Right atrial enlargement.
(2) Right ventricular enlargement.
(3) Left atrial and left ventricular enlargement in tricuspid atresia.
(4) Oligaemia.

TRICUSPID STENOSIS

Congenital tricuspid stenosis is very rare. Cardiac enlargement is due entirely to the large right atrium. The superior vena cava may be dilated. The lungs may appear oligaemic due to the low cardiac output. Acquired tricuspid stenosis is nearly always rheumatic, associated with mitral valve disease, especially stenosis, and aortic valve disease. The diagnosis is suggested when the right atrium is enlarged (Kitchen and Turner, 1964). Tricuspid stenosis may prevent the lung changes of pulmonary venous hypertension in important mitral valve disease (*see Figure 317*), but if the mitral valve offers a greater resistance to flow than the tricuspid, pulmonary hypertension will be seen in the presence of important tricuspid stenosis; it depends on the time relationship between the development of stenosis in each valve (Kitchen and Turner, 1964). Radiologically it may be impossible to tell whether the right atrial dilatation is due to tricuspid valve disease or to pulmonary hypertension. Tricuspid stenosis is occasionally caused by right atrial thrombus or myxoma or by the vegetations of bacterial endocarditis. Other rare causes include systemic lupus erythematosus, carcinoid syndrome and endocardial fibro-elastosis.

TRICUSPID REGURGITATION

Congenital tricuspid regurgitation is rare except for Ebstein's anomaly, only 14 cases having been reported up to 1969 (Antia and Osunkoya). The right atrium and right ventricle dilate, the pulmonary trunk is small and the lungs may be oligaemic, a radiological picture resembling Ebstein's anomaly. The other causes of isolated tricuspid regurgitation are right-sided endomyocardial fibrosis and right atrial myxoma. A few myxomas show visible calcification and, if hard, may destroy the tricuspid valve to produce severe tricuspid regurgitation. If friable, the tumour may embolize to the lung, causing infarction and embolic pulmonary hypertension. Tricuspid endocarditis is common in heroin addicts who use the intravenous route. The diagnosis is suggested by fever, pulmonary infarction and tricuspid regurgitation. Where organic tricuspid regurgitation is rheumatic in origin, it is always associated with involvement of other valves, mitral regurgitation being the most common. All four chambers are enlarged so that the heart is large and globular in shape (*see Figure 19*). Functional tricuspid regurgitation is caused by dilatation of the tricuspid valve ring in the presence of pulmonary hypertension with mitral valve disease. It is impossible to tell from the plain films whether the tricuspid regurgitation is organic or functional, although functional regurgitation is not seen without pulmonary hypertension. It may be difficult to assess the size of the right atrium in the presence of a large left atrium unless two separate contours are clearly defined. The two atrial borders often overlap, and then the presence of right atrial enlargement can only be proved at cardiac catheterization (*see* page 15 for the radiology of right atrial enlargement).

EBSTEIN'S ANOMALY OF THE TRICUSPID VALVE

Ebstein's anomaly (Ebstein, 1886) usually consists of displacement of the attachments of the septal and posterior cusps into the right ventricle; these two cusps are deformed, often with vestigal chordae and papillary muscles (*Figure 299*). The anterior cusp retains all or most of its attachment to the tricuspid valve ring; it is frequently a large sail-like structure and tends to be the only functional portion of the valve. Because of dislocation of the valve into the right ventricle, the effective part of the right ventricle is reduced in size, and its efficiency is often further impaired by muscle loss and fibrosis of the myo-cardium. The right ventricle proximal to the tricuspid valve shows a normal right ventricular electro-cardiogram, but has an atrial pressure and is said to be atrialized. A patent foramen or atrial septal defect is present in about 75 per cent. Ebstein's anomaly is occasionally found in corrected transposition with ventricular inversion. The atrio-ventricular valve regurgitation is then on the left side of the heart and simulates mitral regurgitation.

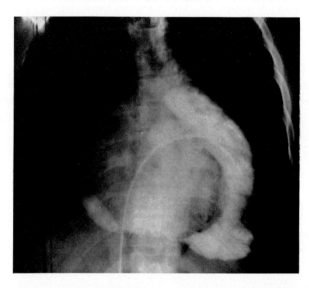

Figure 299. Ebstein's anomaly. Angiogram, anterior view. Tricuspid valve displaced into right ventricle

The incapacity in Ebstein's anomaly depends on the impairment of the right ventricle as a pump, the functional abnormality of the tricuspid valve and the arterial desaturation from a reversed shunt at atrial level. The tricuspid valve may be competent, regurgitant or stenosed, but stenosis is rarely more than mild. The combination of poor right ventricular function and tricuspid regurgitation causes elevation of the right atrial pressure and a right-to-left shunt if there is a defect in the atrial septum. There is a very wide clinical spectrum: cyanosis may be present at birth, appear later or never occur at all; patients have lived to the seventh or eighth decade. Asymptomatic patients may present with a murmur; symptoms include palpitation from paroxysmal dysrhythmia and dyspnoea. Sudden death is not uncommon.

Radiology

Heart size depends almost entirely on the amount of tricuspid regurgitation. The heart may be of normal size at birth but then enlarge quite quickly. In mild cases there may be little or no cardiac enlargement and no right atrial prominence (*Figure 300a*). With severe tricuspid regurgitation, the heart is huge with a very large right atrium (*Figure 300b*). The right atrial border is long and abnormally convex, often forming more than half the vertical height of the mediastinum. Although the functional part of the right ventricle is reduced, the outflow tract is dilated and contracts vigorously. This dilatation may produce a convexity below the pulmonary trunk segment, which resembles a very large left atrial appendix (*Figure 300a*). Although in many cases the ventricular border on the anterior view is typical of

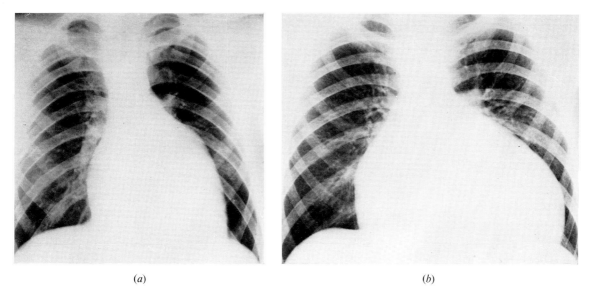

(a)   (b)

Figure 300. Ebstein's anomaly, anterior view. Typical appearances

right ventricular enlargement, this is not always so, and some cases may look more like left ventricular enlargement (*see Figure 32*). The pulmonary trunk is small and usually invisible. The aorta is small in severe cases; its ascending portion may be obscured by a huge right atrium. On the lateral view the heart appears globular and encroaches anteriorly on the retrosternal space. The right atrium may form much of the anterior, inferior and posterior cardiac border.

The hilar arteries are small, and the intrapulmonary vessels are small in cyanotic cases (*Figure 301*): as cyanosis usually occurs with important tricuspid regurgitation, small pulmonary vessels are typically associated with a large heart. In the absence of a right-to-left shunt, vessel size is usually within normal limits, but it may be reduced.

The differential diagnosis includes the following conditions.

    (1) Fallot's tetralogy.
    (2) Pulmonary stenosis and congestive cardiac failure.
    (3) Pericardial effusion.
    (4) Cardiomyopathy.
    (5) Isolated tricuspid regurgitation.
    (6) Chronic rheumatic heart disease.
    (7) Parchment right ventricle (Uhl's anomaly).

Fallot's tetralogy comes seriously into the differential diagnosis of Ebstein's anomaly only in the newborn before the onset of marked cardiac enlargement. Occasionally in the cyanotic Ebstein the heart remains small. The pulmonary trunk is hypoplastic as in Fallot's tetralogy, but the aorta is not enlarged. Pericardial effusion may closely resemble Ebstein's anomaly except that the pulmonary vessels are normal or occasionally dilated in the upper zones; the echocardiogram is decisive. The heart in pulmonary stenosis with congestive cardiac failure may be very large from dilatation of the right atrium and right ventricle, and although the pulmonary trunk is dilated, it may be hidden within a large heart; dilatation of the left pulmonary artery, if present, suggests the diagnosis. Right-sided endomyocardial fibrosis causes dilatation of the right atrium and right ventricle resembling Ebstein's disease. Isolated congenital tricuspid regurgitation and important rheumatic tricuspid valve disease with mild involvement of other valves are rare causes of enlargement of the right-sided chambers. If a penetrated anterior view shows any left atrial enlargement, Ebstein's anomaly is excluded. In the parchment right ventricle or Uhl's anomaly (Uhl, 1952), the right ventricle is dilated because of deficient muscle in its wall. The condition is probably allied to Ebstein's anomaly, but the position of the tricuspid valve at angiography is normal.

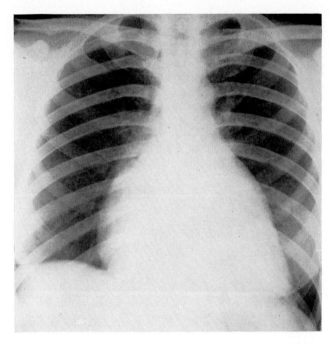

Figure 301. Ebstein's anomaly. Very oligaemic lungs due to right-to-left shunt at atrial level

TRICUSPID ATRESIA

In tricuspid atresia there is an atretic tricuspid valve. Systemic venous blood entering the right atrium crosses the atrial septum, usually through a patent foramen ovale, and survival is dependent on this shunt being adequate (*Figure 302*). The left atrium is the common mixing chamber where systemic

Figure 302. Tricuspid atresia. Right atrial angiogram. Contrast passes from right atrium via left atrium to left ventricle. Triangular defect due to absence of right ventricular opacification

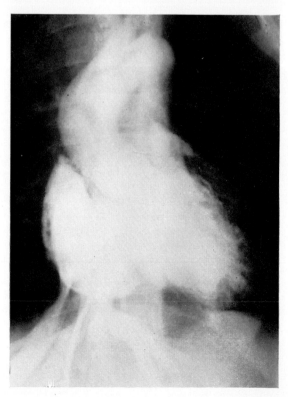

venous blood meets oxygenated blood from the pulmonary veins. Systemic arterial oxygen saturation depends on the relative volumes of systemic and pulmonary venous blood entering the left atrium and, thus, on the pulmonary blood flow. The right ventricle is hypoplastic and the left ventricle is the common ejection chamber maintaining the systemic and pulmonary circulations. Although these features are common to all cases of tricuspid atresia, there is considerable variation in the clinical and radiological manifestations, depending mainly on the pulmonary blood flow.

Obstruction to pulmonary blood flow is present in over 50 per cent of cases; it may be due to stenosis (or atresia) of the pulmonary valve or to subvalvar stenosis, but in non-transposed cases it is more commonly the result of a ventricular septal defect which is too small or a hypoplastic right ventricle. Transposition occurs in 30 per cent. *D*-transposition is more frequent than *l*-transposition (Keith *et al.*, 1967).

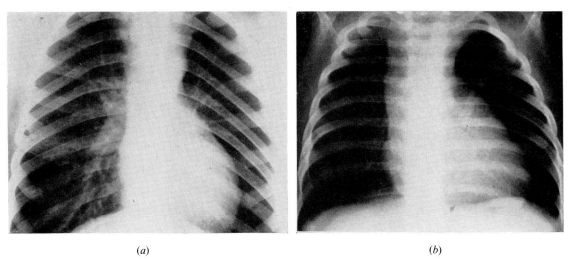

(a)   (b)

Figure 303. Tricuspid atresia. Anterior view. (a) Typical appearances resembling Fallot's tetralogy but with large heart and left ventricular contour. (b) Flat right atrial border

Right ventricular outflow obstruction is commoner with normally related great vessels than with transposition. Pulmonary atresia may occur so that the blood supply to the lungs is via a ductus arteriosus or systemic vessels from the aorta.

Radiology

The commonest finding is a decrease in the size of the hilar and pulmonary vessels with a heart which is normal in size or only slightly enlarged and superficially resembles that seen in Fallot's tetralogy. A concavity may be present in the middle of the left cardiac border due to the smallness of the pulmonary trunk or to its central position in transposition. Below the concavity, however, the contour is more rounded than in Fallot because of enlargement of the left atrium and left ventricle (*Figure 303a*); in the lateral projection this may show as a prominent posterior bulge. A larger and higher bulge may be seen on the anterior view due to left juxtaposition of the atrial appendices; the right atrial appendix extends posteriorly behind the great vessels and lies on the left cardiac border immediately above the left atrial appendix (*see Figure 20*). The presence of the typical bulge of left juxtaposition in a cyanotic patient indicates that complete transposition is present and that, in addition, tricuspid atresia is likely (Elliott *et al.*, 1968). The right atrial border is characteristically flat (*Figure 303b*), particularly with left juxtaposition, when there may also be a concavity in its upper part where the appendix normally lies. If the defect in the atrial septum is small, there may be dilatation of the right atrium and superior vena cava. The aortic arch is right-sided in about 7 per cent (Elliott *et al.*, 1968).

Normal or enlarged pulmonary vessels in tricuspid atresia are more common with transposition than with normally related vessels and a large ventricular septal defect. Rarely plethora may be present if there is a large ductus arteriosus, and very rarely cases may present as the Eisenmenger syndrome with dilatation of the proximal pulmonary arteries.

CHAPTER 24

Pulmonary Obstruction and Regurgitation

INTRODUCTION

The following lesions are described.
(1) Pulmonary stenosis.
(2) Pulmonary regurgitation.
(3) Pulmonary artery stenosis.

Radiological signs which may occur are:
(1) Right ventricular enlargement due to hypertrophy and/or dilatation.
(2) Pulmonary trunk dilatation.
(3) Oligaemia.

PULMONARY STENOSIS

The term pulmonary stenosis is used here to mean obstruction to right ventricular outflow with intact ventricular septum. To maintain a normal cardiac output, the right ventricle generates a high systolic pressure and is hypertrophied as a result of the systolic overload. Right ventricular dilatation occurs only when the diastolic pressure rises in congestive failure. The right atrium also enlarges to overcome the increased filling resistance of the incompliant right ventricle. If the obstruction is severe, the right ventricular pressure may not be high enough to maintain a normal output, particularly on exercise. The right atrial pressure may exceed the left atrial pressure, and if there is a patent foramen ovale or atrial septal defect, a right-to-left shunt occurs at atrial level, causing cyanosis (*see* page 191).

Pulmonary valve stenosis is nearly always congenital. There is fusion of the valve cusps into a dome with a small central or eccentric orifice (*Figure 304*). Muscle hypertrophy involves the infundibulum, and although a subvalvar gradient is rarely found before operation, marked obstruction may follow valvotomy and cause congestive cardiac failure. Lone fixed infundibular stenosis (*Figure 305*) is rare without a ventricular septal defect, which may, however, be so small as to go undetected at catheterization. The obstruction is due to displacement of the parietal and/or septal bands into the right ventricular outflow, which causes constriction at the ostium of the infundibulum several centimetres below the pulmonary valve ring. Beyond the stenosis the infundibulum is typically wide (infundibular chamber, third ventricle—*Figure 305*).

The causes of pulmonary stenosis are as follows.

Congenital isolated
  Valve.
  Infundibular.

Congenital with general disease
  Rubella (Venables, 1965).
  Ullrich's syndrome.

Acquired (Seymour et al., 1968)
  Compression: aneurysm of aorta, aortic sinus or ventricular septum; tumour, pericardial constriction.

222

Infiltration of myocardium: primary or secondary tumours, lymphoma.
Obstruction of lumen: tumours, cysts.
Thickening of myocardium: hypertrophic cardiomyopathy, tumours, cysts, anomalous muscle bundle.
Valve stenosis: carcinoid syndrome, chronic rheumatic heart disease.

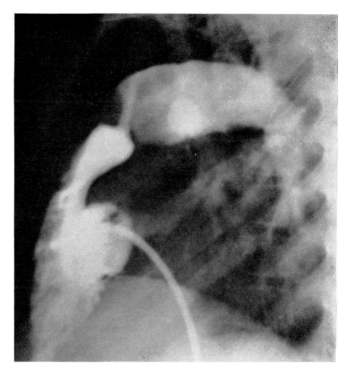

Figure 304. Pulmonary valve stenosis. Right ventricular angiogram. Systole. Lateral view

In the rubella syndrome, pulmonary valve stenosis may be combined with pulmonary artery branch stenosis and ductus arteriosus. Seventy-five per cent of patients with Ullrich's syndrome have pulmonary stenosis, often combined with atrial septal defect. Aneurysms of the ascending aorta are the commonest cause of acquired pulmonary stenosis; the majority are syphilitic in origin, and they may rupture into the right ventricle or the pulmonary trunk (Seymour *et al.*, 1968). They may compress other structures such as the superior vena cava and the bronchial tree. Tumours can cause an abnormal cardiac bulge which may be mistaken for post-stenotic dilatation if situated in the position of the pulmonary artery. Compression of the right ventricular outflow tract by a pericardial band after incomplete resection for constrictive pericarditis was first described by Mounsey (1959). A right ventricular outflow gradient may be found in hypertrophic cardiomyopathy. An anomalous muscle bundle may obstruct the body of the right ventricle to produce a two-chambered right ventricle (Barnes *et al.*, 1971). If the ventricular septum is intact, the features resemble those of pulmonary stenosis (Coates *et al.*, 1964). In the carcinoid syndrome with liver metastases, the commonest valve lesions are pulmonary stenosis and tricuspid regurgitation, but tricuspid stenosis and pulmonary regurgitation can also occur (Aroesty *et al.*, 1966). Rheumatic involvement of the pulmonary valve is found in less than 2 per cent of patients with chronic rheumatic heart disease. A case of combined mitral and pulmonary valve stenosis has been diagnosed in life by McCredie and Richards (1966).

Radiology

The heart is usually normal in size even with severe stenosis, but may be slightly enlarged in childhood as a result of marked hypertrophy of the right ventricle; gross cardiac enlargement is seen only with congestive cardiac failure. The heart is often normal in shape, but its left contour may suggest right ventricular hypertrophy (*see Figure 35*). The right atrium appears prominent only in enlarged hearts.
Post-stenotic dilatation of the pulmonary trunk and/or the left branch occurs in over 90 per cent of

cases with stenosis at valve level. Usually both the pulmonary trunk and the left branch are enlarged, but the pulmonary trunk alone or the left branch alone may be involved (*Figure 306*). In valve stenosis, there is invariably dilatation of the roof of the pulmonary trunk related to where the jet through the pulmonary valve hits the inside of the pulmonary trunk. This superior enlargement may be evident on

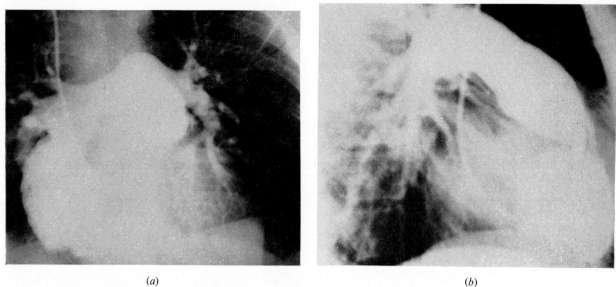

(a)　　　　　　　　　　　　　　　　　　　　(b)

Figure 305. Infundibular stenosis. Right ventricular angiogram. Systole. Stenosis at the ostium of the infundibulum with an infundibular chamber beyond. (a) Anterior view. (b) Lateral view

the plain film; the top of the pulmonary trunk may be so high as partially to overlap the aortic knuckle (*Figure 307*). Dilatation of the left pulmonary artery often extends into the lobar and occasionally into the segmental branches; a characteristic feature is a lower lobe pulmonary artery wider on the left than on the right, a sign present in over 50 per cent of cases (*see Figure 306a*). The right descending pulmonary

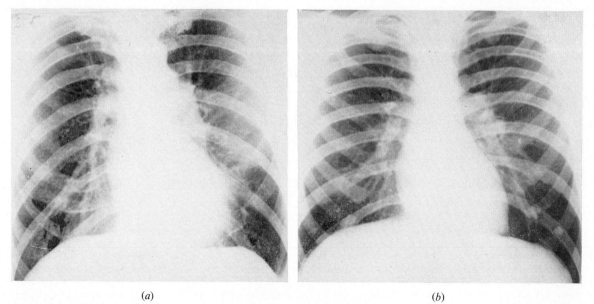

(a)　　　　　　　　　　　　　　　　　　　　(b)

Figure 306. Pulmonary valve stenosis with post-stenotic dilatation. (a) Pulmonary trunk and left pulmonary artery. (b) Left pulmonary artery alone

artery may be normal or, in severe obstruction, narrow. Post-stenotic dilatation may involve the right pulmonary artery, but this is invisible radiologically as it lies entirely within the mediastinum; the dilatation rarely extends into the right lower lobe artery. The absence of visible post-stenotic dilatation of the pulmonary trunk or the left branch does not deny the diagnosis of valve stenosis. If the dilatation involves the roof only, it may be invisible, and occasionally no dilatation is seen on angiography. Dilatation may be absent in the rubella syndrome (*Figure 308*). The degree of post-stenotic dilatation is unrelated to the severity of the stenosis (d'Cruz *et al.*, 1964a). The dilatation tends to be progressive and the largest pulmonary trunks are encountered in the rare middle-aged or elderly patients.

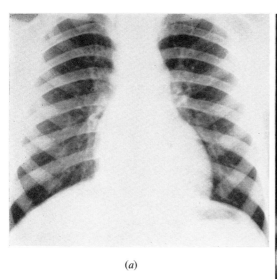

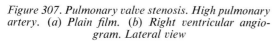

(*a*)

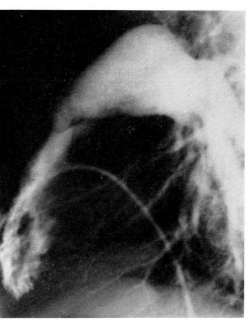

Figure 307. Pulmonary valve stenosis. High pulmonary artery. (a) Plain film. (b) Right ventricular angiogram. Lateral view

(*b*)

A notch or a localized bay between the pulmonary trunk and the ventricular border is sometimes caused by a small valve ring interposed between a large pulmonary trunk above and a large right ventricle below. If present, this is useful in distinguishing pulmonary valve stenosis from a small atrial septal defect, in which the left cardiac border is without an obvious bay. The aorta is normal except in severe obstruction, where it may be small as a result of a low cardiac output. A right aortic arch is

Figure 308. Pulmonary valve stenosis in the rubella syndrome. No post-stenotic dilatation

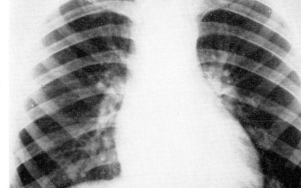

strongly suggestive of associated ventricular septal defect, but has been reported with an intact septum (Hipona, 1965). Calcification of the pulmonary valve may be seen in middle-aged patients and after bacterial endocarditis. The intrapulmonary vessels are normal in mild or moderate cases, but small with severe obstruction (*Figure 309*). Oligaemia is obvious only when a right-to-left shunt is present at atrial level.

The radiological differential diagnosis of the pulmonary valve stenosis is as follows.

    (1) Small atrial septal defect.
    (2) Fallot's tetralogy.
    (3) Idiopathic dilatation of the pulmonary trunk.
    (4) Eisenmenger ventricular septal defect.

The only abnormality in all these may be an enlarged pulmonary trunk. Fallot's tetralogy with post-stenotic dilatation of the pulmonary trunk may exactly resemble pulmonary valve stenosis with an intact septum, but there is usually an enlarged aorta and oligaemia.

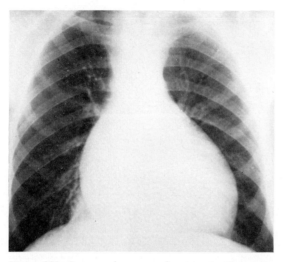

Figure 309. *Severe pulmonary valve stenosis. Congestive failure. Large right atrium and ventricle, the latter hiding the post-stenotic dilatation. The lungs are oligaemic*

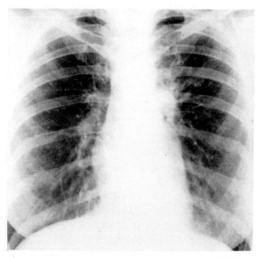

Figure 310. *Infundibular stenosis. Bulge on left cardiac border due to the infundibular chamber*

Pulmonary stenosis may present at any age with cardiac enlargement and congestive heart failure. These patients are usually cyanotic from a right-to-left shunt at atrial level. The right atrium and right ventricle are very large. Post-stenotic dilatation may be hidden by the dilated right ventricular outflow. The lungs are always oligaemic (*Figure 309*). Diagnosis may be difficult radiologically and the appearances may resemble a number of conditions including:

    (1) Ebstein's anomaly.
    (2) Pericardial effusion.
    (3) Cardiomyopathy.
    (4) Tricuspid regurgitation.
    (5) Chronic multivalvar rheumatic heart disease.
    (6) Parchment right ventricle (Uhl's anomaly—*see* Ebstein's anomaly, page 218).

The appearances of the heart and of the lungs are often the same in infundibular as in valve stenosis. The pulmonary trunk, however, is usually normal or small. The infundibular chamber may be large and show as a bulge on the left cardiac border at the level of the left atrial appendix (*Figure 310*). The sinus portion of the pulmonary trunk may be included in the post-stenotic dilatation, which is lower than in valve stenosis and never involves the left pulmonary artery. Below the dilatation there may be an indentation corresponding to the stenotic area. A right aortic arch has been reported in infundibular stenosis without a ventricular septal defect (Kjellberg *et al.*, 1958).

After a successful pulmonary valvotomy, the post-stenotic dilatation of the pulmonary trunk usually becomes less but does not disappear. The heart remains the same and even when markedly large is often unchanged, probably because of irreversible damage to the right ventricular myocardium.

PULMONARY REGURGITATION

Pulmonary regurgitation may be congenital, acquired or functional (Hamby and Gulotta, 1967). The causes are listed below.

Congenital
  Isolated cusp anomaly.
  Associated with ventricular septal defect, pulmonary stenosis, Fallot's tetralogy, idiopathic dilatation of the pulmonary trunk.

Acquired
  After surgery, bacterial endocarditis, rheumatic endocarditis, syphilis, carcinoid syndrome, rubella syndrome, trauma.

Functional
  Secondary to pulmonary hypertension.

Congenital pulmonary regurgitation is rare. It may be due to isolated cusp anomalies, but is usually associated with infundibular stenosis and ventricular septal defect as part of Fallot's tetralogy (Macartney and Miller, 1970); in the latter condition the valve cusps are rudimentary or absent (*see* page 173). Pulmonary regurgitation may result from a dilated ring in idiopathic dilatation of the pulmonary trunk, but not all cases of cusp anomaly or idiopathic dilatation have regurgitation. The commonest acquired cause of pulmonary regurgitation is post-operative. Functional regurgitation is caused by stretching of the valve ring secondary to pulmonary hypertension. It is commonest in the Eisenmenger syndrome, being present in 50–66 per cent of Wood's (1958) 127 cases. The authors' impression is that it occurs more often with a ductus arteriosus than with atrial or ventricular shunts. An early diastolic murmur in rheumatic heart disease with pulmonary hypertension is more often due to aortic than to pulmonary regurgitation (Graham Steell murmur) (Runco *et al.*, 1968).

Radiology

Isolated pulmonary regurgitation is a benign lesion unless associated with pulmonary hypertension (Kelly, 1965). The heart and pulmonary trunk show little or no enlargement, but the ultimate prognosis is uncertain and older patients with severe regurgitation may develop congestive failure. When the pulmonary trunk is large with a normal-sized heart, idiopathic dilatation is the most likely cause of pulmonary regurgitation (*Figure 311*). The diagnosis is confirmed on angiography by showing normal

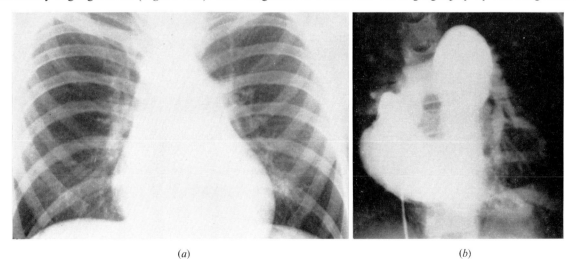

(*a*)   (*b*)

Figure 311. Idiopathic dilatation of pulmonary trunk with pulmonary regurgitation. (a) Plain film. (b) Right atrial angiogram showing uniform dilatation of pulmonary trunk

cusps with uniform dilatation of the pulmonary trunk. The condition differs from the localized dilatation seen beyond a stenotic valve. Surgically induced pulmonary regurgitation, such as occurs after total correction of Fallot's tetralogy, causes cardiac enlargement, particularly if there is pulmonary hypertension. Functional regurgitation in the Eisenmenger syndrome is seen with all grades of enlargement of the pulmonary trunk. Functional pulmonary regurgitation is not encountered in mitral valve disease unless there are radiological signs of a high pulmonary vascular resistance (*Figure 312*).

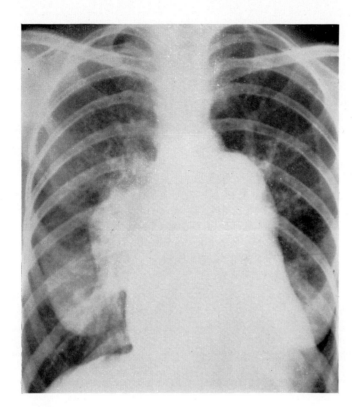

Figure 312. Mitral stenosis with severe pulmonary hypertension and pulmonary regurgitation

PULMONARY ARTERY STENOSIS

Pulmonary artery stenosis may be single or multiple and may lie anywhere in the pulmonary arteries beyond the pulmonary valve. There are three main types (Schlesinger and Meester, 1967).

(1) Single or multiple stenoses in the pulmonary trunk, right or left pulmonary artery or intra-pulmonary arteries.
(2) Stenosis at the bifurcation of the pulmonary trunk.
(3) Supravalvar membranous stenosis.

Stenotic lesions may be short or long, or a combination of both may be seen in the same patient. Localized stenoses tend to have a post-stenotic dilatation. Widespread involvement of the pulmonary arteries causes right ventricular hypertension. About two-thirds of reported cases have congenital heart disease (d'Cruz *et al.*, 1964b), the commonest lesions being pulmonary valve stenosis, ductus arteriosus, ventricular septal defect and Fallot's tetralogy. Pulmonary artery stenosis may be familial and also occurs in the rubella syndrome (*see* page 134), with supravalvar aortic stenosis (*see* page 244) and with hypercalcaemia of infancy.

In the rubella syndrome, peripheral stenoses may be associated with pulmonary valve stenosis, ductus arteriosus, supravalvar aortic stenosis and other stenoses of systemic arteries. Pulmonary artery stenosis, with or without supravalvar aortic stenosis, may be familial and inherited as an autosomal dominant

(McDonald *et al.*, 1969). Pulmonary artery stenosis is occasionally the result of partial lysis or recanalization of pulmonary emboli.

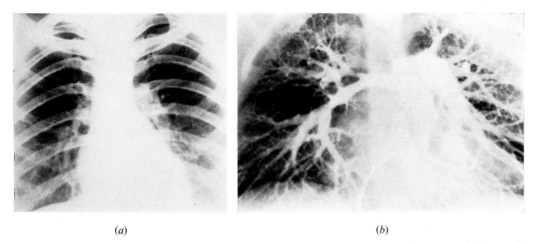

(*a*)   (*b*)

Figure 313. Pulmonary artery stenosis. (a) Plain film. Reduced pulmonary vascularity in right lung with post-stenotic dilatation of two basal segmental arteries. (b) Right ventricular angiogram showing multiple arterial stenoses with post-stenotic dilatation in right lung

Radiology

Multiple pulmonary stenosis may be present yet impossible to detect on the plain film. If it is unilateral, there may be asymmetry in vessel size between the two lungs; if patchy, there may be evidence of uneven perfusion (*Figure 313*). Post-stenotic dilatations are occasionally seen. The pulmonary trunk is small if it contains a stenosis, but is dilated with pulmonary hypertension.

CHAPTER 25

Mitral Obstruction and Regurgitation

INTRODUCTION

The following lesions are described.

(1) Mitral stenosis.
(2) Mitral regurgitation.
(3) Mitral and aortic valve disease.
(4) Mitral and tricuspid valve disease.
(5) Triple valve disease.
(6) Left atrial and pulmonary venous obstruction.

Radiological signs which may occur are:

(1) Cardiac enlargement involving one or both ventricles.
(2) Left atrial enlargement.
(3) Enlargement of the left atrial appendix.
(4) Calcification of the mitral valve.
(5) Calcification of the left atrium.
(6) Upper zone vessel dilatation.
(7) Interstitial oedema.
(8) Alveolar oedema.
(9) Haemosiderosis.
(10) Pulmonary ossific nodules.
(11) Segmental vessel narrowing.
(12) Dilatation of the pulmonary trunk and lobar arteries.

The correlation of some of these signs with the haemodynamics is given in Appendix C.

MITRAL STENOSIS

Mitral stenosis presenting in infancy or early childhood is due to a congenital lesion. As the valve takes many years to stenose after rheumatic fever, symptoms of rheumatic mitral stenosis are rare before adolescence except in the Orient, where the disease takes a more severe form and cases are encountered in children. Congenital mitral stenosis may be an isolated anomaly but is more often associated with other defects, particularly left-sided obstructive lesions, ventricular septal defect and ductus arteriosus. The obstructive lesions include aortic stenosis, aortic atresia and coarctation; they tend to augment the pulmonary venous hypertension. Shone *et al.* (1963) described the combination of parachute mitral valve with a single papillary muscle, supravalvar mitral stenosis, sub-aortic stenosis and coarctation. With a ventricular septal defect or ductus arteriosus, the increased pulmonary flow combined with the pulmonary venous hypertension results in severe arterial pulmonary hypertension. Shunt reversal may occur if the mitral obstruction is severe and the defect large. Mitral stenosis and atrial septal defect (Lutembacher's syndrome—*see* page 144) may coexist, but in this situation the mitral lesion is usually rheumatic.

Mitral obstruction in the adult is rheumatic in origin except for the rare case of atrial myxoma. Following an attack of rheumatic endocarditis, it is probable that the valve becomes progressively narrowed over a long period of time, rarely less than ten years and usually twenty or even thirty years. Fusion occurs at the two concentrations of chordae termed by Brock the critical areas of tendon insertion, which lie 2·5 cm apart on either side of the central orifice. Mild mitral stenosis is present when the opening is about 2·5 × 1·5 cm; a loud first heart sound and an opening snap may be heard, but there are usually no symptoms. Moderate stenosis implies an orifice size of 1·75–1·5 × 0·9–0·75 cm. The mean left atrial pressure is around 10 mm Hg, rising sharply to 30 mm Hg or more on exercise. In addition to the commissure fusion, the cusps and chordae may be fibrosed, thickened and contracted. The cusps are held downwards so that the valve orifice becomes funnel-shaped. Varying degrees of mobility are retained, but in the later stages calcification is common, particularly in the commissures, and is associated with distortion and rigidity of the cusps. The obstruction, together with rheumatic involvement of the atrial wall, causes dilatation of the left atrium which may be slight or moderate but is rarely gross in the absence of regurgitation. The atrial appendix is enlarged and is frequently the site of thrombus formation, especially with atrial fibrillation. Thrombus may also form within the left atrial chamber. Calcification in the left atrium may lie in the wall or in thrombus.

Mitral stenosis produces a pressure load on the left atrium and ultimately on the right ventricle. The primary effect on the circulation is elevation of the left atrial pressure so that a gradient exists between the left atrium and the left ventricle in diastole. When the stenosis is severe, the gradient persists throughout a long diastole, but in mild stenosis it may be present only during the initial phase of rapid ventricular filling or the second phase of rapid flow in late diastole during atrial contraction. Assessment of gradient measurements should always take into account the forward flow, since alterations in flow markedly affect the pressure difference across the stenotic valve. Thus with moderate stenosis the left atrial pressure may be normal at rest but rise abruptly with the increased flow produced by exercise. The heart rate should also be taken into account as the gradient may be present in a short diastole but disappear at the end of a long diastole.

The high left atrial pressure is transmitted to the pulmonary veins and causes a passive rise in the pulmonary arterial pressure. Interstitial oedema occurs when the pressure exceeds the plasma osmotic pressure of 25 mm Hg. An increase in the pulmonary vascular resistance is common with severe stenosis and is due to a combination of vasoconstriction and organic changes in the muscular arteries and arterioles.

Under certain circumstances mitral stenosis has to be differentiated from other causes of left atrial and pulmonary venous obstruction (*see* page 238).

Radiology

In mitral stenosis the heart as a whole may be normal in size, particularly when judged on the anterior view alone (*Figure 314*). However, when assessed on volume measurement, which takes into account the depth of the heart and hence also the left atrial enlargement, it is enlarged in the majority of cases. On these criteria, a completely normal-sized heart is seen in only 10 per cent of patients with critical mitral stenosis. Some correlation probably exists between the size of the heart and the severity of the obstruction in that no patient was encountered with a normal-sized heart and a resting pulmonary venous pressure over 20 mm Hg. The heart is enlarged in older patients and in those with long-standing atrial fibrillation or a high pulmonary vascular resistance.

Left atrial enlargement (*see* page 16 and *Figures 22–27*) is the best known and most obvious sign. The diagnosis of mitral stenosis is, however, a clinical one, and the function of the radiograph is to give help in assessing the severity of the obstruction. It is therefore superfluous for the radiologist to be requested to confirm or exclude left atrial enlargement in order to make the diagnosis except in the very rare patient presenting with severe pulmonary hypertension and inaudible mitral murmurs due to low cardiac output. Left atrial enlargement may be undetectable with mild stenosis, but is absent in only 2 per cent of patients with significant obstruction. In some patients, enlargement of the appendix may be the only clue. Enlargement of the atrium may be slight (62 per cent) or moderate (36 per cent), but is rarely gross in the absence of regurgitation. The degree of enlargement shows no correlation with the severity of the obstruction as judged by the pulmonary venous pressure. Rather surprisingly, the incidence of slight or moderate left atrial enlargement is roughly the same whether the resistance is normal, moderately or greatly raised.

Calcification may be seen in the valve or in the left atrium (*see* pages 59 and 53).

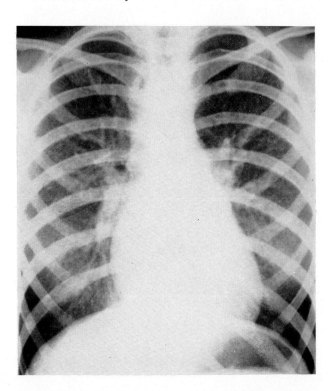

Figure 314. Typical mitral stenosis showing large left atrial appendix and upper zone vessel dilatation

If left atrial enlargement is an unimportant factor in assessing the severity of the obstruction, signs of pulmonary venous hypertension are all important (*see* page 84). Mitral stenosis is rarely severe enough to warrant valvotomy if there is no upper zone vessel dilatation. The only qualification to this statement is where there is lung disease with vascular obliteration in the upper lobes. Upper zone vessel dilatation may be absent in about 6 per cent (Simon, 1972), but this finding is always an indication for reviewing the clinical and haemodynamic data critically before recommending surgery. The correlation between the degree of upper zone vessel dilatation and the pulmonary venous pressure is strong. While with normal pressures at rest the dilatation is slight in about 75 per cent and obvious in 25 per cent, with pulmonary venous hypertension up to 19 mm Hg the incidence changes to 50 per cent slight and 50 per cent obvious, and over 19 mm Hg it is 10 per cent slight and 90 per cent obvious.

Interstitial oedema (*see* page 86 and *Figures 121–127*) is commonly found in mitral stenosis and is a clear indication of severe obstruction and of a raised resting pulmonary venous pressure. Oedema is present in 30 per cent of patients with a pressure up to 19 mm Hg and in 70 per cent of patients with a pressure over 19 mm Hg. Horizontal basal septal lines (Kerley B lines) are the commonest manifestation, and are seen more often and more obviously in mitral stenosis than in the other causes of pulmonary venous hypertension. Other short deep septal lines are also seen, but the long A lines are rare and occur only with severe long-standing obstruction. The lines are usually persistent unless caused by a transient episode of dysrhythmia, especially uncontrolled atrial fibrillation. Other more florid signs such as mottling, hilar oedema and pleural effusions may then develop, but these disappear with medical treatment. Alveolar oedema occurs early in the disease before an increase in pulmonary vascular resistance with its accompanying pericapillary fibrosis, and is classically seen, one hopes with increasing rarity, in pregnancy. Pulmonary haemosiderosis and ossific nodules are other signs of long-standing venous hypertension and more commonly result from mitral stenosis than from any other cause.

Mitral stenosis may be complicated by a raised pulmonary vascular resistance, and a fairly accurate prediction can usually be achieved from the radiograph. The signs in order of appearance are (1) narrowing of the lower lobe segmental arteries, (2) dilatation of the pulmonary trunk, (3) dilatation of the lower lobar arteries (pars interlobaris—*see* page 70), and (4) narrowing of the middle and upper segmental arteries (*see Figure 131*). Tables 10 and 11 give the incidence of these signs and the probabilities of the prediction being accurate in 150 cases of chronic mitral valve disease.

TABLE 10

Incidence of Positive Signs at Various Levels of Pulmonary Vascular Resistance

	PVR		
	< 3	*3–9*	*> 9*
Narrow lower segmental arteries	5%	50%	100%
Dilated pulmonary trunk	5%	65%	85%
Dilated lower lobar arteries	0	45%	100%
Narrow mid and upper segmental arteries	0	0	5%

TABLE 11

Probabilities of Correct Prediction of Pulmonary Vascular Resistance from Radiological Signs

	PVR		
	< 3	*3–9*	*> 9*
Narrow lower segmental arteries:			
Slight	10%	40%	50%
Obvious	0	50%	50%
Dilated pulmonary trunk:			
Slight	10%	70%	20%
Obvious	0	0	100%
Dilated lower lobar arteries	0	40%	60%
Narrow mid and upper segmental arteries	0	0	100%

One should therefore be able correctly to predict a rise in vascular resistance in 9 out of 10 cases, but the degree of rise may be more difficult to assess, particularly if pulmonary trunk dilatation is only slight. Narrowing of the middle and upper segmental arteries is rare and, in practice, occurs only in patients with extreme elevation of the pulmonary vascular resistance and very obvious clinical pulmonary hypertension: the problem may then be more one of detecting mitral stenosis as the underlying cause if the left atrium is small.

It has been stated (Kerley, 1972) that interstitial oedema tends to lessen or disappear with a high vascular resistance. In the authors' experience this is not so. Eighty per cent of patients with severe mitral stenosis and a resistance over 9 units had oedema, compared with 60 per cent with a resistance from 3 to 9 units and 20 per cent with a normal resistance. Figures were not available in patients with resistances greater than 15 units, but quite possibly the statement may hold good for this rather rare group.

MITRAL REGURGITATION

Mitral regurgitation has many causes, which include those listed below.
   (1) Congenital isolated valve abnormality.
   (2) Cleft anterior cusp with atrio-ventricular defects (*see* page 143).
   (3) Rheumatic valve disease.
   (4) Bacterial endocarditis.

(5) Prolapsed mitral cusp (late systolic murmur, mid-systole click), including 'floppy valve syndrome', Marfan's syndrome (*see* page 119), Ehlers–Danlos syndrome (*see* page 126), mucopolysaccharidoses (*see* page 116), osteogenesis imperfecta (*see* page 126).

(6) Ruptured chordae (spontaneous, bacterial endocarditis, rheumatic valve disease).

(7) Ischaemic heart disease (papillary muscle dysfunction or rupture—*see* page 259).

(8) Cardiomyopathy (*see* Chapter 28).

(9) Annular subvalvar aneurysm (*see* page 279).

(10) Corrected transposition (left-sided tricuspid regurgitation with or without Ebstein's anomaly).

(11) Left atrial myxoma (*see* page 281).

(12) Functional, associated with left ventricular dilatation from any cause.

Mitral regurgitation may result from functional or anatomical disturbances of the cusps, the chordae, the papillary muscles or the ring. Congenital mitral regurgitation is usually due to cusp abnormality (clefts, accessory or deficient cusp tissue, double mitral orifice), but may also result from abnormal chordae and papillary muscles. The commonest anomaly is a cleft anterior cusp of the mitral valve in association with an ostium primum atrial septal defect. Regurgitation in rheumatic heart disease is largely due to cusp retraction, but chordal rupture also occurs. In the floppy valve syndrome the posterior cusp is usually involved; the cusps and chordae are stretched, and the cusp balloons into the left atrium in systole. The mitral valve may be competent, and if regurgitation occurs it is usually slight. The condition is benign except in the Marfan syndrome, when regurgitation may be progressive. Prolapse of the posterior cusp may be associated with secundum atrial septal defect, and when mitral regurgitation is present the diagnosis of an ostium primum may be made in error (McDonald *et al.*, 1971). Both conditions show a left axis on the electrocardiogram. Familial cases have been reported (Shell *et al.*, 1969). The characteristic signs are a mid-systolic click and a late systolic murmur. A few patients have chest pain and an electrocardiogram suggesting postero-inferior myocardial ischaemia without coronary atheroma (Barlow *et al.*, 1968); dysrhythmias and sudden death are occasional complications, and subacute bacterial endocarditis may occur. Functional mitral regurgitation from left ventricular dilatation is thought to be due to an abnormal angle of pull and stretching of the papillary muscles more than dilatation of the ring.

Regurgitation may be mild or severe, acute or chronic. There is a volume and pressure load on the left ventricle and left atrium and, in severe regurgitation, a pressure load on the right ventricle. The left atrial pressure is raised intermittently due to transmission of the systolic pressure wave (V wave) of the ventricle to the atrium coinciding with atrial filling from the pulmonary veins. Although the severity of the regurgitation is approximately reflected in the mean left atrial pressure and the height of the V wave, this is often modified by other factors, especially the size and compliance of the left atrium. With a large compliant atrium, the mean pressure and the V wave may be normal in the presence of severe regurgitation; conversely, they may be significantly raised with only moderate regurgitation if the atrium is small and non-compliant. As a general guide, usually the atrium is large and its mean pressure is normal or only slightly raised in chronic rheumatic regurgitation, whereas the atrium is small and its mean pressure is high in the initial period after the onset of acute regurgitation such as occurs with chordal rupture or papillary muscle dysfunction. Thus pulmonary hypertension is seen less frequently in chronic regurgitation than in mitral stenosis, but is the rule in acute regurgitation. Similarly, the pulmonary vascular resistance remains low until late in the disease compared with mitral stenosis, but in long-standing severe cases it is frequently raised. Thus in a series of 80 patients with severe lesions, the incidence and severity of pulmonary vascular disease in dominant stenosis and dominant regurgitation was approximately equal at 60 per cent of cases, of whom 20 per cent had a resistance of over 10 units. Combined stenosis and regurgitation is always due to rheumatic endocarditis except for myxoma and rare anomalies such as the parachute deformity. There is a combination of commissure fusion, fibrous contracture of the cusps and calcification, each of these tending to render the cusps more rigid and to prevent their closing in systole. Retraction of the posterior cusp is particularly common. The subvalvar apparatus may be affected, and chordal rupture is an occasional complication.

Radiology

In mild regurgitation from any cause, the heart is normal in size. Moderate or severe regurgitation is rare with a normal-sized heart except when the onset is acute (*Figure 315*). If the regurgitation is chronic and other lesions, particularly left ventricular disease, can be excluded, the size of the heart is a reasonably reliable guide to the severity of the regurgitation. In chronic regurgitation there is no correlation between heart size and pulmonary venous pressure, but patients with a raised pulmonary vascular

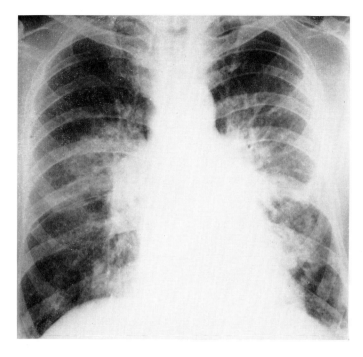

Figure 315. Acute mitral regurgitation—slight cardiac enlargement, obvious pulmonary oedema

resistance have, with rare exceptions, at least moderate cardiac enlargement. The shape of the ventricular border on the anterior view may suggest left ventricular rather than right ventricular enlargement, but it is usually less characteristic than with aortic valve disease or other causes of left ventricular enlargement. Left atrial dilatation is usually obvious, but in rheumatic heart disease the atrial size is related as much to wall disease and length of the history as to severity of regurgitation (*Figure 316*).

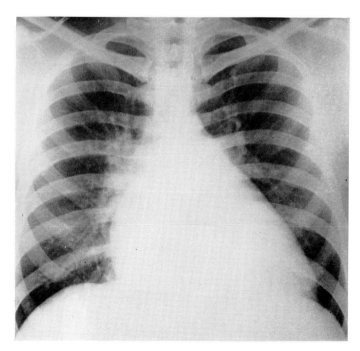

Figure 316. Chronic mitral regurgitation. Left atrium large relative to lung changes

Gross enlargement or aneurysmal left atrium is typically seen with severe chronic rheumatic regurgitation associated with some stenosis (*see Figure 27*). In chronic regurgitation there is no correlation between the size of the atrium and the mean pulmonary venous pressure.

Calcification may be seen in the mitral valve, left atrium or pericardium (*see* pages 59, 53 and 55).

The lung changes are less obvious in mitral regurgitation than in mitral stenosis of comparable severity, excepting again the acute variety in which they are a prominent feature. This is reflected in a significantly lower incidence of upper zone vessel dilatation in patients with a normal resting pulmonary venous pressure. When the pressure is raised, however, the correlation is similar to that seen in mitral stenosis except that the dilatation is less marked at a comparable pressure. Obvious upper zone vessel dilatation is a reliable sign of severe regurgitation with left ventricular failure.

Interstitial oedema is rarely chronic and is seen following the onset of acute regurgitation or with progressive left ventricular failure (*see Figure 315*). Septal lines at the bases are not so obvious compared with other signs such as deep lines, mottling, hilar oedema and parietal effusions. A high pulmonary vascular resistance is uncommon with chronic regurgitation and occurs only if the condition is long-standing and severe. With acute regurgitation the vascular resistance rises rapidly, but this change is not initially accompanied by radiological signs. Where present, the pulmonary changes are similar to those of mitral stenosis, and a prediction of the resistance can be made with a comparable degree of accuracy.

With combined stenosis and regurgitation, the heart is enlarged and left atrial dilatation is obvious. It is sometimes possible to detect that the left ventricle is enlarged from the shape of the left border, but the relative size of each ventricle cannot be determined. It is usually impossible to judge from the chest radiograph which lesion is dominant, but in patients with clinically mixed lesions, dominant stenosis is suggested by a small heart and left atrium relative to the severity of the lung changes (*see Figure 314*), as opposed to dominant regurgitation which is more likely when the heart and left atrium are large and the lung changes are only slight (*see Figure 316*). This is borne out by the figures in Table 12.

TABLE 12

	Dominant stenosis	Dominant regurgitation
Incidence of cardiac enlargement +2 or more	25%	80%
Left atrial enlargement +2 or more	35%	85%
Obvious upper zone vessel dilatation	60%	40%
Interstitial oedema	50%	10%

Mitral valve calcification is very common, and left atrial calcification is more frequently found in combined than in pure lesions. Aneurysmal dilatation of the left atrium is typically associated with a mixed lesion, usually with dominant regurgitation, but has been reported in pure stenosis (*see Figure 27*).

MITRAL AND AORTIC VALVE DISEASE

When more than one valve is affected by rheumatic fever, the commonest combination is that of mitral and aortic valve disease. The mitral valve is often dominantly stenotic and the aortic valve mainly regurgitant. One lesion may mask the other.

Mitral stenosis may mask the auscultatory and electrocardiographic clues to aortic valve disease because of low cardiac output. The ascending aorta is small in mitral stenosis, and any prominence suggests additional aortic valve disease. Calcification of the aortic valve is rare in the presence of an important mitral lesion. A diastolic murmur at the base of the heart in a patient with mitral stenosis is usually due to aortic regurgitation, as the Graham Steell murmur of pulmonary regurgitation occurs only with severe pulmonary hypertension and dilatation of the pulmonary trunk.

Signs of mitral valve disease may also be hidden by important aortic valve disease. A mitral lesion additional to aortic valve disease is suggested by dilatation of the atrial appendix, by more than slight dilatation of the body of the left atrium, by absence of aortic valve calcification with dominant aortic stenosis, and by signs of pulmonary venous hypertension with only moderate aortic valve disease. A mid-diastolic murmur (Austin Flint murmur) may be heard in the mitral area with severe aortic regurgitation and is due to vibration of the anterior mitral cusp between the diastolic inflow from the aorta and the left atrium. The anterior cusp of the mitral valve may be damaged by an aortic regurgitant jet, particularly if infected, and cause secondary mitral regurgitation and left atrial dilatation.

MITRAL AND TRICUSPID VALVE DISEASE

Rheumatic mitral disease may be accompanied by tricuspid valve involvement with regurgitation or stenosis or a combination of both. Regurgitation alone is usually functional, and is assumed to be so when the pulmonary vascular resistance is raised and when the signs disappear with medical treatment. The right ventricle is enlarged, causing dilatation of the tricuspid ring, but the cusps themselves are normal. Organic tricuspid regurgitation is usually associated with mitral regurgitation, the pulmonary vascular resistance is often normal, and signs of tricuspid regurgitation do not disappear on medical treatment. Tricuspid stenosis is always organic, but in practice most organic tricuspid lesions are mixed. Regurgitation produces a volume load on the right ventricle and right atrium, while stenosis produces a pressure load on the right atrium.

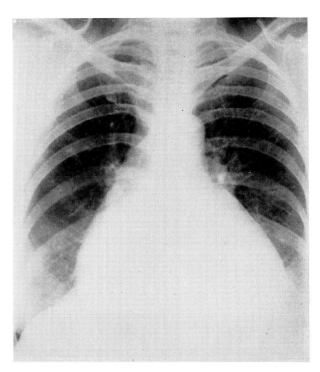

Figure 317. Mitral stenosis with tricuspid stenosis. The signs of pulmonary venous hypertension are masked

The heart is always considerably enlarged, but the specific confirmation or exclusion of tricuspid disease is difficult from the radiograph alone. Definite prominence of the right heart border, extending upwards and continuous with the superior vena cava, and dilatation of the azygos vein are suggestive signs and, when obvious and persistent, usually indicate organic tricuspid involvement (*see Figures 11* and *19*).

The importance of organic tricuspid disease associated with mitral disease is that the lung changes of mitral disease may be masked (*Figure 317*). Important mitral stenosis and/or regurgitation may be present with lungs which show little or no upper zone vessel dilatation and no interstitial oedema.

TRIPLE VALVE DISEASE

The picture is a variable combination of the signs of mitral, aortic and tricuspid valve disease, depending on the severity of each. One of the three lesions is easily missed, but triple valve disease should be suspected if there is a large heart with evidence of four chamber enlargement and severe lung changes.

LEFT ATRIAL AND PULMONARY VENOUS OBSTRUCTION

Left atrial myxoma, cor triatriatum and veno-occlusive disease obstruct the flow of blood into the left heart and must be distinguished from mitral valve stenosis. Rare cases of venous obstruction from mediastinitis, tumour, thrombosis and congenital stenosis (Hudson, 1970) have been described. Obstructed total anomalous pulmonary venous drainage is described on page 202.

Left atrial myxoma

Myxomas are discussed on page 281. The following radiological features, if present, suggest the diagnosis.
(1) Absence of left atrial enlargement with clinically obvious obstruction.
(2) Variable interstitial oedema without obvious cause such as dysrhythmia.
(3) Changes suggesting a rapid rise of pulmonary vascular resistance.
(4) Calcification in the left atrium distinguishable from calcium in the wall, in thrombus and in the mitral valve cusps or ring.

Cor triatriatum

Cor triatriatum is a rare congenital anomaly resulting from incomplete fusion of the common pulmonary vein with the left atrium. A perforated muscular membrane separates the atrium into upper and lower chambers. The pulmonary veins enter the upper chamber, while the lower chamber communicates with the appendix and the mitral valve. The size of the orifice in the membrane determines the degree of obstruction.

Cor triatriatum may be associated with atrial septal defect or with hemi-anomalous pulmonary venous drainage, either of which may dominate the clinical picture and mask the atrial obstruction (Somerville, 1966).

Physiologically the lesion exactly simulates mitral stenosis, but the clue to the diagnosis lies in the radiograph which, in a symptomatic patient, shows signs of pulmonary venous and often arterial hypertension in the absence of any clinical evidence of mitral or left ventricular disease. The left atrium may not be enlarged. An unusual type of obstruction should then be suspected, but pulmonary venous obstruction due to anomalous drainage, mediastinal fibrosis, tumour infiltration or veno-occlusive disease may present in a similar way.

Veno-occlusive disease

Veno-occlusive disease is a condition of unknown cause in which there is thrombosis and thickening of the small intrapulmonary veins, leading to severe chronic pulmonary venous and arterial hypertension. There is dyspnoea due to pulmonary oedema, signs of pulmonary hypertension are present, and death occurs in congestive failure. The chest radiograph shows widespread interstitial oedema. The heart enlarges with marked dilatation of the pulmonary trunk but without left atrial dilatation.

SURGERY IN MITRAL VALVE DISEASE

After a successful valvotomy, repair or valve replacement, the heart usually shows some reduction in size unless irreversible myocardial changes have occurred such as those seen in the elderly, in long-standing disease with a very high pulmonary vascular resistance, or in chronic left ventricular failure. The reduction is least in pure mitral stenosis and may not occur at all in hearts which were only slightly enlarged, whereas it may be spectacular in pure or dominant mitral regurgitation (*Figures 318* and *319*). The left atrium also becomes smaller, roughly paralleling the change in heart size, but its size may be unaltered in atrial fibrillation and with severe rheumatic involvement of the atrial wall. The upper zone vessels show a reduction in calibre (*Figures 318* and *319*) but rarely return to normal except in mitral stenosis with normal pulmonary vascular resistance and in acute mitral regurgitation.

In patients with a high pulmonary vascular resistance, the dilated pulmonary trunk often returns to normal and is an excellent guide to successful surgery (*Figures 318* and *319*). Dilatation of upper zone vessels decreases, but return to normality is exceptional; lower zone narrowing rarely alters as the vascular changes here are largely irreversible. Whereas these alterations in vessel size may continue for weeks or months, interstitial oedema disappears quickly, often in a matter of days. Septal lines may occasionally persist from haemosiderin deposition in the interlobular septa, but they become thinner and better defined.

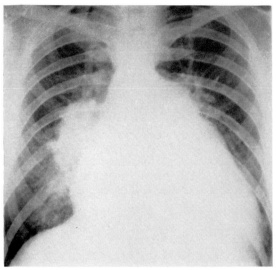
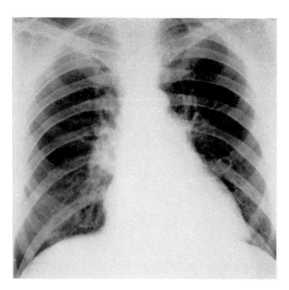

Figure 318. Mitral stenosis and regurgitation with pulmonary hypertension, pre-operative

Figure 319. Same patient after valve replacement. Excellent result

In summary, the best guide to a drop in pulmonary venous pressure after operation is a reduction in the size of the left atrium and upper zone vessels and resolution of interstitial oedema. Decrease in pulmonary vascular resistance is reflected by a reduction in the size of the pulmonary trunk, but other vascular changes are unspectacular, and an abnormal pattern after operation does not necessarily reflect continuing pulmonary hypertension. There is evidence that homograft replacement of the mitral valve leads to more frequent reduction in the size of upper zone vessels than Starr valve replacement and closed mitral valvotomy (Salzmann *et al.*, 1972). This is presumed to be a result of the small gradient across a Starr valve and of some residual obstruction and regurgitation commonly remaining after closed mitral valvotomy. Post-operative pulmonary hypertension may be due to continuing regurgitation or stenosis, or to irreversible myocardial damage (from the disease or during surgery).

CHAPTER 26

Aortic Obstruction and Regurgitation

INTRODUCTION

The following lesions are described.
1. Aortic valve stenosis.
2. Subvalvar stenosis.
3. Supravalvar stenosis.
4. Aortic regurgitation.
5. Aortic stenosis and regurgitation.
6. Coarctation of the aorta.

Radiological signs which may occur are:
1. Left ventricular enlargement due to hypertrophy and/or dilatation.
2. Aortic dilatation.
3. An abnormal aortic knuckle and rib notching in coarctation.
4. Aortic valve calcification.
5. Left atrial enlargement.
6. Pulmonary venous hypertension with interstitial and rarely alveolar oedema.
7. Signs of raised pulmonary vascular resistance (rare).

AORTIC VALVE STENOSIS

Isolated aortic valve stenosis is congenital in origin in over 90 per cent of cases and takes two forms. In the first there is congenital fusion of valve cusps with a stenotic orifice, and patients usually present in infancy or childhood with left ventricular obstruction. The valve is bicuspid with commissure fusion and a slit-like orifice or monocuspid with a central or eccentric orifice. In infantile cases particularly, the valve may be very thick and rigid, causing severe obstruction and left ventricular failure. In childhood the valve is usually mobile, but a few cases present with complex obstruction, which may include supravalvar and subvalvar stenosis in addition to a thickened myxomatous valve (Somerville and Ross, 1971). The valve is characteristically thick in Turner's syndrome.

In the second type of isolated congenital aortic valve stenosis a bicuspid valve, initially non-obstructive, undergoes gradual commissure fusion with calcification, and obstruction is delayed until adult life. A raphe representing the third fused commissure is present in about half the cases and commonly calcifies. A bicuspid valve may become regurgitant due to cusp stretching or endocarditis (*Figure 320*). When a bicuspid valve is associated with coarctation, aortic stenosis may occur earlier and may become manifest after repair of the coarctation. Congenital aortic stenosis may also be associated with ductus arteriosus, ventricular septal defect or pulmonary valve stenosis. When the aortic ring is underdeveloped, aortic stenosis may be part of the hypoplastic left heart syndrome, which includes aortic hypoplasia or atresia and other left-sided obstructive lesions. Isolated pure aortic stenosis of rheumatic origin is rare since regurgitation is usually present. Aortic stenosis due to sclerosis of the valve in the elderly is very occasionally seen. Aortic valve calcification is laid down in the ring and bases of the cusps, which become splinted to cause obstruction; spread of calcification into the anterior mitral cusp or ventricular septum may occur. Subvalvar mitral calcification may also be present (*see* page 61).

In aortic valve stenosis the critical orifice size in an average adult is 0·6 cm², but values up to 1 cm² may produce significant pressure gradients at ordinary rates of flow. The obstruction imposes a pressure load on the left ventricle, which is hypertrophied, but in the absence of failure or regurgitation is not dilated.

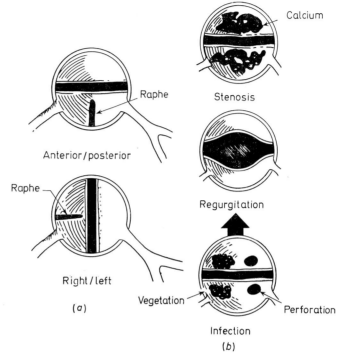

Figure 320. Bicuspid aortic valve. (a) Location of cusps. (b) Complications

Atrial contraction is forceful and is reflected in a large left atrial A wave. If the ventricle fails, there is a sustained increase in end-diastolic pressure which is transmitted to the left atrium and pulmonary veins. The pulmonary arterial pressure rises passively, but an increase in the pulmonary vascular resistance is rare. Post-stenotic dilatation of the ascending aorta is invariably present, but appears to depend more on the duration than on the severity of the obstruction.

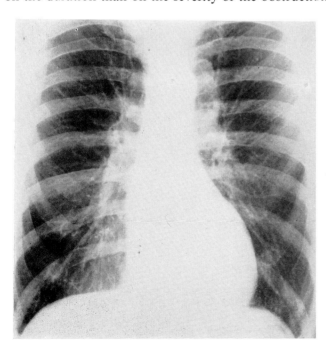

Figure 321. Aortic valve stenosis. Normal heart size, but shape suggesting left ventricular enlargement

Radiology

In aortic valve stenosis, the heart is never more than slightly enlarged unless there is regurgitation, left ventricular failure or another lesion. However, even with a normal-sized heart the shape of the left border is often more rounded or longer than normal with a low apex—a shape characteristic of left ventricular enlargement (*Figure 321*). Post-stenotic dilatation of the aorta is seen as a localized bulge to the right above the right atrium (*Figure 322*). In children, this sign is useful but not always present;

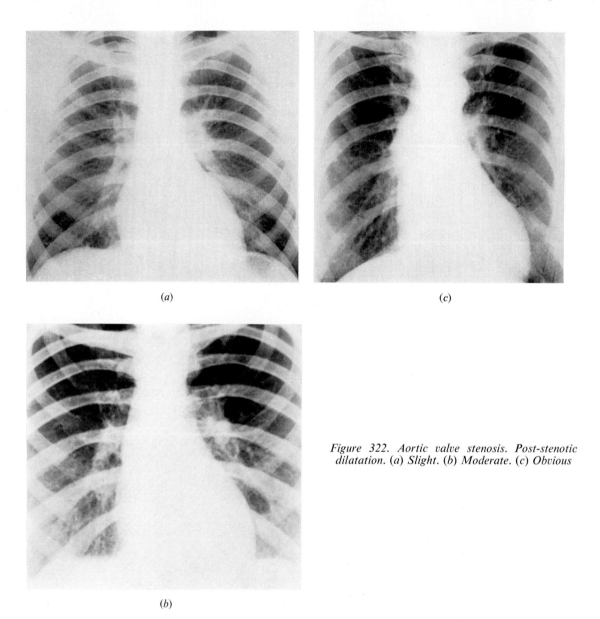

(a)

(c)

(b)

Figure 322. Aortic valve stenosis. Post-stenotic dilatation. (a) Slight. (b) Moderate. (c) Obvious

the aorta may displace the superior vena cava outwards, so that the border is still prominent but has a straight margin and is not so opaque as the aorta (*Figure 323*). In adults, post-stenotic dilatation becomes increasingly difficult to evaluate with advancing age as it may be impossible to differentiate dilatation from elongation. Calcification of the valve (*see* page 57) is almost invariable in males over the age of 40 years, and indeed in this age group the diagnosis is barely tenable if calcification cannot be detected on fluoroscopy. In females, calcification is less common. Obvious calcification under the age of 60 years is an indication that the stenosis is severe (Batson *et al.*, 1972), but over 60 years of age the calcification may be severe with mild obstruction.

The left atrium may show a minor degree of enlargement as a result of the increased pressure needed to fill the hypertrophied and incompliant left ventricle. Left atrial dilatation is more obvious when the end-diastolic pressure is raised, but the heart is then also enlarged and there are signs of pulmonary venous hypertension. With any degree of left atrial enlargement, associated mitral valve disease should be suspected; if the atrial appendix is enlarged, it is almost certain.

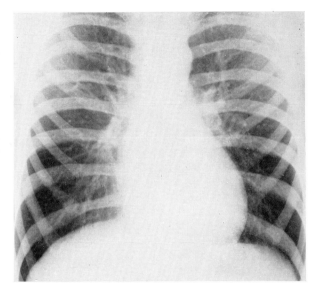

Figure 323. Aortic valve stenosis. Superior vena cava displaced laterally by post-stenotic dilatation of the aorta

SUBVALVAR STENOSIS

In subvalvar aortic stenosis, there is obstruction in the left ventricular outflow below the aortic valve which may be due to:

    (1) A diaphragm.
    (2) A fibro-muscular ring.
    (3) Muscle hypertrophy (hypertrophic cardiomyopathy—*see* pages 264 and 268.
    (4) A redundant anterior mitral cusp.

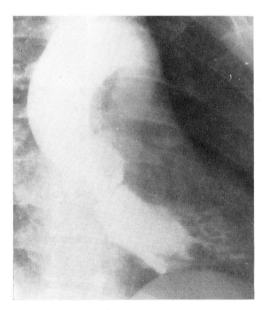

Figure 324. Subvalvar aortic stenosis. Left ventricular angiogram. Diaphragm immediately below the aortic valve

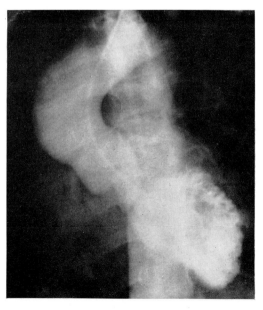

Figure 325. Subvalvar aortic stenosis. Left ventricular angiogram. Fibro-muscular ring 2 cm below the aortic valve

The diaphragm lies immediately below the aortic valve and may take the form of intercommissural webbing or a true diaphragm with a central or eccentric orifice (*Figure 324*). The diaphragm may be adherent to the underside of the cusps, which may be congenitally deformed. The fibro-muscular ring lies lower in the outflow, 1 cm or more below the valve (*Figure 325*). It may be adherent to the anterior cusp of the mitral valve and is occasionally associated with mitral regurgitation. The aortic valve cusps are thickened by the trauma of the ejection jet and, because of this, slight aortic regurgitation is almost

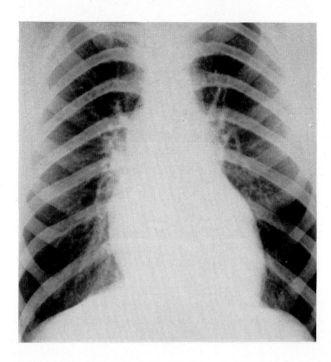

Figure 326. Subvalvar aortic stenosis. Cardiac enlargement and post-stenotic dilatation

invariable. Sub-aortic stenosis is usually an isolated lesion but may be associated with coarctation, with parachute mitral valve and supravalvar ring of the left atrium (Shone *et al.*, 1963), with aortic valve stenosis or with ductus arteriosus. A redundant anterior mitral cusp is a rare deformity in which billowing folds of a large cusp prolapse into the left ventricular outflow in systole, causing obstruction. All types of subvalvar stenosis produce a pressure load on the left ventricle, and any regurgitation causes a volume load in addition. Because the obstruction dates from birth, the left ventricle usually shows severe hypertrophy which on angiocardiography closely resembles hypertrophic cardiomyopathy. It is therefore essential not to miss a fixed subvalvar stenosis which is surgically correctable.

Subvalvar aortic stenosis can rarely be differentiated from valve stenosis on the plain film. The heart is often enlarged because of massive hypertrophy combined with slight regurgitation (*Figure 326*), whereas it is usually normal in valve stenosis. Post-stenotic dilatation of the ascending aorta is seen in both cases (*Figure 326*). As most cases of subvalvar stenosis present in childhood and adolescence, absence of valve calcification is of no significance. The most important differentiating point is a clinical one, namely the absence of an aortic ejection click.

SUPRAVALVAR STENOSIS

Supravalvar aortic stenosis is a narrowing of the ascending aorta beginning at the supravalvar ring at the superior margin of the aortic sinuses. There are three types.

Hour-glass type: a localized obstruction of the supravalvar ring due to overgrowth of the media (*Figure 327*).

Membranous type: an obstructing diaphragm with a small opening.

Hypoplastic type: a long narrow segment of the ascending aorta above the sinuses.

244

In the hour-glass type, which is commonest, there may be some hypoplasia of the rest of the aorta. The aortic cusps may be adherent to the supravalvar ring, and occasionally they are grossly diseased (Somerville and Ross, 1971). The coronary arteries, being proximal to the obstruction, are typically dilated and tortuous.

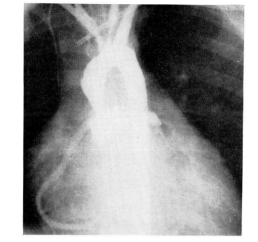

Figure 327. Supravalvar aortic stenosis. Left ventricular angiogram

Supravalvar aortic stenosis may be combined with pulmonary artery stenosis, an association often termed the 'supravalvar aortic stenosis syndrome'. The syndrome may occasionally be more extensive and include pulmonary valve stenosis, aortic valve disease, coarctation, stenosis of the major thoracic and abdominal aortic branches and hypoplasia of the thoracic and abdominal aorta (Ottesen *et al.*, 1966), ventricular septal defect and ductus arteriosus. The syndrome includes different clinical groups (Logan *et al.*, 1965):

(1) Non-familial sporadic—normal face and intelligence.
(2) Familial—normal face and intelligence.
(3) Abnormal face and mental retardation:
    (*a*) Infantile hypercalcaemia in some cases, and normal chromosomes.
    (*b*) Abnormal chromosomes.

Familial cases are genetically determined and evidence suggests that inheritance is by an autosomal dominant trait with variable expression; there is usually pulmonary artery stenosis as well. McDonald *et al.* (1969) reported a family with a 'macaroni arteriopathy' involving the aorta and the pulmonary arteries. The syndrome of 'elfin facies', mental deficiency, large ridged teeth and supravalvar aortic stenosis was first described by Williams *et al.* (1961). The full syndrome with pulmonary artery stenosis was later reported by Beuren *et al.* (1962). Black and Bonham-Carter (1963) and Garcia *et al.* (1964) demonstrated an association with severe infantile hypercalcaemia in some patients. Supravalvar aortic stenosis with pulmonary stenosis has been reported in rubella.

In supravalvar aortic stenosis the ascending aorta is usually hypoplastic and invisible on the plain film (*Figure 328*). No calcification is seen and the heart is normal or slightly enlarged. Pulmonary artery stenosis and pulmonary hypertension may complicate the picture.

AORTIC REGURGITATION

Aortic regurgitation may be due to the following causes.

Lesions of the aortic cusps

Rheumatic endocarditis, bacterial endocarditis, congenital malformation (isolated or with ventricular septal defect or Fallot's tetralogy), syphilis, ankylosing spondylitis, Reiter's disease, rheumatoid arthritis, mucopolysaccharidoses, spontaneous or traumatic rupture, degeneration in the elderly.

Disease of the aortic wall or valve ring causing dilatation and often aortic root aneurysm
Cystic medionecrosis, Marfan's syndrome, aortic dissection, syphilis, systemic hypertension.

Congenital anomalies of the aortic root
Aortic sinus aneurysm, aortic sinus fistula to left ventricle, aorto-left ventricular tunnel.

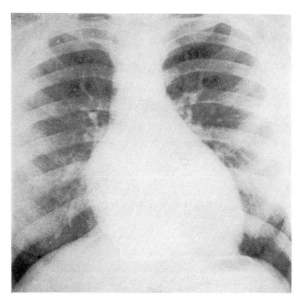

Figure 328. Supravalvar aortic stenosis. Invisible ascending aorta

Aortic regurgitation due to rheumatic heart disease is often associated with stenosis because commissure fusion occurs as well as retraction; either may be dominant. All the other causes listed above produce pure regurgitation of varying severity. Congenital regurgitation is usually due to a bicuspid valve whose cusps elongate or lack support. When associated with a ventricular septal defect (*see* page 153), aortic regurgitation is not congenital in the strict sense since it usually appears after infancy and is progressive; it is due to loss of support of the right coronary and sometimes non-coronary cusps. The right ventricular outflow may be narrowed by cusp prolapse through the ventricular septal defect, or there may be an associated infundibular stenosis. Regurgitation may occur in syphilitic aortitis without aneurysm. In cystic medionecrosis and Marfan's syndrome, regurgitation is due to stretching of the valve ring and may occur before an aneurysm is detectable on the plain film if the dilated aortic root lies entirely within the pericardium. Systemic hypertension may cause dilatation of the aortic root sufficient to cause regurgitation, but this is only seen with any frequency in West Indians.

Aneurysm of an aortic sinus may cause regurgitation before rupture due to mechanical interference with valve closure. Rupture is not usually seen before early adult life. In contrast, aorto-left ventricular tunnel causes severe aortic regurgitation from birth, and surgical correction may be indicated early in life. The tunnel originates above the right coronary sinus, distinguishing it from sinus aneurysm and cusp prolapse, although in all three conditions the right sinus may be dilated. The tunnel typically has a dilated segment proximal to its entry into the ventricular cavity. Because it lies anterior to the aorta, it is best seen on aortography in the lateral projection.

Aortic regurgitation may be acute in bacterial endocarditis, cusp rupture, dissecting aneurysm and aortic sinus fistula, but otherwise it is chronic and usually well tolerated for years until left ventricular failure ensues. It imposes a volume load on the left ventricle, whose stroke volume is augmented by an increase in fibre length. The chamber dilates and there is an increase in muscle mass. With the onset of failure, further but inappropriate dilatation occurs, with elevation of the left ventricular end-diastolic pressure, and the situation may be aggravated by functional mitral regurgitation. The left atrial and pulmonary venous pressures are raised and there may ultimately be a rise in the pulmonary vascular resistance.

Radiology

In acute regurgitation such as follows bacterial endocarditis, the heart may take many months to

246

enlarge. In chronic regurgitation which is more than trivial, cardiac enlargement is almost invariable, particularly when assessed by volume measurement. The ventricle enlarges mainly downwards and may cause no increase in transverse diameter, but yet a significant increase in long axis diameter (*see Figure 11a*). The size of the heart provides a fairly reliable indication of the severity of the regurgitation, but is

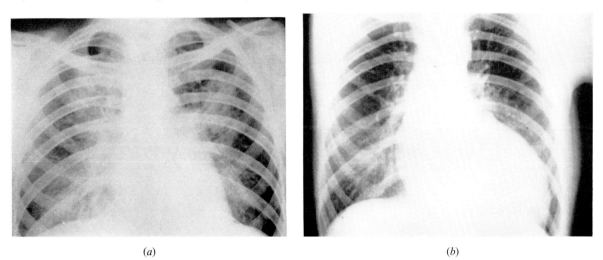

| (a) | (b) |

Figure 329. (a) Acute severe aortic regurgitation. Minor cardiac enlargement. Pulmonary oedema. (b) Chronic aortic regurgitation. Major cardiac enlargement. Dilated aorta

also a reflection of its duration and of the efficiency of left ventricular contraction. Thus with acute severe regurgitation the heart may not be greatly enlarged (*Figure 329a*), but with a chronic lesion and a ventricle beginning to fail, a large heart may be present with only moderate regurgitation (*Figure 329b*). Slight dilatation of the left atrium may occur without failure due to increased resistance to left ventricular filling (*Figure 330*). It is also seen with left ventricular failure, but if left atrial enlargement is more

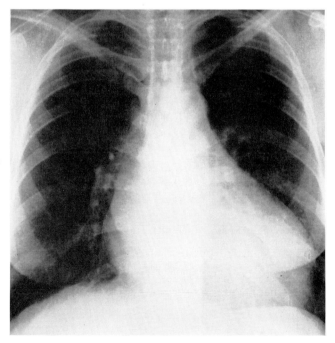

Figure 330. Aortic regurgitation. Minor left atrial dilatation

than slight, an additional mitral valve abnormality should be suspected. This may be due not only to separate organic mitral valve disease but to functional regurgitation or regurgitation due to a jet lesion on the anterior mitral cusp, especially if there is bacterial endocarditis of the aortic valve. A prominent appendix is particularly suggestive of rheumatic mitral valve disease.

Characteristically, dilatation of the ascending aorta is more diffuse than in aortic stenosis (*see Figure 329b*) and may even involve the aortic knuckle. The descending aorta is not dilated but may be elongated in association with systolic hypertension (*Figure 331*). The aorta may be normal in young patients with severe regurgitation who have a normal aortic wall. On the other hand, marked aortic dilatation in the young should suggest the possibility of a congenital anomaly of the aortic root or Marfan's syndrome, and in older patients cystic medionecrosis, syphilis or dissection. Dilatation of the ascending aorta is particularly prominent in young children with aorto-left ventricular tunnel and should suggest the diagnosis (*Figure 332*).

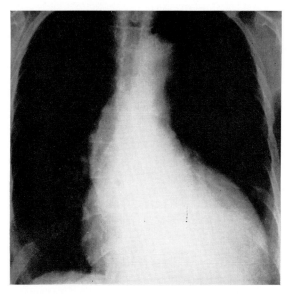

Figure 331. Aortic regurgitation. Elongation of descending aorta seen with systolic hypertension

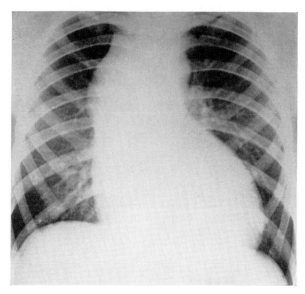

Figure 332. Aorto-left ventricular tunnel. Very large ascending aorta

Calcification of the valve is less common and less extensive with pure regurgitation than with stenosis. A few plaques are occasionally seen, but obvious calcification almost always means a mixed lesion with dominant stenosis.

AORTIC STENOSIS AND REGURGITATION

In combined aortic stenosis and regurgitation, the increased stroke volume resulting from regurgitation produces a higher systolic gradient than would be present with stenosis alone at a comparable orifice size. The high diastolic pressure gradient between the aorta and the left ventricle also allows a large volume of blood to regurgitate through a comparatively small orifice. Moderate mixed lesions therefore impose a considerable volume and pressure load on the left ventricle, which is always hypertrophied and dilated. Pulmonary venous hypertension and a raised pulmonary vascular resistance are more frequently encountered in mixed than in pure aortic lesions.

With mixed aortic stenosis and regurgitation in the absence of failure, cardiac enlargement is dependent on the relative importance of regurgitation and stenosis, the trend of which is shown in Table 13.

TABLE 13

	Heart volume		
	Normal	*Up to 700 ml/m²**	*Over 700 ml/m²*
Dominant stenosis	27%	63%	10%
Dominant regurgitation	2%	61%	37%
Mixed lesions	0	55%	45%

*Square metre body surface.

248

The figures must not be assumed to show the absolute incidence of the heart size in the various groups as this depends on the proportion of mild lesions included; in this particular group there were none. Calcification of the aortic valve is common when stenosis is dominant and rare when there is important regurgitation.

Mitral valve involvement with aortic valve disease is described on page 236.

SURGERY IN AORTIC VALVE DISEASE

Reduction in heart size after successful aortic valve replacement is usually greater than after mitral valve replacement except in pure aortic stenosis without much pre-operative cardiac enlargement. Signs of pulmonary venous hypertension disappear, but the aorta rarely changes. Persistent cardiac enlargement implies poor left ventricular function or regurgitation.

COARCTATION OF THE AORTA

Coarctation is a congenital narrowing of the aortic lumen in the region of the isthmus (the junction of the aortic arch and the descending thoracic aorta). Stenosis may occur distal to the isthmus in the thoracic or the abdominal aorta; the narrowing may be localized or diffuse, or occasionally at multiple sites. As many of these lesions are probably acquired, the term coarctation of the aorta is best reserved for isthmic narrowing.

Coarctation can be divided into two types.

Pre-ductal
Proximal to the ductus or the ligamentum arteriosum. Keith *et al.* (1967) found three variations:
(1) A localized constriction just above the ductus in 40 per cent; 16 per cent had other major defects.
(2) A narrowed segment from the left subclavian artery to the ductus in 40 per cent; 28 per cent had other major defects.
(3) A narrowing involving the aortic arch and extending to the ductus in 20 per cent; 80 per cent had other major defects.

Post-ductal
Distal to the ductus or the ligamentum arteriosum.

In 1903 Bonnet divided coarctation into infantile and adult types, the infantile being pre-ductal and the adult post-ductal. This division is confusing as one-third of infants seen in the first year of life have the adult type (Keith *et al.*, 1967) and the infantile may not present until well after infancy.

When coarctation presents in the first year of life, two-thirds of the cases are pre-ductal; cardiac failure is common and the high mortality is often attributable to the major associated cardiac anomalies, including ductus arteriosus (64 per cent), ventricular septal defect (32 per cent), transposition (10 per cent) and atrial septal defect (6·5 per cent) (Keith *et al.*, 1967). Aortic stenosis is infrequent except in Turner's syndrome. The infants are usually acyanotic, but cyanosis is seen with transposition and in the lower limbs if the coarctation is pre-ductal with severe pulmonary hypertension (reversed differential cyanosis).

If a coarctation presents after the first year of life, patients are usually symptom free and the lesion is discovered because of hypertension, a murmur or an abnormal chest radiograph. Except for the rare case in late infancy or childhood, the coarctation is post-ductal (adult type). The ductus is patent in 20 per cent of children, but is almost invariably closed in the adult. In contrast to pre-ductal coarctation, major associated anomalies are usually absent, except that a bicuspid aortic valve is frequent. Its reported incidence varies from 27 to 85 per cent (Edwards *et al.*, 1965). A bicuspid valve may produce no haemodynamic abnormality but usually leads to premature aortic valve disease, either regurgitation or stenosis with calcification (*see Figure 256*). Important aortic stenosis may prevent upper limb hypertension with severe coarctation; it may also cause symptoms after relief of the coarctation. The subclavian arteries may be abnormal. The right artery may arise distal to the coarctation, so that the radial pulse and rib notching are absent on this side. The left may be atretic or may arise beyond the coarctation, causing an absent radial pulse and no rib notching on the left side. A combination of the two gives rise to absent or reduced pulses in all four limbs but bounding pulses in the neck. Coarctation was reported in association with sub-aortic stenosis, supravalvar ring in the left atrium and parachute mitral valve by Shone *et al.* (1963). Some of the anomalies associated with pre-ductal coarctation in infants are occasionally seen in later life.

Complications of coarctation are subacute bacterial endocarditis, dissecting aneurysm proximal or distal to the coarcted segment, aortic sinus aneurysm, circle of Willis berry aneurysm, intercostal aneurysm and aortic valve disease. Rupture of the aorta, subarachnoid haemorrhage and congestive failure are the usual causes of death.

Coarctation causes a systolic overload on the left ventricle with hypertension in the upper part of the body. There is an additional volume overload if aortic regurgitation is present.

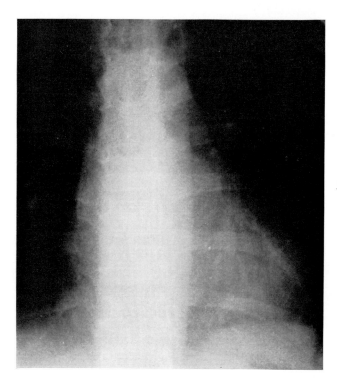

Figure 333. Coarctation. Descending aorta abnormally far to the left in an infant

Radiology

In infants it is not possible to distinguish pre-ductal from post-ductal coarctation. The heart enlarges in the early weeks after birth and may become very large if there is heart failure. An abnormal aortic knuckle is not seen, but the descending aorta may lie abnormally far to the left of the spine (*Figure 333*). With the onset of left ventricular failure, the lungs show upper zone vessel dilatation and sometimes oedema. Plethora with or without oedema suggests a shunt in addition to coarctation.

The most important radiological sign in the older child and adult is an abnormal contour to the left upper mediastinum in the region of the aortic knuckle. It usually takes one of four forms.

Double knuckle, in which the upper bulge is formed by the left subclavian artery and/or the aortic arch and the lower bulge by post-stenotic dilatation of the descending aorta ('figure three' appearance—*Figure 334a, b*).

High knuckle, formed by the left subclavian artery and/or arch without appreciable post-stenotic dilatation (*Figure 334c*).

Low knuckle, formed by post-stenotic dilatation but without prominence of the left subclavian artery or aortic arch (*Figure 334d*).

Flat knuckle, due to any combination of absent left subclavian artery, small aortic arch, narrow isthmus and absent post-stenotic dilatation (*Figure 334e, f*).

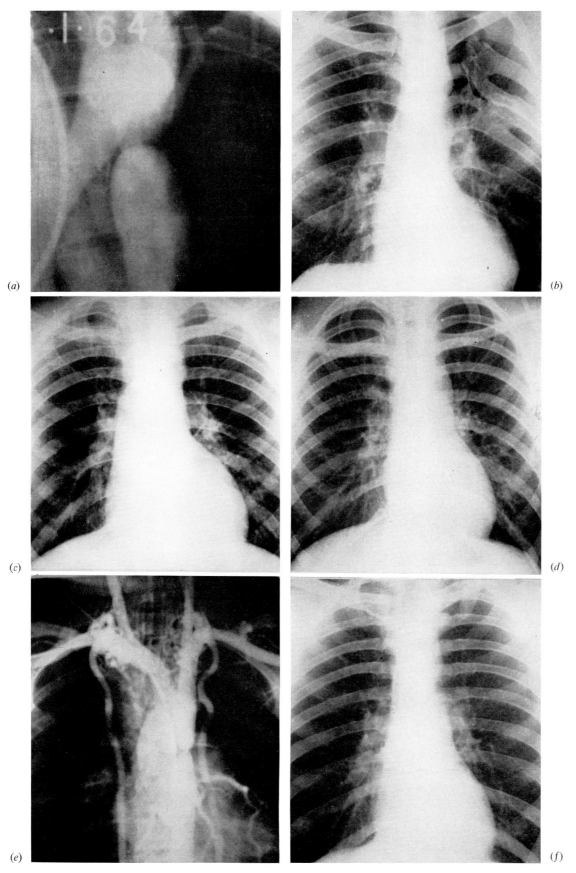

Figure 334. Coarctation. (a) Double knuckle. Aortogram. (b) Double knuckle. (c) High knuckle. (d) Low knuckle. (e) Flat knuckle. Aortogram. (f) Flat knuckle

251

Even with a flat knuckle, the lateral border of the aorta may show a medial indentation due to inward and backward kinking of the aorta at the level of the ligamentum arteriosum. An abnormal knuckle is almost invariable in adults and is often detectable in quite young children. If the coarctation is unusually high, the post-stenotic dilatation is also high and may be mistaken for a normal aortic knuckle. Barium swallow may be helpful by showing two indentations in the region of the aortic knuckle, the upper and smaller one being the aortic arch and the lower and larger one the post-stenotic dilatation. The whole oesophagus may be displaced to the right if dilatation of the descending aorta is marked. The ascending

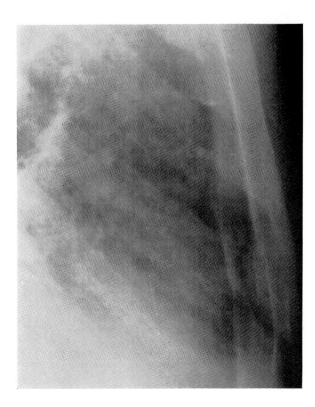

Figure 335. Coarctation. Lateral view. Retrosternal soft tissue shadow due to dilated internal mammary arteries

aorta is sometimes dilated even in the absence of aortic valve disease. The descending aorta is sometimes seen unusually far to the left beyond the spine, and this abnormal position is a valuable sign in children (*see Figure 333*). The heart is normal in size in adult coarctation without aortic valve disease, other associated anomalies or heart failure, but is quite often enlarged in children due to left ventricular hypertrophy. Its shape may suggest left ventricular enlargement whether there is cardiac enlargement or not. The left atrial dilatation is seen more often in children than in adults and occurs with left ventricular failure. Rib notching is indirect evidence of the collateral circulation and develops only when the obstruction is severe (*see* page 105). Dilated internal mammary arteries may be seen on the lateral view as a soft tissue shadow with a tortuous posterior margin up to 1 cm in width behind the sternum (*Figure 335*).

A particularly large ascending aorta or obvious post-stenotic dilatation of the descending aorta suggests an aneurysm. Rarely an intercostal aneurysm may be visible. Cardiac enlargement in adult coarctation suggests aortic valve disease from a bicuspid valve which may show calcification even in early adult life.

SECTION VII
Myocardial and Pericardial Disease

CHAPTER 27

Ischaemic Heart Disease

The term ischaemic heart disease, used in its widest sense, implies insufficient oxygenation of heart muscle from any cause including the following.

Congenital anomalies of the coronary arteries
Coronary artery fistula (*see* page 167).
Origin of left coronary artery from pulmonary trunk (*see* page 165).
Coronary artery aneurysm.

Acquired coronary artery disease
Atherosclerosis.
Syphilitic ostial stenosis.
Polyarteritis nodosa.

Coronary artery embolism

Diminished coronary perfusion
Aortic stenosis.
Aortic regurgitation.
Mitral stenosis.
Severe pulmonary hypertension.

Relative myocardial ischaemia in cardiac hypertrophy

Anaemia

Impaired liberation of oxygen from haemoglobin
Abnormal oxygen dissociation curve (Eliot and Bratt, 1969).

This chapter is concerned with coronary atherosclerosis and its effect on the heart and lungs. Coronary artery calcification is discussed on page 62.

CORONARY ARTERY ANATOMY

The anatomy of the coronary arteries is illustrated in *Figures 336–341*. The left coronary artery arises from the left posterior aortic sinus and passes to the left behind the pulmonary trunk to divide into two major branches. Its length before division is variable and may be less than 5 mm; in these circumstances selective coronary arteriography and coronary perfusion at surgery are more difficult in that one or other of the major branches only is likely to be entered. The anterior descending branch of the left coronary artery turns forward and to the left and runs in the anterior interventricular groove. It has at least one diagonal branch which passes to the left on the surface of the left ventricle. The other important branches are the anterior septal branches or perforators, which arise at right angles to supply the anterior and major part of the ventricular septum. The main anterior descending branch may bifurcate and rarely trifurcate, so that the main trunk distally may be difficult to identify with certainty. It runs to the apex of the heart, but rarely if ever extends for any distance on to the inferior surface. It supplies the antero-lateral and apical portions of the left ventricle and the major part of the ventricular septum.

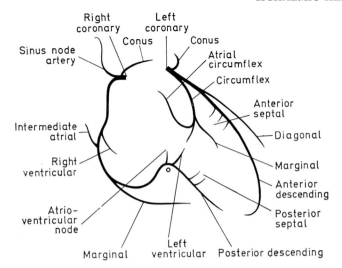

Figure 336. Coronary artery anatomy. Anterior view

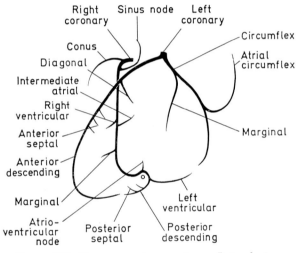

Figure 337. Coronary artery anatomy. Lateral view

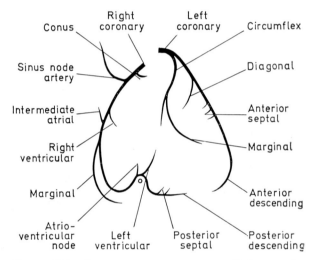

Figure 338. Coronary artery anatomy. Right anterior oblique

Figure 339. Coronary artery anatomy. Left anterior oblique

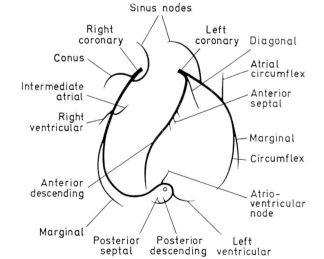

256

The circumflex branch of the left coronary artery passes downward and backward in the left atrio-ventricular groove. It gives off a left marginal branch which may be larger than the continuation of the circumflex and supplies the lateral and posterior portions of the left ventricle.

The right coronary artery arises from the anterior aortic sinus, passing forward and then downward in the right atrio-ventricular groove. The conal branch arises close to its origin and passes forward and to the left around the right ventricular outflow. In 40 per cent of cases the conal artery has a separate origin from the aortic sinus. The right coronary artery gives off a right marginal and other branches to the atria and the right ventricular myocardium before passing around the lower margin of the heart.

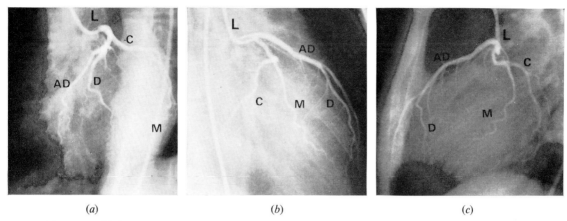

(a) (b) (c)

Figure 340. Normal left coronary arteriogram. (a) Left anterior oblique. (b) Right anterior oblique. (c) Left lateral

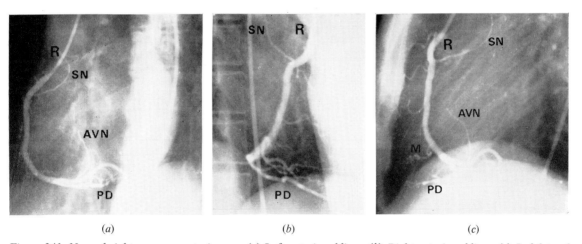

(a) (b) (c)

Figure 341. Normal right coronary arteriogram. (a) Left anterior oblique. (b) Right anterior oblique. (c) Left lateral

R = right coronary artery	AVN = atrio-ventricular node artery	C = circumflex artery
L = left coronary artery	AD = anterior descending artery	D = diagonal branch
SN = sinus node artery	PD = posterior descending artery	M = marginal branch

The postero-inferior surface of the left ventricle is supplied by the posterior descending artery, which begins at the crux of the heart (the point at which the atrio-ventricular and interventricular grooves meet) and runs forward in the posterior interventricular groove. This artery is a continuation of the distal right coronary artery in 90 per cent of cases, and in these circumstances the right coronary is said to be dominant. The posterior descending artery gives off posterior septal branches to the ventricular septum. The distal branches of the right coronary artery supply the posterior papillary muscle, usually with a contribution from the circumflex artery. Left dominance is present when the posterior descending artery arises from the circumflex branch of the left coronary artery. The posterior descending artery often divides into two or more branches.

The sinus and atrio-ventricular node arteries usually arise from the dominant coronary artery. The sinus node artery is thus a proximal branch of either the right or the circumflex branch of the left coronary artery. Rarely it arises from the main left coronary artery. The atrio-ventricular node artery arises from the posterior descending artery close to the crux and ascends in the ventricular septum.

The right and left atrial circumflex branches are inconstant and arise from the right coronary artery and the circumflex branch of the left coronary artery respectively.

ACUTE MYOCARDIAL INFARCTION

Bennett and Rees (1973) found a good correlation between the left ventricular end-diastolic pressure and the radiological signs of pulmonary venous hypertension in acute myocardial infarction. They studied radiographs with simultaneous pressure recordings. The pulmonary artery diastolic pressure, assumed to reflect left ventricular end-diastolic pressure (Forsberg, 1971), was compared with the radiological changes, which were assessed without knowledge of the haemodynamics. Absence of upper zone vessel dilatation on the chest radiograph indicated that the pressure was below 15 mm Hg unless it was elevated from another cause such as pulmonary embolism. Radiological signs of pulmonary venous hypertension usually indicated a pressure above 15 mm Hg, the discrepancies being due to a time lag between fall of pressure and radiological improvement. Occasionally, however, severe pulmonary oedema may be present without any pressure rise, the reasons for this being obscure. Subjective assessment of heart size also correlated well, and patients with cardiac enlargement had significantly higher

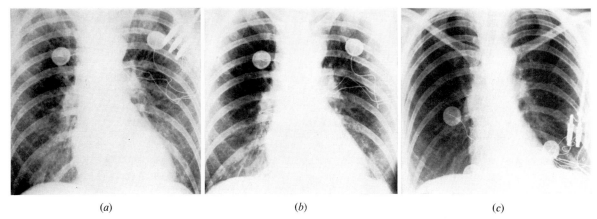

(a)   (b)   (c)

Figure 342. Acute myocardial infarction. (a) Interstitial oedema (pulmonary artery diastolic pressure (40 mm Hg). (b) Still upper zone vessel dilatation oedema clearing (pulmonary artery diastolic pressure 25 mm Hg). (c) Lungs now normal (pulmonary artery diastolic pressure 10 mm Hg)

pressures. It is apparent, therefore, that useful information may be obtained from a technically satisfactory portable film taken in the semi-erect position (*Figure 342*).

About 60 per cent of patients in a coronary care unit have a normal chest radiograph throughout their clinical course. Cardiac enlargement and signs of an elevated left ventricular end-diastolic pressure may last for only a few days. In extensive infarction the heart enlarges and the lungs are invariably abnormal; the cardiac enlargement usually persists and may be due to generalized left ventricular dilatation, left ventricular aneurysm (*see* page 261), ruptured ventricular septum or mitral regurgitation.

Sequelae of Myocardial Infarction

Ruptured ventricular septum

The rupture occurs in the muscular ventricular septum within two weeks of infarction following a major occlusion, usually of the anterior descending branch of the left coronary artery (*Figure 343*). There may be more than one defect. Perforation is commonest in first infarcts and with hypertension. The shunt is frequently large, and the pulmonary venous pressure rises as a result of the high pulmonary flow and left ventricular dysfunction. The perforation is frequently complicated by a left ventricular aneurysm or mitral regurgitation. The heart suddenly enlarges and the lungs show interstitial or alveolar oedema with pleural effusion. Pulmonary oedema often hides the pulmonary vessels, but when they become visible they appear dilated in the upper zones and the appearances are indistinguishable at this

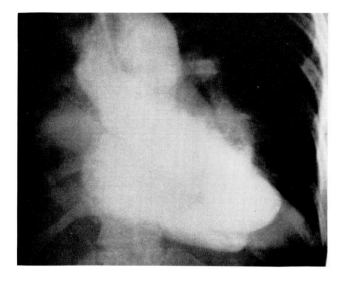

Figure 343. Ruptured ventricular septum with apical aneurysm. Left ventricular angiogram, anterior view

stage from those of acute mitral regurgitation. If the patient survives, evidence of pulmonary venous hypertension becomes less striking and the picture ultimately suggests a shunt, but the upper zone vessels may remain larger than the lower (*see Figure 216*).

Mitral regurgitation

Mitral regurgitation after acute infarction may be:
    (1) Transient.
    (2) Due to established papillary muscle dysfunction.
    (3) Due to papillary muscle rupture.
The signs of regurgitation are frequently transient and are probably due to temporary papillary muscle ischaemia or to acute dilatation of the left ventricle with altered angle of pull of the papillary muscles. Established mitral regurgitation occurs when the blood supply to the papillary muscles is permanently compromised by ischaemia or infarction. The posterior papillary muscle is usually affected, probably because the anterior papillary muscle has the better collateral blood supply. The infarction is inferior or posterior and follows occlusion of the right coronary artery or the circumflex branch of the left coronary artery. Regurgitation is caused by failure of papillary muscle contraction and later by fibrosis and contracture; regurgitation may also result if a papillary muscle is attached to an infarct of the free wall or to a left ventricular aneurysm. Its degree depends on the extent of the damage to the papillary muscle or the surrounding myocardial wall. It usually begins in the first week after infarction and, if important, results in congestive cardiac failure.

The heart may show little or no increase in size, and the left atrium is initially normal and may be only slightly enlarged even after weeks or months. Because of the small incompliant left atrium, the systolic wave is transmitted directly to the pulmonary veins and the lungs show evidence of a high venous pressure with upper zone vessel dilatation, pulmonary oedema and pleural effusion. If the pulmonary vascular resistance rises, the pulmonary trunk may enlarge. The early appearances are indistinguishable from those of a ruptured ventricular septum, and clinical differentiation may also be difficult.

Complete rupture of a papillary muscle produces catastrophic mitral regurgitation with acute pulmonary oedema. Death usually occurs within 24 hours unless the mitral valve is replaced.

Other complications of myocardial infarction

Chronic left ventricular failure may develop after infarction without perforation of the ventricular septum or papillary muscle dysfunction. Occasionally the infarct may be clinically silent, and the radiological features then suggest a cardiomyopathy.

Pulmonary emboli are common after infarction. They are usually small and give rise to no symptoms. They show as small band-like shadows at the bases, often horizontal but sometimes angled or even vertical (*see Figure 141*). Effusions may not be present. Less often large infarcts cause pleural effusion and congestive failure.

The post-myocardial infarction syndrome, possibly a hypersensitivity reaction to necrotic cardiac muscle, consists of pericardial pain with pericarditis, sometimes with pericardial effusion, pleural effusion and pneumonitis. It occurs weeks or months after infarction, with which it must not be confused, and may recur. Occasionally the syndrome appears earlier, and it should be suspected if signs of pericarditis last for more than one week after infarction. Pericardial effusion may also arise from haemorrhage in a patient on anticoagulants.

CHRONIC ISCHAEMIC HEART DISEASE

This is manifested clinically as angina of effort, with or without evidence of previous infarction. Rarely patients present with dysrhythmia or congestive failure without angina.

The pain may be stable, may slowly diminish due to the establishment of an intercoronary collateral circulation, or may get worse as a result of progressive arterial narrowing (*Figure 344*). The heart is

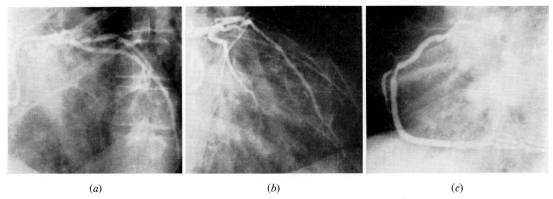

(a) (b) (c)

Figure 344. Coronary atherosclerosis. (a). Anterior descending block—left anterior oblique. (b) Anterior descending block—right anterior oblique. (c) Right coronary stenosis—left anterior oblique

enlarged in about 30 per cent of patients in whom angina is of sufficient severity to warrant coronary angiography with a view to surgical treatment (Gahl *et al.*, 1973). This is a selected group, and the incidence of cardiac enlargement in unselected patients is much lower. Systemic hypertension and previous cardiac infarction are, however, important factors predisposing to cardiac enlargement.

Radiological changes in the size and shape of the heart in chronic ischaemic heart disease are discussed below in relation to fluoroscopy, left ventricular cine-angiography, haemodynamics, and surgical and autopsy findings. Alterations in left ventricular contraction as seen on cine-angiography show various patterns (Gahl *et al.*, 1973).

Localized dyskinesis (diminished inward systolic movement—*Figure 345*) involves a limited area of myocardium, most commonly at the apex but also on the antero-lateral or postero-inferior surface or any combination of the three. Localized dyskinesis is rarely associated with ventricular enlargement or with elevated end-diastolic pressure. The plain film is normal, but the dyskinetic area may be seen on fluoroscopy. On left ventricular angiography, a localized dilatation is seen in systole which is not apparent in diastole and reflects deficient ventricular contraction. Rarely more than one-third of the chamber outline is involved. Dyskinetic areas may contain viable but ischaemic muscle or a mixture of muscle and fibrous tissue, so that surgical resection would seem inappropriate; indeed, they may not be detected by the surgeon at all. Gorlin *et al.* (1967) called them 'functional aneurysms', a term recommended by Raphael *et al.* (1972).

With generalized dyskinesis (*Figure 346*), the left ventricle shows a uniform increase in systolic and diastolic volumes and the end-diastolic pressure is elevated. The appearances resemble congestive cardiomyopathy. Radiologically the heart is enlarged and the lungs show evidence of pulmonary venous hypertension.

Akinesis (total lack of inward systolic movement) or paradoxical pulsation (outward systolic movement) means that a true fibrous aneurysm is nearly always present.

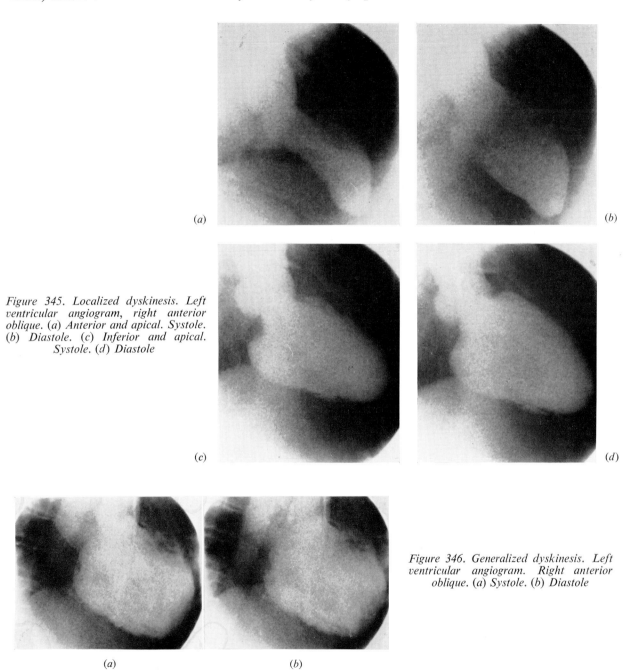

(a)

(b)

Figure 345. Localized dyskinesis. Left ventricular angiogram, right anterior oblique. (a) Anterior and apical. Systole. (b) Diastole. (c) Inferior and apical. Systole. (d) Diastole

(c)

(d)

(a)

(b)

Figure 346. Generalized dyskinesis. Left ventricular angiogram. Right anterior oblique. (a) Systole. (b) Diastole

Left ventricular aneurysm has been defined as 'A protrusion of a localized portion of the external aspect of the left ventricle beyond the remainder of the cardiac surface with simultaneous protrusion of the cavity itself. . . .' (Edwards, 1961). An alternative and perhaps simpler definition is a localized dilatation of the left ventricle with akinesis which is seen in systole and nearly always in diastole as well (*Figure 347*). A dyskinetic area (functional aneurysm) shows only in systole and is not apparent in diastole. Fibrous aneurysm usually involves the apex and includes at least one-third of the ventricular

261

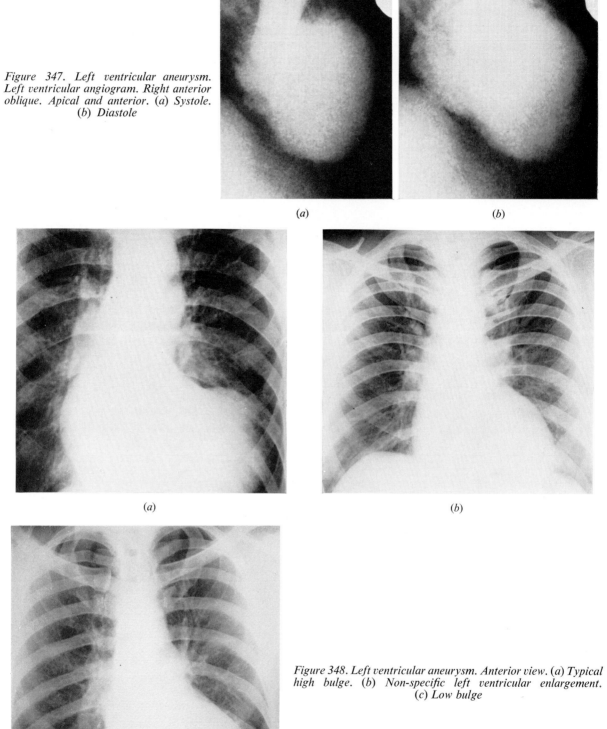

Figure 347. Left ventricular aneurysm. Left ventricular angiogram. Right anterior oblique. Apical and anterior. (a) Systole. (b) Diastole

(a)

(b)

(a)

(b)

Figure 348. Left ventricular aneurysm. Anterior view. (a) Typical high bulge. (b) Non-specific left ventricular enlargement. (c) Low bulge

(c)

outline. It may extend on to the antero-lateral surface; inferior aneurysms are less common, and posterior aneurysms are very rare. An antero-septal aneurysm may accompany a ruptured ventricular septum, and inferior aneurysms cause mitral regurgitation from involvement of the posterior papillary muscle. It is unusual to see a well-defined neck on angiography: if present, it is broad and best seen in systole. At surgery, however, a clear zone of demarcation is visible when the aneurysm is a month or two old. In a typical case the sub-aortic area of the ventricle contracts vigorously but may be dyskinetic in severely affected ventricles. Coronary arteriography shows an occlusion or severe proximal stenosis of the anterior descending branch of the left coronary artery, with or without disease of other arteries.

Radiologically the classical left ventricular aneurysm presents as a localized bulge on the left border of the heart (*Figure 348*). It is most easily seen when situated high up below the left atrial appendix. Most aneurysms, however, do not show this typical contour, and the commonest appearance is that suggesting non-specific left ventricular enlargement or a smooth elongation of the left ventricular border with a low apex. These types of heart shape are seen when the aneurysm is apical or antero-lateral (*Figure 348*). Inferior aneurysms may also give this appearance by displacing the left ventricular border outwards. Antero-lateral or lateral aneurysms may cause a more rounded appearance with elevation of the apex. Apical aneurysms and those arising inferiorly may not produce any alteration in heart size or shape, but careful fluoroscopy should reveal a lack of pulsation in the appropriate areas. An inferior aneurysm may be visible below the diaphragm if the fundus of the stomach is distended with air.

Most patients with an aneurysm causing cardiac enlargement show evidence of pulmonary venous hypertension, but a few with quite large aneurysms, particularly if healed and calcified, have normal lungs. Those with a normal-sized heart tend to have normal lungs, but there are exceptions.

CHAPTER 28

Cardiomyopathy

PRIMARY CARDIOMYOPATHY

Goodwin and Oakley (1972) have defined cardiomyopathy as 'a disorder of heart muscle of unknown cause or association'. They suggest that the term secondary cardiomyopathy, which implies that other organs are involved and the aetiology is clear, should be abandoned and the lesion classified according to the underlying disease—for example amyloid disease, haemochromatosis or sarcoidosis. The above definition serves to emphasize that cardiomyopathy is apparently a primary disorder of heart muscle, but it does not state that sometimes there is endocardial and pericardial involvement which is of clinical importance.

For the purposes of this discussion, the terms primary and secondary cardiomyopathy will be retained and three haemodynamic types distinguished:

Congestive, characterized by poor systolic contraction; predominantly left-sided.

Hypertrophic, characterized by impaired diastolic filling with or without outflow obstruction; predominantly left-sided.

Restrictive, characterized by impaired diastolic filling; right or left sided.

It must be emphasized that the three types are not always clear-cut and one may change into another. For example, some cardiomyopathies may show congestive or restrictive features, and the hypertrophic type may eventually develop impairment of left ventricular systolic contraction as in congestive cardiomyopathy.

Congestive cardiomyopathy

Congestive cardiomyopathy is characterized by impairment of myocardial contractility of unknown cause. There is dilatation of the affected ventricle, but some hypertrophy is usual. Endocardial thrombosis, systemic embolism and atrial fibrillation occur. As the left ventricle is affected more often than the right, left ventricular failure is common, and finally congestive failure with mitral and tricuspid regurgitation terminates the illness. Primary myocardial disease is frequently reported from Africa, the West Indies, India and South America, but is probably not much less frequently seen in the so-called developed societies (Goodwin and Oakley, 1972). Angiocardiography shows a large ventricular systolic and diastolic volume with poor contraction and a reduced ejection fraction (*Figure 349*). Coronary artery disease without angina diffusely affecting the myocardium may show similar clinical and angiocardiographic features; moreover, 10 per cent of patients with congestive cardiomyopathy experience angina, and some show ECG changes suggesting infarction (Goodwin and Oakley, 1972). Coronary arteriography is therefore necessary to exclude coronary artery disease; the term ischaemic cardiomyopathy should not be used. Hypertensive heart disease with failure may also be difficult to separate from cardiomyopathy, as at this stage the blood pressure may be normal. Retinal artery changes and a prominent aorta on the chest radiograph may suggest the diagnosis.

Hypertrophic cardiomyopathy

This is an inherited disorder (either dominant or recessive) of unknown cause in which the left ventricle loses its distensibility due to an incompliant thick muscle wall predominantly involving the septum. The result is inflow obstruction. Outflow obstruction is a variable feature of the disease: it tends to be present in patients with marked septal hypertrophy, and may not occur with more symmetrical muscle thickening. It may disappear in the terminal stages of the disease. Mitral regurgitation

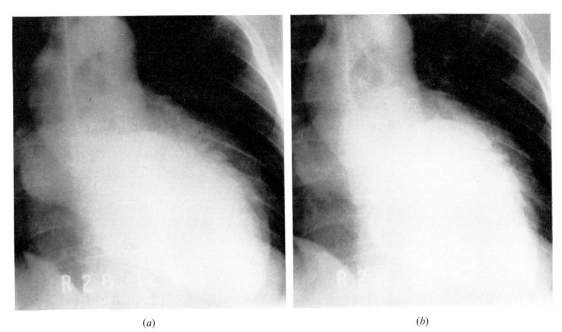

Figure 349. Congestive cardiomyopathy. Left ventricular angiogram. (a) Systole. (b) Diastole

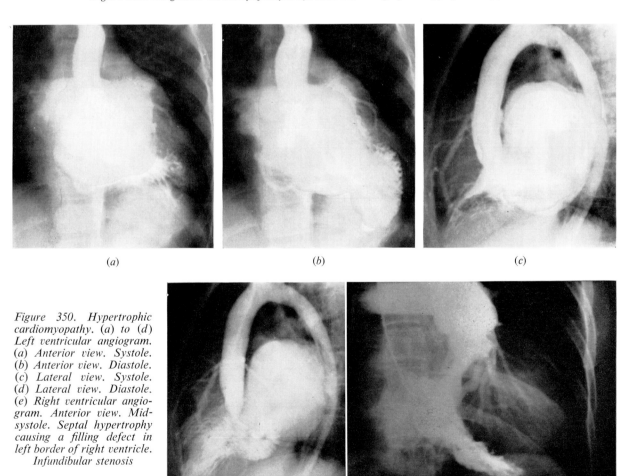

Figure 350. Hypertrophic cardiomyopathy. (a) to (d) Left ventricular angiogram. (a) Anterior view. Systole. (b) Anterior view. Diastole. (c) Lateral view. Systole. (d) Lateral view. Diastole. (e) Right ventricular angiogram. Anterior view. Midsystole. Septal hypertrophy causing a filling defect in left border of right ventricle.
Infundibular stenosis

is usually associated with outflow obstruction since both are caused by a common mechanism. In mid-systole the anterior cusp of the mitral valve is pulled into the left ventricular outflow towards the septum by hypertrophy and an altered angle of pull of the papillary muscles; the result is obstruction between the hypertrophied septum and the anterior cusp of the mitral valve. At the same time the mitral orifice is kept open, allowing mitral regurgitation. Outflow obstruction and mitral regurgitation occur during the second half of systole and result in a late systolic murmur. Gradients due to muscle hypertrophy may be found in the right ventricular outflow.

The pathological anatomy is well illustrated by angiocardiography (*Figure 350*). Septal hypertrophy causes a concave filling defect, seen in the anterior wall of the left ventricle on the lateral view (*Figure 350c*) and in the left lateral wall of the right ventricle on the anterior view (*Figure 350e*); Severe septal thickening elevates the floor of the left ventricle. Thickening of the free wall of the left ventricle, its trabeculae and its papillary muscles is usually striking and best seen in systole (*Figure 350a, c*). Left ventricular cavity size may be normal in diastole, but in severe cases it is reduced (*Figure 350b*). Systolic films show complete or partial obliteration of the apical portions of both ventricles (*Figure 350c, e*); high pressures may be recorded from these areas, but represent wall tension rather than true gradients. Contrast medium may also be squeezed out of the left ventricular cavity between the hypertrophied papillary muscles. During the second half of systole, a narrowing may be evident between the anterior mitral cusp and the thickened ventricular septum, together with mitral regurgitation; both these changes are best seen in the lateral view (*Figure 350c*).

The left ventricular outflow immediately below the aortic valve remains widely patent: this differentiates hypertrophic cardiomyopathy from fixed fibro-muscular sub-aortic stenosis, which involves this area (*Figure 350a*). With marked septal hypertrophy the outflow tract of the right ventricle may be narrowed and a gradient recorded in systole; the stenosis is lower in position and more irregular than in congenital infundibular stenosis (*Figure 350e*). The coronary arteries may be wider than normal. Similar angiocardiographic changes are seen in severe fixed obstruction to left ventricular outflow in children, but here the appearances represent florid concentric hypertrophy and can be differentiated by the pathologist from those of cardiomyopathy (Van Noorden *et al.*, 1971). Hypertrophic cardiomyopathy is occasionally seen in Ullrich's syndrome (*see* Chapter 14) and is an important feature of lentiginosis. The latter is a condition in which pigmented spots on the skin are not related to sunlight exposure (unlike freckles). The patients may show short stature and a diagnosis of von Recklinghausen's disease may be made in error. Hypertrophic cardiomyopathy may present in the first year of life and the right side of the heart may be more severely affected than the left, so that the first diagnosis is often one of pulmonary stenosis (Somerville and Bonham-Carter, 1972).

Hypertrophic cardiomyopathy may remain stable for many years. The prognosis is worse in patients with a short history and a high left ventricular end-diastolic pressure; sudden death is also related to these parameters, but not to the degree of left ventricular outflow obstruction (Goodwin, 1970). Progression of the disease is manifested by angina and by left ventricular failure. The situation is exacerbated by atrial fibrillation, which removes the force of atrial systole in overcoming inflow obstruction. Eight out of 41 deteriorating patients followed by Goodwin over five years showed loss of outflow obstruction (Goodwin, 1970); the systolic murmur became less or disappeared. The heart enlarged, and atrial fibrillation was common and often caused systemic emboli. Five patients died from congestive failure.

Restrictive cardiomyopathy

Restrictive cardiomyopathy is the least frequent of the three types of cardiomyopathy and is caused by disease processes which infiltrate the myocardium and endocardium. Many cases simulate constrictive pericarditis clinically and congestive cardiomyopathy radiologically. Others, especially cases of endomyocardial fibrosis, are characterized by marked cavity obliteration resulting from endocardial thickening and atrio-ventricular valve regurgitation. The right or left side or both sides of the heart may be involved. Unlike the congestive and hypertrophic forms, restrictive cardiomyopathy is usually secondary to a recognizable disease process.

RADIOLOGY

Congestive cardiomyopathy

In congestive cardiomyopathy the heart is invariably enlarged and may be huge. The ventricular border on the anterior view often suggests left ventricular enlargement (*Figure 351*). In large hearts all four chambers may be dilated and assessment of their relative size may be difficult (*Figure 352*). Functional tricuspid and mitral regurgitation occur, but the atria do not reach the proportions they do in chronic rheumatic heart disease. Quite rapid reduction in heart size may occur in response to treatment,

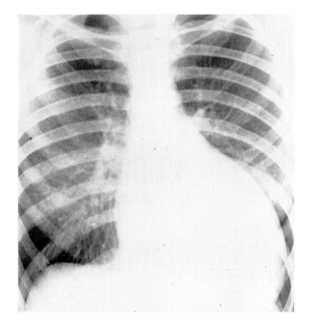

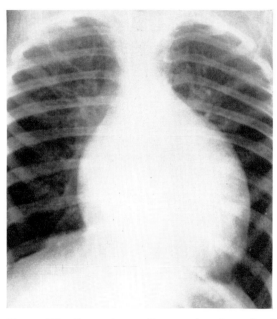

Figure 351. Congestive cardiomyopathy. Enlarged left ventricle

Figure 352. Congestive cardiomyopathy. Generalized cardiac enlargement

but return to normal is rare. Cardiac enlargement may progress rapidly or be static for years. In long-standing cases the aortic knuckle may appear small, presumably due to a restricted cardiac output.

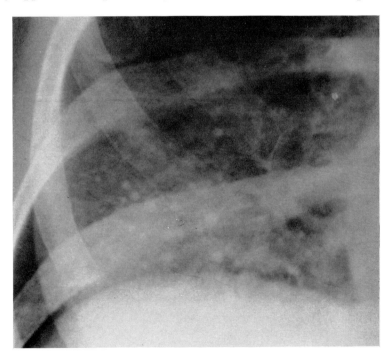

Figure 353. Pulmonary ossific nodules in long-standing congestive cardiomyopathy

As the left side is usually more affected than the right, the lungs show evidence of pulmonary venous hypertension in those cases in which the left ventricular end-diastolic pressure is elevated. Chronic or recurrent pulmonary venous hypertension is usually associated with a heart which is at least moderately enlarged. Pulmonary ossific nodules, similar to those seen in mitral stenosis, are occasionally present in patients who live for years with long-standing pulmonary venous hypertension (*Figure 353*). The lungs, however, are normal (or possibly oligaemic) in cases of right-sided congestive cardiomyopathy.

Differentiation of congestive cardiomyopathy from pericardial effusion may be difficult. In both conditions there is deficient pulsation on fluoroscopy. The diagnosis is made particularly difficult by the fact that pericardial effusion is common in congestive cardiomyopathy. Echocardiography is necessary for confirmation. The lungs are usually normal in patients with large hearts which are due to pericardial effusion, and signs of pulmonary venous hypertension favour cardiomyopathy. A few patients with ischaemic heart disease give no history of angina, show uniform enlargement of the left ventricle without aneurysm, and may have functional mitral regurgitation. The only clue on the plain films may be coronary artery calcification. However, these patients can only be distinguished with certainty from cases of congestive cardiomyopathy by means of coronary angiography. As mentioned above, patients with hypertensive heart disease whose blood pressure is no longer elevated may show similar radiological findings. An elongated or dilated thoracic aorta may suggest the diagnosis.

Hypertrophic cardiomyopathy

The overall heart size is normal in about half the patients with hypertrophic cardiomyopathy when they first present with the disease. This is particularly so in the asymptomatic patient who is found to have a systolic murmur. Although the heart may be normal in size, its shape may suggest left ventricular enlargement (*Figure 354*). The upper part of the ventricular border may show a rather localized bulge

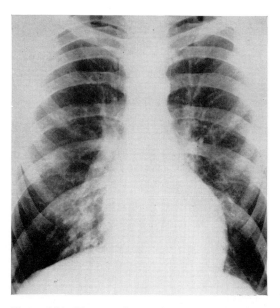

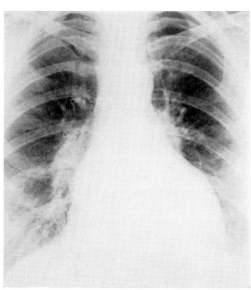

Figure 354. Hypertrophic cardiomyopathy. Normal-sized heart with shape suggesting enlargement of left ventricle

Figure 355. Hypertrophic cardiomyopathy. Bulge or shelf on left cardiac border

or shelf, probably due to thickening of the upper part of the ventricular septum (*Figure 355*). In the patients with progressive disease (10–15 per cent of Goodwin's (1970) series followed up for an average of four years), the heart enlarges. The configuration suggests left ventricular enlargement, but when congestive failure occurs the heart may be globular, suggesting enlargement of all chambers, the appearances resembling those of congestive cardiomyopathy. With important mitral regurgitation, the left atrium dilates but is rarely very large and the appendix does not bulge (*Figure 356*). The lungs show evidence of pulmonary venous hypertension in cases with severe left ventricular inflow obstruction (*Figure 357*); with atrial fibrillation and congestive failure the heart is always enlarged. The onset of atrial fibrillation may precipitate pulmonary oedema.

The aorta is not dilated in hypertrophic cardiomyopathy, and absence of post-stenotic dilatation

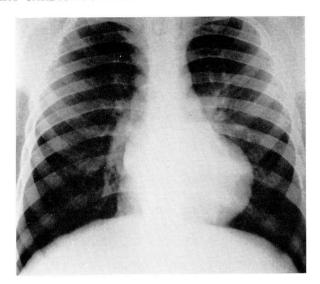

Figure 356. Hypertrophic cardiomyopathy.
Left atrial enlargement

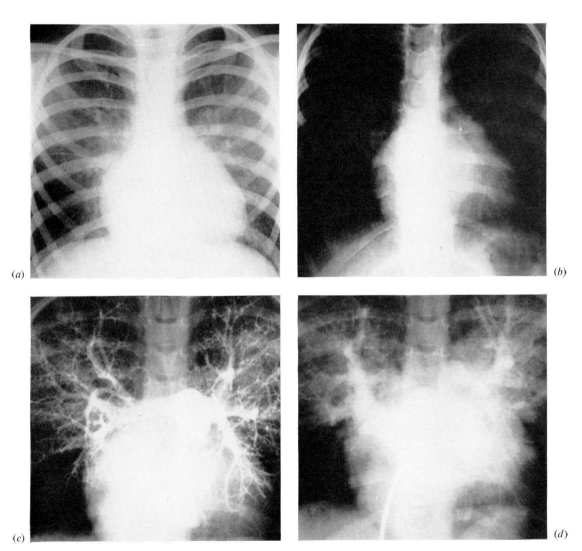

(a)

(b)

(c)

(d)

Figure 357. Hypertrophic cardiomyopathy with severe left ventricular inflow obstruction. (a) Plain film.
Upper zone vessel dilatation. (b) Penetrated film. Left atrial dilatation. (c) and (d) Pulmonary arteriogram.
Arterial and venous phases. Marked flow diversion to upper zones

helps to differentiate this condition from other causes of left ventricular outflow obstruction. Nevertheless, a prominent ascending aorta is very occasionally seen, apparently due to buckling of the ascending aorta from enlargement of the left ventricle in its long axis and elevation of the aortic valve. Fixed sub-aortic stenosis cannot be distinguished from hypertrophic cardiomyopathy on plain films except that any prominence of the ascending aorta makes the former much more likely. In patients with left atrial enlargement, the radiological appearances are indistinguishable from those of mitral regurgitation.

Restrictive cardiomyopathy

In this condition the heart may be either normal in size or enlarged. There may be features suggesting tricuspid or mitral regurgitation. Endocardial thickening is characteristic of some forms and may occasionally calcify. The lungs are normal or oligaemic if the changes are predominantly right-sided, but signs of pulmonary venous hypertension indicate important left-sided involvement.

Endocardial fibro-elastosis and endomyocardial fibrosis merit individual description because each forms a well-defined clinico-pathological entity.

Endocardial fibro-elastosis

Endocardial fibro-elastosis is a congenital lesion involving the left side of the heart, possibly due to foetal myocarditis or some other insult, and leading to congestive failure in the first year of life. There is diffuse thickening of the endocardium with hypertrophy and dilatation of the left ventricle. The papillary muscles tend to be incorporated in the thickening and give rise to short thick chordae, the mitral cusps are shortened, and the result is that mitral regurgitation is common. Angiocardiography shows a thick, poorly contracting, smooth-walled, dilated left ventricle with mitral regurgitation. Rarely the left ventricle is thick but small and the disease is referred to as the contracted type of endocardial fibro-elastosis. Patients usually die in infancy. Endocardial thickening is found in association with congenital heart disease, especially obstructive lesions in the left heart. Fibro-elastosis in the adult is probably the result of myocarditis with secondary endocardial thickening (Amplatz, 1969).

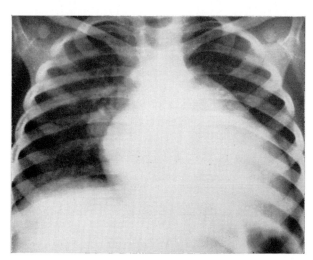

Figure 358. Endocardial fibro-elastosis. Marked cardiac enlargement with left atrial dilatation

Radiologically there is considerable cardiac enlargement with left atrial dilatation, suggesting a left-sided lesion (*Figure 358*). Depending on the severity of the condition, the lungs may appear normal or may show evidence of pulmonary venous hypertension or oedema. It is important to exclude congenital heart disease in the infant, particularly aortic stenosis or coarctation. Other lesions which may be indistinguishable on the plain film include myocarditis, glycogen storage disease, and origin of the left coronary artery from the pulmonary trunk.

Endomyocardial fibrosis

This is an acquired disease usually affecting children and young adults. It is endemic in hot, humid climates, particularly in Uganda and Southern India, but has been reported from many countries; it attacks all races, and any person living in an endemic zone may contract the disease. The main feature is fibrosis of the endocardium and to a lesser extent of the myocardium, involving one or both ventricles. The lesion usually begins in the apex of the ventricle and leads to progressive obliteration of its inflow portion with obstruction to diastolic filling. Tricuspid and mitral regurgitation occur due to involvement of the subvalvar apparatus and later the cusps. Clinical, haemodynamic and radiological features depend on the severity of the right or left ventricular disease; when both ventricles are involved, right-sided signs usually dominate the picture.

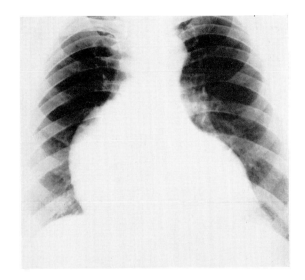

Figure 359. Right-sided endomyocardial fibrosis

Right-sided endomyocardial fibrosis presents with ascites, raised venous pressure and liver enlargement. Angiocardiography may show stasis of medium in the enlarged right atrium due to increased right ventricular filling resistance, obliteration of the inflow portion of the right ventricle and dilatation of the outflow, thrombus in the right atrial appendix and pericardial effusion. The plain film shows cardiac enlargement, which may be gross (*Figure 359*). It is due to either right atrial dilatation or pericardial effusion or to a combination of the two. The right ventricular outflow may be prominent, but is sometimes hidden by the pericardial effusion. A dilated azygos vein is often visible on the penetrated view. Linear calcification in the endocardium of the right ventricle is rare. The lungs are strikingly oligaemic in the advanced case.

Left-sided endomyocardial fibrosis presents clinically as dyspnoea with signs of pulmonary hypertension and left ventricular failure. Angiography shows obliteration of the apex of the left ventricle, poor contraction, and mitral regurgitation with a wide jet (in contrast to rheumatic mitral regurgitation, where the jet is usually localized to some extent because of cusp fusion). The plain film is often indistinguishable from that of mitral regurgitation. Pericardial effusion is rare. Right atrial enlargement with signs of pulmonary venous hypertension suggests biventricular disease.

Two other tropical cardiomyopathies, Chagas' disease and primary heart muscle disease, must always be considered in the differential diagnosis.

SECONDARY CARDIOMYOPATHY

Diseases affecting the myocardium for which a specific aetiology can be determined form a large and heterogeneous group of disorders which have been termed the secondary cardiomyopathies (Goodwin, 1967). They cause disease indistinguishable from primary congestive or restrictive cardiomyopathy of unknown cause. The usual presentation is that of congestive cardiomyopathy, but some cases—namely amyloid, sarcoid, haemochromatosis, polyarteritis nodosa, Loeffler's syndrome and tumour infiltration of the myocardium—may show evidence of restriction. Acute rheumatic fever is included here as it is a pancarditis, and it is primarily the endocardial involvement which determines the subsequent course of the disease. Hypertrophic cardiomyopathy is usually a primary cardiomyopathy and should not be confused with muscle hypertrophy secondary to left ventricular obstruction or systemic hypertension. The following is a list of conditions which may cause or be associated with a cardiomyopathy.

Infective
    Streptococcal (acute rheumatic fever).
    Viral (Coxsackie B, rubella, etc.).
    Septic (subacute bacterial endocarditis).
    Diphtheritic.
    Parasitic (Chagas' disease, trichiniasis).

Endocrine and metabolic
    Myxoedema.
    Thyrotoxicosis.
    Acromegaly.
    Phaeochromocytoma.
    Nutritional deficiency (beriberi, kwashiorkor).
    Anaemias.
    Glycogen storage disease.
    Haemochromatosis.
    Mucopolysaccharidosis (Hurler's syndrome).

Toxic and drug sensitivity
    Alcohol.
    Cobalt (in beer).
    Emetine.
    Antimony and arsenic poisoning.
    Nor-adrenaline.
    Sulphonamides.
    Penicillin and other antibiotics.

Collagen disease and granulomas
    Lupus erythematosus.
    Polyarteritis nodosa.
    Scleroderma.
    Dermatomyositis.
    Sarcoidosis.

Neuro-muscular
    Progressive muscular dystrophy.
    Friedreich's ataxia.
    Myotonia atrophica.
    Polymyositis.

Amyloidosis

Peripartum

Tropical pulmonary oesinophilia

Radiation

Tumour infiltration

Infections

Acute rheumatic fever is a pancarditis in which the endocardial involvement primarily determines the subsequent course of the disease. The illness is now believed to be a hypersensitivity reaction to the streptococcus and is usually preceded by a streptococcal sore throat or scarlet fever. Clinical features include fever, leucocytosis, raised ESR and polyarthritis, which characteristically respond to salicylates;

Jaccoud's arthritis (*see* Chapter 13) is a rare joint sequela. Subcutaneous nodules are very suggestive of the diagnosis, but are also seen in Still's disease and rheumatoid arthritis. Rheumatic pneumonia is a doubtful entity, but pleural effusion may accompany pericardial effusion. Erythema marginatum, a recurring circular erythematous rash, occurs in 10–15 per cent of cases. Chorea, characterized by loss of co-ordination and multiple involuntary movements, has less severe cardiac sequelae than rheumatic fever and is not accompanied by arthritis.

Early involvement of the mitral valve is indicated by a short soft mitral diastolic murmur (Carey Coombs murmur). This is usually heard when the heart size is normal; it may disappear leaving no abnormality, or mitral stenosis may develop later. A pansystolic murmur indicates mitral regurgitation, which is more likely to become established if the murmur is loud. Aortic systolic and diastolic murmurs may be transient or indicate permanent damage.

Cardiac enlargement is due to pericardial effusion or heart failure. Distinction between the two may be difficult, but effusion appears within the first month of the illness, whereas failure is uncommon before three months (Wood, 1968). Heart failure is rarely caused by a simple carditis and is nearly always accompanied by serious valve lesions and signs of pulmonary venous hypertension.

The relative frequency of valve involvement is: mitral 85 per cent, aortic 44 per cent, tricuspid 10–16 per cent, and pulmonary 1–2 per cent (Cabot, 1926). This corresponds to the natural mechanical stress to which each valve is subjected (Wood, 1968). For example, the mitral valve has to withstand the systemic systolic pressure, whereas the pulmonary valve has to withstand only the pulmonary diastolic pressure. Cardiac involvement is more severe following rheumatic fever in childhood than in adolescence or later. Rheumatic valve disease may also follow chorea, but the lesions tend to be milder than those which develop after rheumatic fever. Severe cardiac damage occurs with failure or pericarditis and after recurrent attacks and is most often seen in undernourished communities, particularly in the Far East. Regurgitant lesions reflect severe rheumatic damage and are established from the time of the acute attack. Dominant stenosis, on the other hand, follows milder rheumatic fever or chorea and usually takes ten years or more to develop. Pericarditis leaves no clinical sequelae, but areas of adherent pericardium may show calcified plaques which are visible on the radiograph and may be mistakenly diagnosed as lying in a valve. Constrictive pericarditis is very rare. Rheumatic carditis affects the atrial wall and is probably the single most important factor in left atrial dilatation; endocardial lesions in the left atrium predispose to thrombus formation. A myocardial factor, resulting from rheumatic involvement of the ventricles, has been invoked in patients who have cardiomegaly of a degree that cannot be accounted for by the severity of the valve lesions.

Viruses can cause a myocarditis, often with pericardial and occasionally with endocardial involvement. There may be merely transient cardiac enlargement during a febrile illness, dysrhythmias or progressive dilatation ending in congestive failure and death. Rarely a patient with quite a large heart becomes clinically and radiologically normal.

Chagas' disease is caused by blood-borne infection with *Trypanosoma cruzi*, which enters either by the bite of a triatome or by simultaneous defaecation and scratching. The bug infests the roofs of mud huts in rural areas of central and southern America and the south-west of the United States. The infection starts in childhood and initially is usually silent, but rarely there is a severe constitutional upset with meningo-encephalitis, myocarditis and sometimes pericarditis (Puigbo, 1968). The mortality varies from 2 to 10 per cent in patients with clinical evidence of the disease (Reeder and Simão, 1969). The heart is probably involved in virtually all cases, but the involvement goes unrecognized until later in life. In acute Chagas' myocarditis, the plain film shows a variable degree of cardiac enlargement with or without left ventricular failure, the features being similar to those of any acute congestive cardiomyopathy. After the initial infection there is a latent period of 10 to 20 years—less in severe cases—when clinically silent but progressive cardiac damage is occurring. Towards the end of this period electrocardiographic, radiological and haemodynamic abnormalities may be shown although the patient is symptom free. Finally patients present with chronic Chagas' disease.

The clinical and radiological findings depend on the amount of myocardial damage, but the prognosis is bad as about 20 per cent of patients are dead within two years of diagnosis. Heart block and other dysrhythmias are common and may be the cause of sudden death. The apices of the ventricles show the greatest loss of muscle, sometimes with the formation of aneurysms, these appearances being diagnostic on angiography (*Figure 360*) but not detectable on plain films. The remainder of the ventricle may be

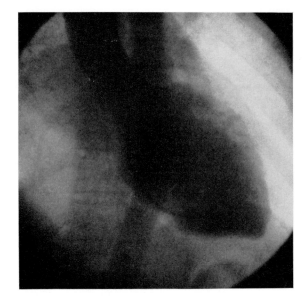

Figure 360. Chagas' disease. Left ventricular angiogram. Apical aneurysm

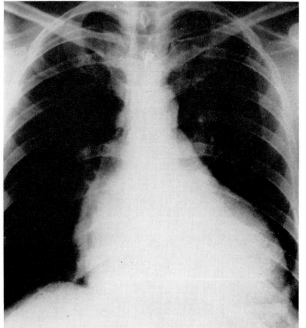

Figure 361. Chagas' disease. Gross cardiac enlargement and normal lungs

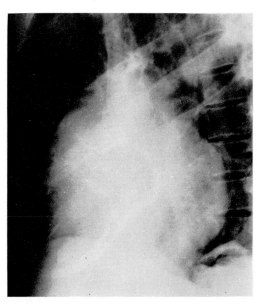

Figure 362. Chagas' disease. Left anterior oblique view showing dilatation of right atrial appendix and left ventricular enlargement

hypertrophied. Thrombus may be present in the ventricles and in the right atrial appendix; pulmonary and systemic emboli are common in patients with congestive failure. In advanced cases the radiological appearances resemble those of any congestive cardiomyopathy, but the right side of the heart is characteristically more severely involved than the left, with the result that the lungs may be normal in conjunction with important cardiac enlargement (*Figure 361*). Dilatation of the right atrial appendix, best seen in the left anterior oblique view, is helpful in early diagnosis of chronic Chagas' cardiomyopathy (Morales *et al.*, 1962) and is characteristic of the disease when combined with left ventricular enlargement (*Figure 362*). Parasites destroy ganglion cells of the peripheral autonomic nervous system, and oesophageal changes resembling achalasia of the cardia are seen. In some endemic areas the oesophagus is not dilated but shows lack of peristalsis with stasis of barium in the supine position, while in other areas (Brazil for example) it may attain a large size. Other hollow viscera such as the stomach, duodenum, colon and ureters may also show dilatation (Reeder and Simão, 1969).

Endocrine and metabolic disorders

Cardiac enlargement in myxoedema is usually due to pericardial effusion (*Figure 363a*). Patients are mostly female and middle-aged or over. Myxoedema should be suspected when there is a combination of cardiac enlargement, normal lungs and an ECG showing low voltage R waves and flat T waves. Occasionally the pericardial effusion is large enough to cause tamponade. Dilatation of the heart also occurs (*Figure 363b*). The pericardial and myocardial changes are reversible with thyroxine treatment. It is possible that there is an increased susceptibility to coronary artery disease.

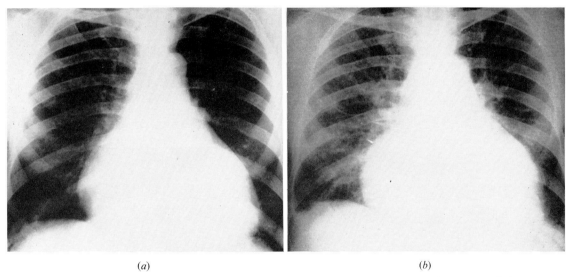

(a)   (b)

Figure 363. Myxoedema. (a) Pericardial effusion. (b) Dilatation of the heart and congestive failure

Slight cardiac enlargement has been described in uncomplicated cases of thyrotoxicosis (Evans, 1949). Patients rarely present with cardiac symptoms before the age of 40 years. Clinical manifestations of thyrotoxicosis may be occult with no weight loss, eye signs or goitre. Atrial fibrillation, a high output circulatory state or congestive failure with cardiac enlargement may be present (*Figure 364*).

In acromegaly, cardiac enlargement may be due to myocardial fibrosis and hypertrophy resulting from growth hormone stimulus or due to systemic hypertension, and coronary artery disease appears frequent. Patients usually die from heart disease.

Beriberi is caused by a diet deficient in thiamine. It is associated with general malnutrition in the tropics, but in the West is most commonly seen in the male alcoholic. Clinically the patient presents in a high output state with raised jugular venous pressure and peripheral oedema; occasionally there is a low cardiac output. The heart may show any degree of enlargement with or without signs of an elevated pulmonary venous pressure. Clinical and radiological improvement in response to thiamine is rapid. The heart may remain enlarged after irreversible myocardial changes have occurred.

Anaemia, particularly that found in the tropics in association with malaria or hookworm disease, may cause a high output state with congestive failure. Sickle cell anaemia may similarly be found with a high cardiac output, but also may cause pulmonary hypertension and coronary artery disease due to blockage of the small pulmonary and coronary arteries by the abnormal red cells.

Glycogen storage disease is an autosomal recessive disorder in which abnormal amounts of glycogen accumulate in skeletal and cardiac muscle due to the absence of a specific enzyme. The disease presents in infancy, and death generally occurs before the age of one year. There is muscular weakness, feeding difficulty and congestive failure. Massive cardiac enlargement is caused by extreme thickening of the left ventricular wall, which may compress the right ventricle. As the left ventricle usually contracts well, cardiac pulsation is normal.

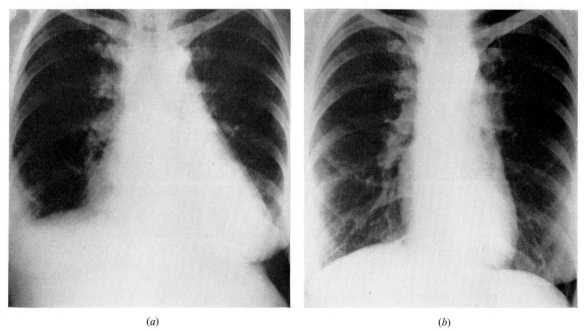

(a)   (b)

Figure 364. Thyrotoxicosis. (a) Congestive failure and atrial fibrillation. (b) Treated. Heart returns to normal size

The triad of cirrhosis of the liver, diabetes mellitus and skin pigmentation which develops in haemo-chromatosis is caused by deposition of iron in the liver, pancreas and skin. The disease is found predominantly in middle-aged men. Iron deposits in the heart cause a cardiomyopathy from which one-third to half the patients die. There is cardiac enlargement, heart block and other dysrhythmias, and congestive failure. Occasionally patients present with heart disease before the skin changes and diabetes become manifest.

Alcohol and cobalt poisoning

Alcohol is considered to be an important cause of non-coronary heart disease in this country (Brigden and Robinson, 1964). Three mechanisms have been invoked: direct toxic action on the myocardium, beriberi due to thiamine deficiency, and cobalt poisoning. Cobalt was used as a stabilizer of froth to promote a good head on beer by breweries in Canada, Belgium and possibly elsewhere. It produced a congestive cardiomyopathy, frequently with pericardial effusion and sometimes with pulmonary hypertension, in patients who took beer as their major source of calories (Sullivan *et al.*, 1969).

Patients with alcoholic heart disease present with dysrhythmias, particularly atrial fibrillation, or with congestive failure. Partial reversibility is sometimes seen following abstinence, but this is often difficult to achieve.

Other conditions associated with cardiomyopathy

Collagen diseases and granulomas may involve the myocardium, pericardium, endocardium, conducting tissue and coronary arteries, so that clinical and radiological manifestations are variable. In addition, some of these disorders cause diffuse lung disease and cor pulmonale.

Cardiomyopathy of the congestive type develops sooner or later in over half the patients with progressive muscular dystrophy, Friedreich's ataxia and myotonia atrophica and may occasionally antedate the other manifestations.

Cardiac amyloidosis is usually primary and confined to the heart; it presents as congestive failure in patients over 70 years of age and occasionally earlier. Heart block and other dysrhythmias are common. The heart may not be very large, but it shows a striking reduction in pulsation. There may be involvement of valves, coronary arteries and pulmonary arteries causing murmurs, angina and pulmonary hypertension. Pleural effusion may occur. Amyloid disease secondary to chronic infection or myelomatosis affects the heart less commonly.

Peripartum cardiomyopathy is primary myocardial disease occurring in the last trimester of pregnancy or within three months of delivery in the absence of toxaemia, hypertension or other known heart disease (Hughes et al., 1970). If these rigid criteria are observed, the disease is rare and it is quite possible that all cases are really unrecognized cases of heart disease brought to light by pregnancy. The condition has been reported more frequently in the tropics, where malnutrition probably plays an important part. Mortality as high as 60 per cent has been reported, and if the patient survives, recurrence at the next pregnancy is usual.

Tropical eosinophilia (Loeffler's disease) is characterized by endocardial thickening of the ventricles with secondary involvement of myocardium, chordae and papillary muscles. Left ventricular disease and mitral regurgitation are more common than right-sided changes, and there may be endocardial thrombosis and systemic emboli. Aetiologically this condition is considered to be a hypersensitivity reaction, possibly to filaria. The clinical features are similar to those of restrictive cardiomyopathy, and radiologically the heart is normal or slightly enlarged.

CHAPTER 29

Cardiac Aneurysm, Tumour and Cyst

CARDIAC ANEURYSM

Aneurysm of the heart is most commonly due to ischaemic heart disease (*see* page 261). Other types are rare and include congenital, surgical, infective and annular subvalvar. An aneurysm usually involves the left ventricle, less often the right ventricle and rarely the atria. Aneurysms may be true or false. A true ventricular aneurysm is a localized dilatation of the ventricular wall and contains thinned myocardium, some of which is replaced by fibrous tissue. A false aneurysm has no myocardium in its wall and arises as a result of deficiency, incision or necrosis of the ventricular muscle, the blood being contained by the endocardium, fibrous tissue or pericardium. A ventricular aneurysm may have a broad or a narrow neck. An aneurysm of the membranous septum is occasionally seen with ventricular septal defect; in some cases it appears to form during spontaneous closure of the defect. It may cause pulmonary stenosis by protruding into the right ventricular outflow tract. Other conditions associated with septal aneurysm include anomalies of the aortic root, sub-aortic stenosis, coarctation, and bacterial endocarditis of the aortic valve with weakening of the septum by the infected regurgitant jet. Aneurysm of the left atrium is seen in chronic rheumatic heart disease (*Figure 365*), and a congenital aneurysm of the right atrium has been reported (Morrow and Behrendt, 1968).

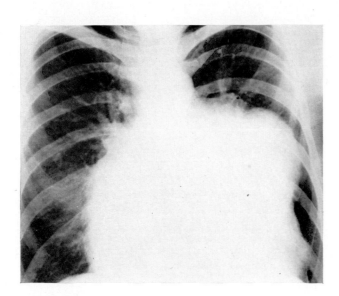

Figure 365. Aneurysm of left atrium (not left atrial appendix)

A congenital aneurysm may contain all layers of the ventricular myocardium (true aneurysm), in which case it contracts in systole and is called a congenital diverticulum. A congenital aneurysm may arise from any part of the myocardium, but one variety originates in relation to the mitral valve ring and another from the apical region in association with defects of the pericardium, diaphragm or abdominal wall. An aneurysm may complicate the origin of the left coronary artery from the pulmonary trunk.

A surgical aneurysm is most often seen after reconstruction of the right ventricular outflow with a pericardial patch or an aortic homograft in Fallot's tetralogy or pulmonary atresia (*Figure 366*). Predisposing causes are incomplete relief of outflow stenosis, residual ventricular septal defect and pulmonary regurgitation (Anderson *et al.*, 1965). A true or false aneurysm may rarely follow left ventriculotomy (*Figure 367*).

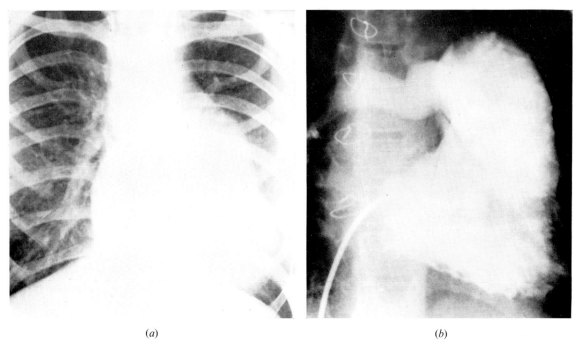

(a) (b)

Figure 366. Aneurysm of right ventricle after surgical reconstruction of its outflow in severe Fallot's tetralogy. (a) Plain film. (b) Right ventricular angiogram

An infective aneurysm is most commonly due to bacterial endocarditis of the aortic valve and involves the free wall or the septum. Mycotic aneurysm has been reported following osteomyelitis (Beare, 1967).

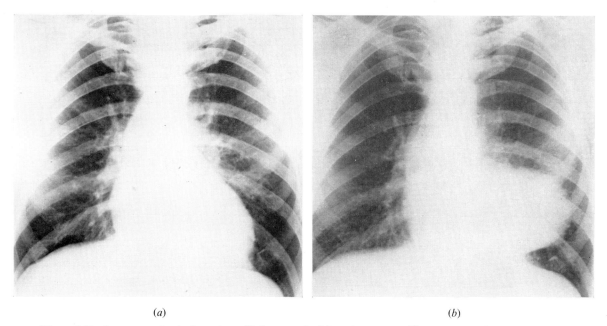

(a) (b)

Figure 367. Aneurysm of apical portion of left ventricle. (a) Pre-operative. (b) Aneurysm after ventriculotomy

Syphilis, tuberculosis and mediastinal abscess have also been quoted as causes. In Chagas' disease an aneurysm may form at the apex of the ventricle but is not detectable on the plain film.

Special mention must be made of annular subvalvar left ventricular aneurysm. This arises below and close to the mitral or less often the aortic valve ring; it has a narrow neck, may be multilocular, and in the sub-mitral position may attain a very large size. Distortion of the mitral or aortic ring can cause regurgitation. An aneurysm may dissect through the myocardium or protrude into the left atrium. Patients may show S–T segment depression, possibly due to stretching of the circumflex branch of the left coronary artery. Thrombosis occurs within the aneurysm but systemic embolism is rare, probably because of the narrow neck. Death results from congestive failure or rupture. The cause of these aneurysms is uncertain, but they probably occur because of congenital or acquired weakness at the junction of the myocardium and the fibrous skeleton of the heart. The disease is almost entirely confined to Africans, but has been reported in white people. It is most common in young adults. In the African it has to be differentiated from endomyocardial fibrosis and primary heart muscle disease.

With a small sub-aortic aneurysm, there is no cardiac enlargement unless distortion of the aortic ring has caused aortic regurgitation. The aneurysm itself is not large enough to be visible as an abnormal bulge. With sub-mitral aneurysm, cardiac enlargement is usually progressive but may regress after treatment of congestive failure. Typically there is a bulge on the left cardiac border, but if the aneurysm is posterior it may show only as a double shadow on the penetrated view. There may be more than one bulge. The heart may be grossly enlarged with a bizarre shape due to the presence of a large aneurysm and its displacement of cardiac chambers. When viewed tangentially on fluoroscopy, the aneurysm shows paradoxical pulsation unless it contains extensive thrombus or calcification in the wall. Calcification is curvilinear and may completely surround an aneurysm or one of its loculi. It was seen in 13 of 46 cases reported by Cockshott et al. (1967), mainly in symptomless patients—a possible reason is that with a rigid or obliterated aneurysm, the load on the left ventricle is less than if the aneurysm expands with each systole. The lungs may show evidence of pulmonary venous hypertension. Complications include thrombo-embolism, dysrhythmia, congestive failure and rupture.

The differential diagnosis of annular subvalvar aneurysm includes the following conditions.

(1) Cardiomyopathy: endomyocardial fibrosis and heart muscle disease in the African.

(2) Other causes of cardiac aneurysm. Coronary artery disease is uncommon in the African. Annular subvalvar aneurysms have a narrow neck and may be multilocular, unlike those due to coronary occlusion.

(3) Other causes of mitral regurgitation.

(4) Other causes of aortic regurgitation, particularly those with abnormalities of the aortic root such as aneurysm of the sinus of Valsalva.

(5) Other causes of cardiac calcification.

CARDIAC TUMOUR

Primary tumours are rare, and 80 per cent of them are benign. Myxomas make up about 50 per cent of primary tumours and usually present in adults between the ages of 30 and 60 years; they are intra-cavitary and pedunculated, and are rarely found elsewhere than in the atria. Other benign tumours usually occur in infants or children, involve the left ventricle or its septum, and are intramural in position. Being mesenchymal in origin, they are variously described as fibromas, rhabdomyomas, teratomas or angiomas. Fifty per cent of rhabdomyomas of the heart are associated with tuberous sclerosis. Calcification is seen in about 10 per cent of myxomas and in nearly 20 per cent of benign tumours in children (Davis et al., 1969).

Twenty per cent of primary tumours are malignant and comprise various types of sarcoma such as rhabdomyosarcoma, fibrosarcoma and angiosarcoma. They are commonest in children and young adults and involve the right atrium and right ventricle, where they are more often intramural than pedunculated. Intraluminal tumours may arise from the endocardium or rarely from the pulmonary artery or one of the valves. Sarcoma in the left atrium has been reported as causing systemic effects similar to those of myxoma (Raftery et al., 1966).

Secondary tumours are 20–40 times more common than primary tumours. They are either metastic (blood-borne) or involve the heart by direct infiltration or by venous invasion. Metastases are most common in the left heart, probably because the coronary flow is greater than on the right side, and occur late in malignant disease. Melanoma has the highest incidence of cardiac involvement, but other tumours prone to metastasize to the heart include carcinoma of the thyroid, kidney, liver, uterus and lung

(Berge and Sievers, 1968). Carcinoma of the lung and mediastinal tumours may directly infiltrate the heart. Invasion along a vein, sometimes from a distant site, occurs in systemic more often than in pulmonary veins. In general, a blood-borne metastasis tends to involve the wall of the left ventricle, whereas direct invasion of the heart by a malignant tumour usually extends into an atrial cavity.

The clinical and radiological presentation of cardiac tumours is extremely variable and depends to some extent on whether the tumours occupy an intracavitary, an intramural or an epicardial position. They may present as follows:

Intracavitary tumours
    Valve disease.
    Constrictive pericarditis.
    Constitutional disturbance.
    Systemic emboli.
    Syncope.
    Sudden death.

Intramural tumours
    Congestive failure.
    Restrictive cardiomyopathy.
    Dysrhythmias.
    Abnormal heart shape.
    Sudden death.

Epicardial tumours
    Abnormal heart shape.
    Pericardial effusion or tamponade.

It is often impossible to tell whether a tumour is benign or malignant except in the case of myxoma, which is the commonest of all cardiac tumours as well as being benign and surgically curable.

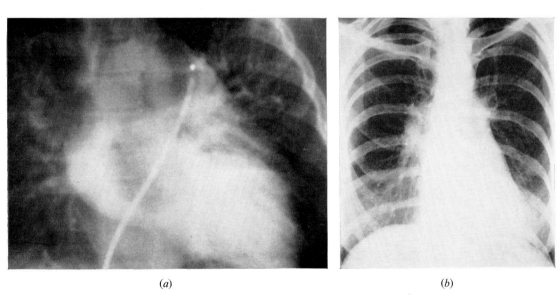

(a)   (b)

Figure 368. Left atrial myxoma. (a) Pulmonary arteriogram. Tumour demonstrated in left atrium during laevo-cardiogram. (b) Plain film. Enlarged left atrial appendix (confirmed by operation) and upper zone vessel dilatation (mean left atrial pressure 15 mm, rising to 30 mm on exercise)

A myxoma is a pedunculated tumour arising from the atrial septum (*Figure 368a*). Seventy-five per cent are found in the left atrium and 25 per cent in the right atrium. Very occasionally they are found in both atria together or in the ventricles. They usually present between the ages of 30 and 60 years, and are rare in children. They typically cause obstruction to the mitral or tricuspid orifice, but interference with valve closure or destruction of cusp tissue by a calcified tumour can lead to regurgitation. Both obstruction and regurgitation may be intermittent, producing variable physical signs, particularly with posture. Sudden obstruction causes syncope. A left atrial myxoma may simulate rheumatic mitral valve disease, while a right atrial myxoma may mimic Ebstein's disease (Oliver and Missen, 1966) or constrictive pericarditis (Emanuel and Lloyd, 1964). A right-to-left shunt has been reported through a patent foramen ovale as a result of right-sided obstruction (Miller *et al.*, 1968). Tumours are friable, so that pulmonary and systemic embolism is common. Systemic emboli are more apparent because of their more dramatic clinical presentation. Embolic pulmonary hypertension has been reported (Heath and Mackinnon, 1964). There may be a history of constitutional disturbance for many months, sometimes before the tumour is large enough to exert any mechanical effects; the features include fever, weight loss, fatigue, anaemia, finger clubbing, joint pain, polyneuritis and hypergammaglobulinaemia.

Radiologically left atrial myxoma may present a whole spectrum of appearances from a normal heart without left atrial enlargement to considerable cardiac enlargement with dilatation of the left atrium, left ventricle and right ventricle. The lungs usually show evidence of venous and arterial hypertension, so that the picture is indistinguishable from that of mitral valve disease with pulmonary hypertension (*Figure 368b*), but the appearances may change for no apparent reason. Right atrial myxoma may cause right atrial dilatation and right ventricular enlargement as well if tricuspid regurgitation is important. There may be evidence of pulmonary emboli. Approximately 10 per cent of myxomas contain calcification dense enough to be visible on plain films. Fluoroscopy may demonstrate calcium that was invisible on plain films because of motional blurring.

Intramural tumours usually present radiologically as an abnormal heart shape or non-specific cardiac enlargement due to tumour infiltration or pericardial effusion. Calcification is seen in 20 per cent of benign tumours in children. Intramural and epicardial tumours cannot be distinguished on plain films from primary or secondary pericardial tumours. Mediastinal neoplasms, especially ectopic thymic tumours, may closely apply themselves to the pericardium and also be indistinguishable.

CARDIAC CYST

Pericardial cyst is considered on page 289. Hydatid cyst in the heart is usually primary and solitary and grows in the myocardium. After 1–5 years, rupture occurs into ventricle, atrium or pericardium unless the cyst dies. Secondary cysts may then grow in multiple distant sites—brain, lung or abdomen—or locally in the heart or pericardium. Cysts in the left side of the heart may cause death from rupture into the ventricle, massive embolism or anaphylactic shock. A ruptured cyst may calcify. Secondary cysts in the heart or pericardium may in turn rupture in the circulation with death of the patient.

As with metastatic tumours, the site of the primary blood-borne hydatid cyst is most commonly in the left ventricle, where an abnormal bulge may be visible radiologically. Dead cysts may show calcification. Multiple cardiac bulges may be seen with secondary cysts together with evidence of hydatid disease elsewhere.

CHAPTER 30

The Pericardium

INTRODUCTION

The pericardium surrounds the heart and covers the proximal half of the ascending aorta, the pulmonary trunk nearly to its bifurcation, and the pulmonary and systemic veins. It consists of a visceral and a parietal layer, between which is the pericardial cavity, a potential space lined with a smooth serous membrane. The visceral pericardium is also termed the epicardium. Areolar tissue, coronary vessels and nerves lie between the epicardium and the myocardium. Fat accumulates, particularly in the obese, in this sub-epicardial space and may be visible as a relatively translucent curved band, 1–2 mm thick, just inside the left lower cardiac border. The soft tissue shadow between the sub-epicardial fat and the air in the adjacent lung represents the two layers of the pericardium and the mediastinal pleura and normally does not exceed 2 mm. Pericardial or mediastinal effusion or thickening broadens this shadow if the sub-epicardial fat layer can be demonstrated on plain films or on tomography.

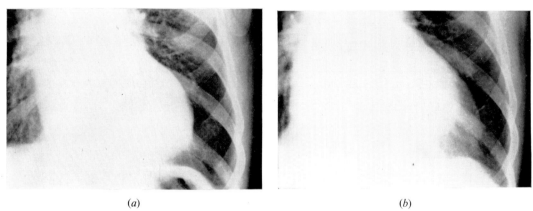

(a)   (b)

Figure 369. Apical fat pad. (a) Small pad. (b) Increase in size with obesity

The parietal pericardium is continuous with the adventitia of the great vessels and is densely adherent to the central tendon of the diaphragm. A layer of fat, however, may separate the pericardium from the mediastinal pleura, being visible on the anterior view as a radiolucent rim between the ventricular border of the heart and the lung. This extrapericardial fat is broader than the sub-epicardial variety and non-uniform in width, and larger triangular collections of fat in the costo-phrenic angles are very common in obese patients of middle age or beyond (*Figure 369*). They are usually on the left side, where they surround the apex of the heart and may simulate cardiac enlargement, but a penetrated view will separate them from the heart itself as they are less dense. On the right side they present with a slightly convex border upwards and outwards towards the lung. On the lateral view they are seen as triangular opacities in the anterior costo-phrenic angle. Pericardial cyst and omental hernia through the foramen of Morgagni may closely resemble extrapericardial fat, and the differential diagnosis is considered below under the heading of pericardial cyst. Occasionally extrapericardial fat may cause prominence in the region of the right atrium and superior vena cava (Cohen, 1953).

PERICARDIAL EFFUSION

The diagnosis of pericardial effusion is often difficult by plain radiography, but is readily confirmed by echocardiography (Pridie *et al.*, 1972). In certain cases, however, particularly where the collection of fluid is asymmetrical, the plain radiograph may be very suggestive of the diagnosis.

The pericardial cavity normally contains 15–30 ml of fluid, and an effusion of between 250 and 500 ml must accumulate before any change in heart size or shape can be detected. The single most important sign of pericardial effusion is a rapid alteration in heart size or shape without lung changes (*Figure 370*). In contrast to constriction, an effusion rarely impedes filling of the left heart, and signs of pulmonary venous hypertension are uncommon unless the collection of fluid is rapid or the effusion is huge.

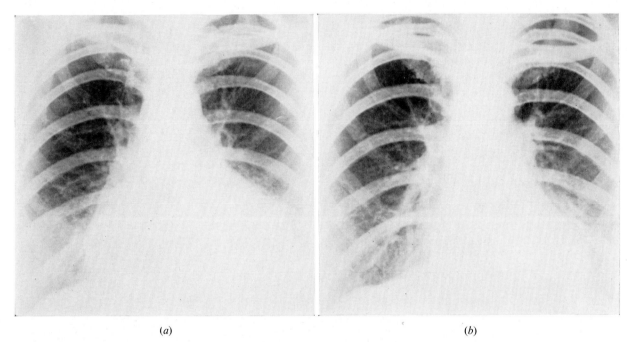

(*a*)   (*b*)

Figure 370. (a) Pericardial effusion. (b) One week later—rapid change in heart size

Similarly, obstruction of systemic venous return is less common than in constriction, so that superior vena caval dilatation is not seen unless tamponade is present. With an acute effusion the heart may enlarge only slightly before tamponade occurs as it takes time for the parietal layer to stretch, but with subacute or chronic effusions the heart may attain a large size before any increase in filling resistance develops. Fluid first accumulates in the most dependent part, the diaphragmatic recess, and later in the anterior and lateral recesses. The distribution may be symmetrical so that on the anterior view the heart appears triangular, pear-shaped or globular (*Figure 371*). The normal contours may be effaced even by small effusions, and filling in of the middle of the left border may be mistaken for dilatation of the left atrial appendage or the right ventricular outflow tract. Acute cardio-phrenic angles have been described as a typical sign; in the authors' experience they are not infrequently normal with effusion and acute with cardiac dilatation. If the accumulation is mainly unilateral the heart shows an asymmetrical bulge to one side, although a dominant collection on the right is rare (*Figure 372*). Anterior collection shows on the lateral view as increased contact of the heart with the sternum and, when larger, as filling in of the retrosternal air space. There is less room posteriorly for any major accumulation of fluid because space is restricted by the pulmonary veins (*see Figure 371b*). Thus marked posterior convexity is rarely seen, but the postero-inferior part of the heart may be prominent due to accumulation of fluid in the posterior part of the diaphragmatic recess. On the anterior view there is broadening of the vascular pedicle caused by accumulation of fluid around the ascending aorta and the pulmonary trunk. The aortic knuckle is extrapericardial and remains visible immediately above the widened cardiac shadow. Alteration in the shape of the heart with changes in posture is often helpful, and with a small heart broadening of the base in a supine film may be a decisive sign. When the heart is large, cardiac dilatation and pericardial effusion tend to produce similar postural changes in contour.

On fluoroscopy, diminished or absent pulsation over the ventricular border of the heart may be helpful in the case of small effusions, but is also seen in constrictive pericarditis and ischaemic heart disease.

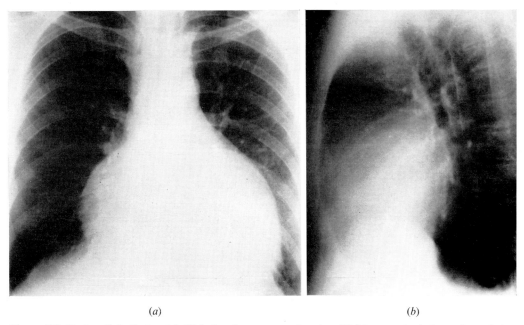

(a)   (b)

Figure 371. Pericardial effusion. (a) Globular shape on anterior view. (b) No posterior bulge on lateral view

With large effusions, pulsation is diminished, but similar appearances are found in cardiomyopathy, Ebstein's anomaly and congestive failure from any cause.

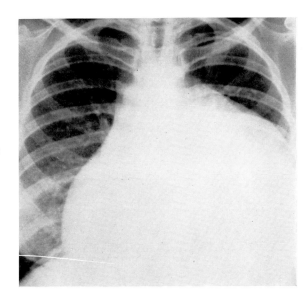

Figure 372. Pericardial effusion, predominantly on left side

Signs of pericardial effusion

The following is a summary of the most important signs of pericardial effusion.
(1) Rapid change in heart size and shape with normal lungs.
(2) Absence of pulmonary venous hypertension and superior vena caval dilatation with a large heart.
(3) Loss of normal cardiac contours with only slight or moderate cardiac enlargement.
(4) Dominant enlargement of the heart laterally and anteriorly but not posteriorly.

(5) Alteration of heart shape with posture.

(6) Diminished or absent pulsation with only slight or moderate cardiac enlargement.

Causes and associated conditions

The causes of pericardial effusion are as follows.

(1) Acute non-specific pericarditis: viral pericarditis—Coxsackie B, mumps, glandular fever, etc.

(2) Tuberculosis.

(3) Post-cardiotomy and post-myocardial infarction syndromes.

(4) Malignant disease: carcinoma of bronchus, etc.

(5) Post-radiation therapy.

(6) Rheumatic fever.

(7) Collagen disorders: rheumatoid arthritis, lupus erythematosus, scleroderma, polyarteritis nodosa.

(8) Myxoedema.

(9) Bacterial infection.

(10) Uraemia.

(11) Chronic anaemia.

(12) Mechanical: trauma, rupture of heart or dissecting aneurysm.

Pericardial effusion may be associated with pleural effusion in non-specific pericarditis, tuberculosis, collagen disease and other auto-immune disorders. In tuberculous pericarditis, pulmonary lesions are not seen, but a calcified mediastinal gland may be identified as the source of infection. Areas of basal pneumonitis are found with non-specific pericarditis and with post-cardiotomy and post-myocardial infarction syndromes. In malignant effusion, a mediastinal mass is sometimes difficult to identify.

Differential diagnosis

The following is the differential diagnosis of pericardial effusion.

(1) Cardiomyopathy.

(2) Ebstein's anomaly: parchment right ventricle (Uhl's anomaly).

(3) Severe chronic rheumatic heart disease.

(4) Severe pulmonary stenosis.

(5) Congestive cardiac failure from any cause.

The appearances of the lungs are often of help in separating these lesions. In cardiomyopathy sometimes, and in chronic rheumatic heart disease nearly always, there will be evidence of pulmonary venous hypertension. In Ebstein's anomaly, Uhl's anomaly and severe pulmonary stenosis, oligaemia in association with the large heart may be striking. In pericardial effusion the pulmonary vascular pattern is nearly always normal. Left atrial enlargement or valvar calcification may be visible in chronic rheumatic heart disease on the penetrated anterior and lateral views.

CONSTRICTIVE PERICARDITIS

Pericardial constriction is a complication which may arise during the healing phase of any type of pericarditis, particularly tuberculosis. Organization of the pericardial exudate leads to fibrous contraction and calcification which impedes filling of the heart. Thickening and contraction are usually maximal in the atrio-ventricular grooves and the adjoining parts of the ventricles. Dominant thickening on the right causes inflow obstruction to the right heart and, less commonly, left-sided thickening results in inflow obstruction to the left heart. Thickening around the right and left ventricular outflow tracts of sufficient severity to cause outflow obstruction has been reported (Mounsey, 1959).

The onset of constriction usually occurs while the heart is still large, and only a minority of patients present with a normal-sized heart (Shawdon and Dinsmore, 1967). The outline may be indistinct due to mediastinal pleural involvement. The cardiac shape is always abnormal and depends upon the sites of constriction, but the right atrial border is typically flat (*Figure 373*).

Calcification is best seen on the lateral view and is detected on plain films in about 50 per cent of patients. The distribution in general corresponds to the areas of maximal fibrosis and constriction, and the calcification is most commonly found in the atrio-ventricular grooves (*see Figure 83*).

If restriction of diastolic filling is predominantly right-sided, then dilatation of the superior vena cava and the azygos vein may be detected and the lungs will be normal or even oligaemic (*Figure 374*).

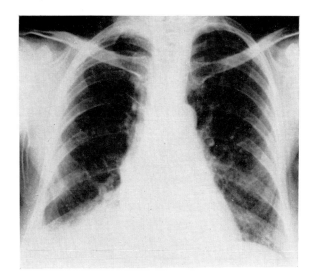

Figure 373. Constrictive pericarditis. Flat right atrium

If it is left-sided, dilatation of the left atrium and signs of pulmonary venous hypertension are usually present and the appearances may resemble those of mitral valve disease (*Figure 375*). Pleural effusions are extremely common.

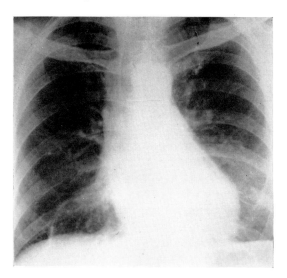

Figure 374. Constrictive pericarditis. Dilated superior vena cava

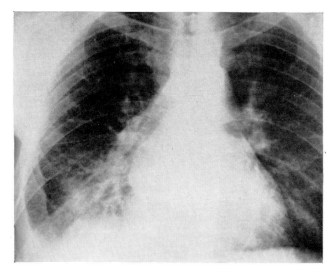

Figure 375. Constrictive pericarditis. Interstitial and alveolar oedema with pericardial calcification

On fluoroscopy the 'diastolic shock' is often a striking feature. Pulsation may be reduced locally over areas of restriction or may be generally diminished (Cornell and Rossi, 1968), but if the calcification and thickening lie in the grooves only, leaving the atria and ventricles free, pulsation may be normal.

ADHERENT PERICARDIUM

After any type of pericarditis, local areas of visceral and parietal pericardium may thicken and adhere. These plaques may calcify without causing any haemodynamic abnormality. In approximately 5 per cent of cases of chronic rheumatic heart disease, calcified plaques may be identified on plain radiographs (*see Figure 84*). Their importance lies in the fact that they must be distinguished from calcification of the aortic and mitral valves and left atrium. Constriction is extremely rare after rheumatic pericarditis.

PERICARDIAL DEFECTS

Pericardial defects are of three types.

Congenital absence of pleuro-pericardium

This can be subdivided as follows.

Partial: right or left (*Figure 376a*).

Complete: right, left or bilateral (*Figure 376b*).

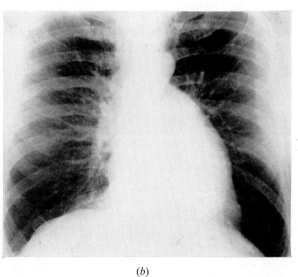

(b)

Figure 376. Left pericardial defect. (a) Partial. (b) Complete

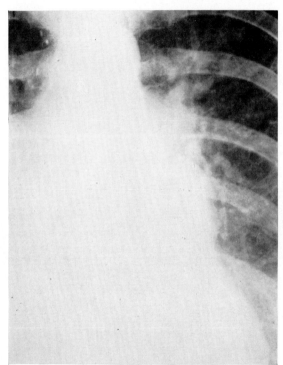

(a)

Congenital absence is usually left-sided, and the complete variety is more common than the partial. A recent review of the literature (Hudson, 1970) showed that 20 per cent of pericardial defects are associated with other congenital anomalies including ductus arteriosus, atrial septal defect, sequestrated lung segment and bronchogenic cyst. Obscure chest pain is sometimes associated with unilateral complete defects, but no serious complications are reported. Partial defects involve the upper part of the pericardium anterior to the hilum. The left atrial appendix and sometimes the pulmonary trunk herniate through left-sided defects and the right atrial appendix through right-sided defects. Enlargement of either atrial appendix in the absence of an obvious cause, and particularly without enlargement of the whole atrium, suggests a partial pericardial defect (Deutsch *et al.*, 1970). Left-sided partial herniation may resemble dilatation of the pulmonary trunk and simulate pulmonary stenosis, small atrial septal defect, pulmonary hypertension and idiopathic dilatation of the pulmonary trunk, but the bulge is usually too low in position to be pulmonary trunk alone. Thrombo-embolism and partial strangulation are possible complications (Tubbs and Yacoub, 1968).

Complete defects are nearly always left-sided, probably because early atrophy of the left duct of Cuvier interferes with obliteration of the left pleuro-pericardial canal. The heart is often slightly enlarged and always shifted to the left, while the trachea remains central. On the left cardiac border the demarcation between the aortic knuckle, the pulmonary trunk and the ventricular border is unusually distinct and the pulmonary trunk appears dilated. Tubbs and Yacoub (1968) mention blurring of the ventricular border as a constant sign, probably due to increased mobility of the apical portion of the heart. Backward displacement of the heart is seen on the lateral view. Left-sided pericardial defect may be mistaken for atrial septal defect as there may be an ejection systolic murmur, a loud pulmonary component of the second heart sound, right axis deviation on the electrocardiogram, a dilated pulmonary trunk and displacement of the heart to the left.

An artificial left pneumothorax, with films taken in the erect and left lateral decubitus positions, will confirm the diagnosis.

Congenital deficiency of septum transversum: defect in central tendon with diaphragmatic hernia

This lesion presents with cardio-respiratory difficulty in infancy. Abdominal contents are seen in the thorax.

Acquired defects after intrapericardial pneumonectomy and trauma

Acquired defects are important as they may allow herniation of the heart with strangulation and death (Borrie, 1969). Radiologically they may be similar to complete congenital defects.

PERICARDIAL CYSTS

The following is suggested as a classification of cystic lesions in and around the pericardium.

True intrapericardial cyst

Pleuro-pericardial cyst, probably arising from a dislocated pleuro-pericardial or pericardial lacuna. This is also described as a pericardial coelomic cyst.

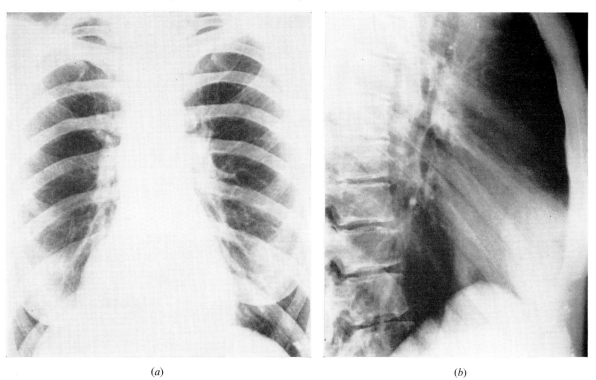

(a)   (b)

Figure 377. Pericardial cyst in right cardio-phrenic angle. (a) Anterior view. (b) Lateral view

Spring-water or lymphangiomatous cyst, arising from lymphatic elements in or adjacent to the pericardium.

Pericardial diverticulum, due to either congenital or acquired weakness of the fibrous layer of the parietal pericardium with herniation of the serosa.

289

True intrapericardial cyst is inseparable from the heart shadow and presents as a bulge usually in the right or left cardio-phrenic angle (*Figure 377*). The other cystic lesions are adjacent to the heart shadow, but can be largely separated from it in tangential projections. They most frequently lie in the cardio-phrenic angles, usually the right, but may also arise anywhere around the pericardium. They are oval with a smooth, clear-cut edge. Extension into the greater fissure, producing a 'tear-drop' appearance, may be seen on the lateral view. Cysts are lax and change their shape with posture and respiration, tending to be longer and narrower in inspiration. Pericardial diverticula may empty into the pericardium in the supine position, but a reduction in their size is often difficult to differentiate from a change in their shape; they fill with air from a pneumopericardium unless the neck is obstructed. Acquired diverticula are probably the result of a previous effusion and may show calcification.

Other cystic lesions around the pericardium such as bronchogenic cyst, teratoma, hydatid cyst and loculated pericardial effusion may closely resemble pericardial cyst. A pericardial fat pad may also be confused with a pericardial cyst, but tends to have a flat rather than a round posterior contour and is less dense because of its fat content. An omental hernia through the foramen of Morgagni presents as an opacity similar to a pericardial cyst in the right cardio-phrenic angle anteriorly. Barium enema examination shows an elevated transverse colon pulled up by the herniated greater omentum.

APPENDICES

APPENDIX A

Radiographic Technique

The National Heart Hospital radiographic technique is as follows.

All new patients have postero-anterior, penetrated postero-anterior and right lateral films. At subsequent visits, patients have a single postero-anterior film unless further views are indicated.

Kodak RP film is used, processed in a 90-second high temperature X-omat automatic processor.

TABLE 14

Radiographic Technique for Adults

Subject	Projection	kV	Maximum mAs with Siemens Iontomat phototimer	FFD	Screens	Grid
Adult male	PA	60–65	30	5 ft (1·5 m)	Standard	—
	Penetrated PA	100	15	40 in (1 m)	Fast	Lysholm Schonander 6·5:1
	Right lateral	110	40	48 in (1·2 m)	Fast	Lysholm Schonander 6·5:1
Adult female	PA	55–60	20	5 ft (1·5 m)	Standard	—
	Penetrated PA	100	15	40 in (1 m)	Fast	Lysholm Schonander 6·5:1
	Right lateral	105	35	48 in (1·2 m)	Fast	Lysholm Schonander 6·5:1

Arbitrary exposure figures are difficult to quote for radiography of children as much depends on their age, size and co-operation. However small, the child must be erect and preferably postero-anterior. Generally it may be said that the smaller the child, the greater the exposure required in relation to size and the less the difference between postero-anterior and lateral exposures. It may not always be necessary to use stationary grids or grid cassettes for the penetrated postero-anterior and right lateral films. A phototimer is not used.

Some exposures suitable for the average child are suggested in Table 15.

TABLE 15

Suggested Exposures for Average Children

Subject	Projection	kV	mAs	FFD	Screens	Grid
Child aged 3 months: Height 60 cm Weight 6 kg	PA	55	12	5 ft (1·5 m)	Standard	—
	Penetrated PA	70	4	40 in (1 m)	Standard	G.E.C. Lucidex
	Lateral	75	16	48 in (1·2 m)	Standard	G.E.C. Lucidex
Child aged 2 years: Height 90 cm Weight 13 kg	PA	55	12	5 ft (1·5 m)	Standard	—
	Penetrated PA	75	4	40 in (1 m)	Standard	G.E.C. Lucidex
	Lateral	75	16	48 in (1·2 m)	Standard	G.E.C. Lucidex
Child aged 6 years: Height 120 cm Weight 20 kg	PA	55	12	5 ft (1·5 m)	Standard	—
	Penetrated PA	75	4	40 in (1 m)	Standard	G.E.C. Lucidex
	Lateral	78	20	48 in (1·2 m)	Standard	G.E.C. Lucidex

APPENDIX B

Material

The observations in this book are based on a study of the following material. All cases had cardiac catheterization data and the diagnosis was verified by angiocardiography and/or surgical findings. Autopsy data were available in a small number of cases.

TABLE 16

Diagnosis	Number of cases
Aortic sinus fistula	12
Aortic valve disease	150
Aorto-pulmonary septal defect	3
Atrial septal defect (primum)	40
With pulmonary hypertension	11
With pulmonary stenosis	2
Atrial septal defect (secundum)	119
With Eisenmenger reaction	26
With mitral valve disease	24
With partial anomalous pulmonary venous drainage	21
With pulmonary hypertension (acyanotic)	20
With pulmonary stenosis	25
Atrio-ventricular canal	13
With hyperkinetic pulmonary hypertension	3
With Eisenmenger reaction	3
With pulmonary stenosis	3
Cardiomyopathy: Congestive	47
Hypertrophic	25
Coarctation	45
Constrictive pericarditis	14
Coronary artery disease	160
Coronary artery fistula	7
Cor triatriatum	1
Ductus arteriosus	39
With Eisenmenger reaction	25
With hyperkinetic pulmonary hypertension	10
Ebstein's anomaly	7
Fallot's tetralogy: Cyanotic	89
Acyanotic	11
With aortic regurgitation	5
Infundibular stenosis	7
Left ventricular/right atrial shunt	5
Mitral valve disease	150
Myxoma	6
Pericardial effusion	13
Pulmonary artery stenosis	5
Pulmonary atresia: With ventricular septal defect	30
With intact septum	2
Pulmonary valve stenosis	61
Single atrium	8
Single ventricle	3
Subvalvar aortic stenosis	19
Supravalvar aortic stenosis	8
Total anomalous pulmonary venous drainage	3
Transposition: Complete	14
Corrected	18
Tricuspid atresia	13
Tricuspid valve disease	40

TABLE 16—*continued*

Diagnosis	Number of cases
Truncus arteriosus	6
Two-chambered right ventricle	2
Ventricular septal defect	89
Acquired	5
With aortic regurgitation	10
With double outflow right ventricle	11
With ductus arteriosus	10
With corrected transposition	11
With Eisenmenger reaction	30
With hyperkinetic pulmonary hypertension	19
With right aortic arch	2

APPENDIX C

Computer Correlations

Correlations of pressures and flows with radiological signs were obtained in the common lesions, including atrial septal defect, ventricular septal defect, ductus arteriosus, Fallot's tetralogy, mitral valve disease and aortic valve disease. In lesions with a left-to-right shunt, the pulmonary to systemic (P/S) flow ratio and the pulmonary artery systolic pressure were correlated with the authors' subjective assessment of heart, right atrial, left atrial, pulmonary trunk and aortic arch size and with the degree of plethora; in Fallot, the systemic oxygen saturation was correlated with aortic size and the degree of oligaemia; and in mitral and aortic valve disease, the pulmonary venous pressure and pulmonary vascular resistance were correlated with heart, left atrial, pulmonary trunk and lobar artery size, upper zone vessel dilatation, lower zone vessel narrowing and pulmonary oedema. The significance of the correlations was determined using the chi-squared test. An example is shown in Table 17.

TABLE 17

Correlation of Pulmonary Venous Pressure and Upper Zone Vessel Dilatation in Chronic Valve Disease

Pulmonary venous pressure (mm Hg)	Upper zone vessel dilatation			
	Absent	Slight	Obvious	Total
	Observed frequency:			
< 10	69	20	5	94
10–19	14	35	36	85
> 19	3	18	82	103
Total	86	73	123	282
	Expected frequency:			
< 10	28·67	24·33	41·00	
10–19	25·92	22·00	37·07	
> 19	31·41	26·67	44·93	

Chi-squared = 161·428. This indicates very strong evidence of correlation ($p = < 0·001$).

In some cases, compression of the gradings was required to establish a correlation. Many statements and conclusions in the text are based on the correlations or on percentages taken from the actual observed frequency tables, selected examples of which are given.

Selection of patients with valve disease

Patients were selected with chronic disease of one valve only, either mitral or aortic, of sufficient severity to require surgical treatment. The diagnosis, and especially the assessment of the relative severity of stenosis and regurgitation, was based on catheter, angiocardiographic and surgical findings. Where these findings disagreed, the case was excluded.

Three disease groups were collected for each valve, with 50 cases in each group. These were as follows.

(1) Stenosis without or with only trivial regurgitation.
(2) Regurgitation without or with only trivial stenosis.
(3) Truly mixed lesions with significant stenosis and regurgitation.

Computer analysis was carried out on each group separately and also on groups 1 and 3 combined (stenosis with or without regurgitation) and groups 2 and 3 combined (regurgitation with or without stenosis). It was also done for all mitral disease, for all aortic disease, and for the whole group of 300 cases of aortic and mitral disease.

Grading of radiological signs

For the purposes of the correlations, the radiological signs were graded as follows.

Heart size (*see* Chapter 1)	Normal (equivalent to CTR* 50 per cent or less, or to a volume of 550 ml/m²† in males and 500 ml/m² in females, or less)
	Slight enlargement (equivalent to CTR up to 55 per cent or a volume up to 700 ml/m²)
	Obvious enlargement (equivalent to CTR over 55 per cent or a volume over 700 ml/m²)
Right and left atrial size	Normal
	Slight enlargement
	Obvious enlargement
Pulmonary trunk size	Normal
	Slight enlargement
	Obvious enlargement
Ascending aorta size	Normal
	Large
Aortic arch size	Normal
	Small
	Large
Oligaemia	None
	Slight
	Obvious
Upper zone vessel size	Normal
	Slight dilatation
	Obvious dilatation
Pulmonary oedema	Absent
	Present
Lower segmental artery size	Normal
	Slight narrowing
	Obvious narrowing
Right lower lobar artery size (reflects degree of plethora in left-to-right shunts)	Normal
	Slight enlargement
	Obvious enlargement

Grading of catheterization data

Pulmonary flow	P/S ratio 1·1 to 2
	P/S ratio over 2
Pulmonary artery systolic pressure	Under 31 mm Hg
	31 to 50 mm Hg
	Over 50 mm Hg
Pulmonary venous pressure	Under 10 mm Hg
	10 to 19 mm Hg
	Over 19 mm Hg
Pulmonary vascular resistance	Under 3 units
	3 to 9 units
	Over 9 units
Systemic oxygen saturation	Under 80 per cent
	80 to 90 per cent
	Over 90 per cent

* Cardio-thoracic ratio.   † Square metre body surface.

298

Grading of defect size

In children, this was corrected according to the body surface area.

Atrial septal defect	Small = maximum diameter 3·0 cm
Ventricular septal defect	Small = maximum diameter 1·5 cm
Ductus arteriosus	Small = maximum diameter 0·7 cm

Significance of correlations

+ + + = Very strong evidence of correlation ($p = <0·001$).

+ + = Strong evidence of correlation ($p = <0·01$).

+ = Some evidence of correlation ($p = <0·05$).

o = No evidence of correlation, but no evidence that no correlation exists ($p = >0·05$).

− = Insufficient data, indicating that one or more of the elements in the observed frequency table is less than 5; again, this is not evidence that no correlation exists.

Correlation tables

In the following Tables, the figures in parentheses refer to numbers of patients.

TABLE 18

Correlation of Pulmonary Flow with Radiological Signs in Left-to-right Shunts

	Cardiac enlargement	Right atrial enlargement	Left atrial enlargement	Pulmonary trunk enlargement	Reduction in aortic arch size	Right lower lobe artery dilatation
All shunts (321)	+ + +	+ +	0	+ + +	+ + +	+ + +
Atrial septal defect (114)	0	0	−	0	−	0
Ventricular septal defect (79)	+ + +	+	0	+	−	+ + +

Comment

The striking feature is the lack of correlation between flow and radiology in atrial septal defect. This may be partly due to the inclusion of a number of pulmonary hypertensives (not Eisenmenger) in whom the heart and vessels are large but the flow is not proportionately increased. Even so, the correlation is lacking and the authors' impression is that there really is no correlation with heart size, but that while obvious enlargement of the right lower lobe artery without pulmonary hypertension means a large shunt, slight enlargement can occur with any size of shunt. The correlations for ventricular septal defect are as expected except for left atrial enlargement, in which the figures do show a trend in the expected direction which is not statistically significant. Catheter data were not available in a sufficient number of patients with ductus arteriosus for inclusion.

TABLE 19

Correlation of Pulmonary Artery Systolic Pressure with Radiological Signs in Left-to-right Shunts

	Cardiac enlargement	Right atrial enlargement	Left atrial enlargement	Pulmonary trunk enlargement	Reduction in aortic arch size	Right lower lobe artery dilatation
All shunts (401)	+ + +	0	+ + +	+ + +	+ + +	+ + +
Atrial septal defect (117)	+ + +	0	−	+ + +	−	+
Ventricular septal defect (85)	+ + +	0	+ +	+ +	−	+ + +

Comment

The correlations in the large group of 401 cases with left-to-right shunts (excluding cyanotic heart disease) are as expected. The correlation with the aortic arch refers to a reduction in size so that statistically the higher the pulmonary artery pressure, the smaller the aortic arch. The lack of correlation with right atrial enlargement underlines the difficulty of estimating the right atrial size. The data are insufficient on the left atrium and the aortic arch in atrial septal defect because these were normal and small respectively in almost all cases. The correlation of right lower lobe artery dilatation in atrial septal defect is not as strong as with other shunts, confirming the authors' impression that this artery is often quite large without much rise in pulmonary artery pressure. Catheter data were not available in a sufficient number of patients with ductus arteriosus for inclusion.

TABLE 20

Correlation of Defect Size with Radiological Signs in Left-to-right Shunts

	Cardiac enlargement	Right atrial enlargement	Left atrial enlargement	Pulmonary trunk dilatation	Reduction in aortic arch size	Right lower lobe artery dilatation
Atrial septal defect (79)	0	−	−	−	−	−
Ventricular septal defect (48)	0	0	0	+	0	+ +
Ductus arteriosus (44)	+ + +	0	0	0	−	−

Comment

The arbitrary division of atrial septal defect above and below a maximum diameter of 3 cm produced very few small defects, so these correlations are lacking in data. A glance at the figures actually suggests a reverse correlation of larger hearts with small defects, etc. The lack of correlation between defect size in ventricular septal defect is rather surprising: the figures show a trend in the expected direction which is not statistically significant. Possibly the division into large and small at 1·5 cm was unrealistic and contrasts with the critical size chosen for a ductus, which produced a very strong correlation. There is an obvious difference in plethora and, to a lesser extent, in pulmonary trunk size in small and large ventricular septal defects.

TABLE 21

Correlation of Systemic Oxygen Saturation with Radiological Signs in Fallot's Tetralogy (63 Cases)

Enlargement of ascending aorta	Enlargement of aortic arch	Oligaemia
0	+	+ +

Comment

The size of the ascending aorta is more difficult to assess than that of the aortic arch, and this no doubt accounts for the lack of correlation. The correlation with oligaemia is as expected.

TABLE 22

Correlation of Pulmonary Venous Pressure with Radiological Signs in Mitral Valve Disease

	Left atrial enlargement	Upper zone vessel dilatation	Pulmonary oedema
Mitral stenosis (50)	0	+ + +	+ +
Mitral regurgitation (50)	−	+	+ + +
Mitral stenosis with or without regurgitation (100)	0	+ + +	+ + +
Mitral regurgitation with or without stenosis (100)	0	+ +	+ + +
Combined mitral stenosis and regurgitation (50)	−	−	+ +
All mitral valve disease (150)	0	+ + +	+ + +

Comment

There were insufficient numbers of small left atria in pure mitral regurgitation and in the combined lesions. In other groups the correlations show no relation between left atrial size and pulmonary venous pressure. The lung signs correlate as expected, more closely with stenosis than with regurgitation.

APPENDIX C

TABLE 23

Correlation of Pulmonary Vascular Resistance with Radiological Signs in Mitral Valve Disease

	Cardiac enlargement	Left atrial enlargement	Upper zone vessel dilatation	Pulmonary oedema	Pulmonary trunk dilatation	Right lower lobe artery dilatation	Segmental artery narrowing
Mitral stenosis (50)	0	0	+ +	+ + +	+ + +	−	+ + +
Mitral regurgitation (50)	−	−	+ +	+	−	−	−
Mitral stenosis with or without regurgitation (100)	0	0	+ + +	+ + +	+ + +	+ + +	+ + +
Mitral regurgitation with or without stenosis (100)	0	0	+ + +	+ + +	+ + +	+ + +	+ + +
Combined mitral stenosis and regurgitation (50)	−	−	−	+ +	+	−	+ + +
All mitral valve disease (150)	+	0	+ + +	+ + +	+ + +	+ + +	+ + +

Comment

There appears to be no correlation between heart or left atrial size and the vascular resistance. The lung changes, including those in the pulmonary trunk, show close correlations where there were sufficient data.

TABLE 24

Correlation of Pulmonary Venous Pressure with Radiological Signs in Aortic Valve Disease

	Cardiac enlargement	Left atrial enlargement	Upper zone vessel dilatation	Pulmonary oedema
Aortic stenosis (50)	−	−	−	−
Aortic regurgitation (50)	0	−	+ + +	−
Aortic stenosis with or without regurgitation (100)	+ +	+ + +	+ + +	+ + +
Aortic regurgitation with or without stenosis (100)	0	+ +	+ + +	+ + +
Combined aortic stenosis and regurgitation (50)	+ +	−	+ + +	+ + +
All aortic valve disease (150)	+ +	−	+ + +	+ + +

Comment

There were insufficient numbers of patients with pure aortic stenosis and left ventricular failure to draw any conclusions, but in aortic stenosis with or without regurgitation the correlations were strong for all the parameters. There was no correlation between heart size and pulmonary venous pressure in both the aortic regurgitation groups, suggesting that the onset of failure may not result in much increase in heart size. The lung changes show strong correlations throughout where the numbers were sufficient.

TABLE 25

Correlations in Mixed Valve Disease

	Cardiac enlargement	Left atrial enlargement
Mitral disease:		
Degree of regurgitation with dominant stenosis (100)	+ + +	+ + +
Degree of stenosis with dominant regurgitation (100)	0	0
Aortic disease:		
Degree of regurgitation with dominant stenosis (100)	+ + +	0
Degree of stenosis with dominant regurgitation (100)	0	0

Comment

As would be expected, increasing regurgitation in the presence of stenosis produces a larger heart and, in the case of mitral disease, a larger left atrium. Conversely, varying degrees of stenosis with regurgitation have no effect on heart or left atrial size.

References

Achard, C. (1902). 'Arachnodactylie.' *Bull. Mém. Soc. med. Hôp. Paris* **19**, 834.

Albright, F., Smith, P. H. and Fraser, R. (1942). 'A syndrome characterised by primary ovarian insufficiency and decreased stature. Report of 11 cases with a digression on hormonal control of axillary and pubic hair.' *Am. J. med. Sci.* **204**, 625.

Amplatz, K. (1969). 'Endocardial fibroelastosis.' *Semin. Roentgenol.* **4**, 360.

Anderson, I. M., Newman, C. G. H. and Urquhart, W. (1965). 'Fallot's tetralogy—some radiological and other findings in the first few years after total correction.' *Br. J. Radiol.* **38**, 81.

Anderson, R. E., Grondin, C. and Amplatz, K. (1968). 'The mitral valve in Marfan's syndrome.' *Radiology* **91**, 910.

Andren, L. and Hall, P. (1961). 'Diminished segmentation or premature ossification of the sternum in congenital heart disease.' *Br. Heart J.* **23**, 140.

Anselmi, G., Munoz, S., Blanco, P., Machado, I. and de la Cruz, M. V. (1972). 'Systematisation and clinical study of dextroversion, mirror-image dextrocardia and laevoversion.' *Br. Heart J.* **34**, 1085.

Antia, A. U. (1971). 'Familial skeletal cardiovascular syndrome (Holt–Oram) in a polygamous African family.' *Br. Heart J.* **32**, 241.

— and Osunkoya, B. O. (1969). 'Congenital tricuspid incompetence.' *Br. Heart J.* **31**, 664.

Aroesty, J. M., DeWeese, J. A. and Hoffman, M. J. (1966). 'Carcinoid heart disease. Successful repair of the valvular lesions under cardiopulmonary bypass.' *Circulation* **34**, 105.

Ascenzi, A. and Marinozzi, V. (1958). 'Sur le "crane en brosse" au cours de polyglobulies secondaires à l'hypoxémie chronique.' *Acta haemat.* **19**, 253.

Ashworth, H. and Morgan-Jones, A. (1946). 'Aneurysmal dilatation of the left auricle with erosion of the spine.' *Br. Heart J.* **8**, 207.

Astley, R. (1963). 'Chromosomal abnormalities in childhood, with particular reference to Turner's syndrome and mongolism.' *Br. J. Radiol.* **36**, 421.

Baer, R. W., Taussig, H. B. and Oppenheimer, E. H. (1943). 'Congenital aneurysmal dilatation of the aorta associated with arachnodactyly.' *Bull. Johns Hopkins Hosp.* **72**, 309.

Barlow, J. B., Bosman, C. K. and Pocock, W. A. (1968). 'Late systolic murmurs and non-ejection ("mid-late") systolic clicks. An analysis of 90 patients.' *Br. Heart J.* **30**, 203.

Barnes, R. J., Kwong, K. H. and Cheung, A. C. S. (1971). 'Aberrant muscle bundle of the right ventricle.' *Br. Heart J.* **33**, 546.

Bartram, C. and Strickland, B. (1971). 'Pulmonary varices.' *Br. J. Radiol.* **44**, 927.

Batson, G. A., Urquhart, W. and Sideris, D. A. (1972). 'Radiological features of aortic stenosis.' *Clin. Radiol.* **23**, 140.

Beare, M. S. (1967). 'Mycotic aneurysm of the left ventricle.' *Thorax* **22**, 70.

Bennett, D. and Rees, S. (1973). 'Correlation of radiological changes and haemodynamics in acute myocardial infarction.' In the press.

Berge, R. and Sievers, J. (1968). 'Myocardial metastases: a pathological and electrocardiographic study.' *Br. Heart J.* **30**, 383.

Besterman, E. (1961). 'Atrial septal defect with pulmonary hypertension.' *Br. Heart J.* **23**, 587.

— (1972). Personal communication.

Beuren, A. J., Apitz, J. and Koncz, J. (1962). 'Die diagnose und Beurteilung der verschiedenen Formen der supravalvulären Aortenstenosen.' *Z. Kreislaufforsch.* **51**, 829.

Birch-Jensen, A. (1949). *Congenital Deformities of the Upper Extremities.* Odense, Denmark: Andelsbogtrykeriet.

Black, J. A. and Bonham Carter, R. E. (1963). 'Association between aortic stenosis and facies of severe infantile hypercalcaemia.' *Lancet* **2**, 745.

Blalock, A. and Taussig, H. B. (1945). 'The surgical treatment of malformations of the heart in which there is pulmonary stenosis or pulmonary atresia.' *J. Am. med. Ass.* **128**, 189.

Bland, J. W., Edwards, F. K. and Brinsfield, D. (1969). 'Pulmonary hypertension and congestive heart failure in children with chronic upper airways obstruction. New concepts of etiological factors.' *Am. J. Cardiol.* **23**, 830.

Boerger, F. (1914). 'Ueber zwei Fälle von Arachnodaktylie.' *Z. Kinderheilk.* **12**, 161.

Bonham Carter, R. E., Capriles, M. and Noe, Y. (1969). 'Total anomalous pulmonary venous drainage: a clinical and anatomical study of 75 children.' *Br. Heart J.* **31**, 45.

Bonnet, L. M. (1903). 'Sur la lesion dite stenose congenitale de l'aorte dans la region de l'isthme.' *Revue méd., Paris* **23**, 108, 255, 335, 419, 481.

Boone, M. L., Swenson, B. E. and Felson, B. (1964). 'Rib notching: its many causes.' *Am. J. Roentg.* **91**, 1075.

Borrie, J. (1969). 'Congenital complete absence of left pericardium.' *Thorax* **24**, 756.

Brigden, W. W. and Robinson, J. F. (1964). 'Alcoholic heart disease.' *Br. med. J.* **2**, 1283.

Brock, R. C. (1950). 'The nomenclature of bronchopulmonary anatomy.' *Thorax* **5**, 222.

Burrows, B., Fletcher, C. M., Heard, B. E., Jones, N. L. and Wootliff, J. S. (1966). 'The emphysematous and bronchial types of chronic airways obstruction. A clinico-pathological study of patients in London and Chicago.' *Lancet* **1**, 830.

REFERENCES

Bywaters, E. G. L. (1950). 'The relationship between heart and joint disease including "rheumatoid heart disease" and chronic post-rheumatic arthritis (type Jaccoud).' *Br. Heart J.* **12**, 101.

Cabot, R. C. (1926). *Facts on the Heart*. Philadelphia and London: W. B. Saunders.

Caffey, J. and Ross, S. (1956). 'Mongolism (mongoloid deficiency) during early infancy—some newly recognized diagnostic changes in the pelvic bones.' *Pediatrics* **17**, 642.

Caflisch, A. (1952). *Das Pterygium*. M.D. Thesis, University of Zürich.

Carey, L. S. and Edwards, J. E. (1965). 'Roentgenographic features in cases with origin of both great vessels from the right ventricle without pulmonary stenosis.' *Am. J. Roentg.* **93**, 269.

Carson, N. A. J. and Neill, D. W. (1962). 'Metabolic abnormalities detected in a survey of mentally backward individuals in Northern Ireland.' *Archs Dis. Childh.* **37**, 505.

Chang, C. H. (1962). 'The normal roentgenographic measurement of the right descending pulmonary artery in 1,085 cases.' *Am. J. Roentg.* **87**, 929.

— (1967a). 'Holt–Oram syndrome.' *Radiology* **88**, 479.

— (1967b). 'Radiological considerations in pulmonary embolism.' *Clin. Radiol.* **18**, 301.

Chesshyre, M. H. and Braimbridge, M. V. (1971). 'Dysphagia due to left atrial enlargement after mitral Starr valve replacement.' *Br. Heart J.* **33**, 799.

Chrispin, A. R., Goodwin, J. F. and Steiner, R. E. (1963). 'The radiology of obliterative pulmonary hypertension and thromboembolism.' *Br. J. Radiol.* **36**, 705.

Clarke, M. (1972). 'Calcific tricuspid incompetence in childhood.' *Br. Heart J.* **34**, 859.

Coates, J. R., McClenathan, J. E. and Scott, L. P. (1964). 'The double chambered right ventricle—a diagnostic and operative pitfall.' *Am. J. Cardiol.* **14**, 561.

Cockshott, W. P., Antia, A. and Ikeme, A. (1967). 'Annular subvalvar left ventricular aneurysms.' *Br. J. Radiol.* **40**, 424.

Cohen, S. L. (1953). 'The right pericardial fat pad.' *Radiology* **60**, 391.

Cole, R. B., Muster, A. J., Lev, M. and Paul, M. H. (1968). 'Pulmonary atresia with intact ventricular septum.' *Am. J. Cardiol.* **21**, 23.

Coleman, E. N., Barclay, R. S., Reid, J. M. and Stevenson, J. G. (1967). 'Congenital aorto-pulmonary fistula combined with persistent ductus arteriosus.' *Br. Heart J.* **29**, 571.

Collett, R. W. and Edwards, J. E. (1949). 'Persistent truncus arteriosus: a classification according to anatomic types.' *Surg. Clins N. Am.* **29**, 1245.

Cornell, S. H. and Rossi, N. P. (1968). 'Roentgenographic findings in constrictive pericarditis—analysis of 21 cases.' *Am. J. Roentg.* **102**, 301.

Cronk, E. S., Sinclair, J. G. and Rigdon, R. H. (1951). 'An anomalous coronary artery arising from the pulmonary trunk.' *Am. Heart J.* **42**, 906.

Criscitiello, M. G., Ronan, J. A. Jnr. and Besterman, E. M. (1965). 'Cardiovascular abnormalities in osteogenesis imperfecta.' *Circulation* **31**, 255.

Currarino, G. and Silverman, F. N. (1958). 'Premature obliteration of the sternal sutures and pigeon breast deformity.' *Radiology* **70**, 532.

Dalith, F. (1961). 'Calcification of the aortic knob; its relationship to the fifth and sixth aortic arches.' *Radiology* **76**, 213.

Datey, K. K., Deshmukh, M. M., Engineer, S. D. and Dalvi, C. P. (1964). 'Straight back syndrome.' *Br. Heart J.* **26**, 614.

Davies, H. (1959). 'Chest deformities in congenital heart disease.' *Brit. J. Dis. Chest* **53**, 151.

— and Dow, J. (1971). 'Differential pulmonary vascularity and the orientation of the right ventricular outflow tract with special reference to corrected transposition.' *Br. J. Radiol.* **44**, 258.

— Williams, J. and Wood, P. (1962). 'Lung stiffness in states of abnormal pulmonary blood flow and pressure.' *Br. Heart J.* **24**, 129.

Davis, G. D., Kincaid, O. W. and Hallermann, F. J. (1969). 'Roentgen aspects of cardiac tumors.' *Semin. Roentgenol.* **4**, 384.

Dayem, M. K. A., Preger, L., Goodwin, J. F. and Steiner, R. E. (1967). 'Double outlet right ventricle with pulmonary stenosis.' *Br. Heart J.* **29**, 64.

d'Cruz, I. A., Arcilla, R. A. and Agustsson, M. H. (1964a). 'Dilatation of the pulmonary trunk in stenosis of the pulmonary valve and of the pulmonary arteries in children.' *Am. Heart J.* **68**, 612.

— Agustsson, M. H., Biscoff, J. P., Weinberg, M. and Arcilla, R. A. (1964b). 'Stenotic lesions of the pulmonary arteries—clinical and haemodynamic findings in 84 cases.' *Am. J. Cardiol.* **13**, 441.

DeBakey, M. E., Henley, W. S., Cooley, D. A., Morris, G. C., Crawford, E. S. and Beall, A. C. (1965). 'Surgical management of dissecting aneurysms of the aorta.' *J. thorac. cardiovasc. Surg.* **49**, 130.

de Nef, J. J. E., Varghese, P. J. and Losekoot, G. (1971). 'Congenital coronary artery fistula—analysis of 17 cases.' *Br. Heart J.* **33**, 857.

Deutsch, V., Yahini, J. H., Shem-Tov, A. and Neufeld, H. N. (1970). 'Congenital pericardial defect.' *Br. J. Radiol.* **43**, 67.

Dollery, C. T., West, J. B., Hugh-Jones, P. and Wickens, D. E. L. (1961). *Ciba Foundation Study Group No. 8: Problems of Pulmonary Circulation*. Boston: Little, Brown.

Dow, Jean (1971). 'Homocystinuria.' Personal communication.

Ebstein, W. (1866). 'Über einen sehr seltenen Fall von Insufficienz der Valvula tricuspidalis, bedingt durch eine angeborene hochgradige Missbildung derselben.' *Arch. Anat. Physiol.* **33**, 238.

Edholm, O. G. and Howarth, S. (1953). 'Studies on the peripheral circulation in osteitis deformans.' *Clin. Sci.* **12**, 277.

— Howard, S. and McMichael, J. (1945). 'Heart failure and bone blood flow in osteitis deformans.' *Clin. Sci.* **5**, 249.

Edwards, J. E. (1961). *An Atlas of Acquired Diseases of the Heart and Great Vessels*. Philadelphia: Saunders.

— Carey, L. S., Neufeld, H. N. and Lester, R. G. (1965). *Congenital Heart Disease*. Philadelphia: Saunders.

Eisenmenger, V. (1897). 'Die angeborenen Defecte der Kammerscheidewand des Herzens.' *Z. klin. Med.* **32**, Suppl. p. 1.

Eldridge, R. (1964). 'The metacarpal index: a useful aid in the diagnosis of the Marfan syndrome.' *Archs intern. Med.* **113**, 248.

REFERENCES

Eliot, R. S. and Bratt, G. C. (1969). 'Paradox of myocardial ischemia and necrosis in young women with normal coronary arteriograms—relationship to abnormal hemoglobin–oxygen dissociation.' *Am. J. Cardiol.* **23**, 633.

Elliot, F. M. and Reid, L. (1965). 'Some new facts about the pulmonary artery and its branching pattern.' *Clin. Radiol.* **16**, 193.

Elliott, L. P. and Amplatz, K. (1966). 'Angiocardiographic observations in the post-rubella syndrome.' *Am. J. Roentg.* **97**, 164.

— Anderson, R. C. and Edwards, J. E. (1964). 'The common cardiac ventricle with transposition of the great vessels.' *Br. Heart J.* **26**, 289.

— Van Mierop, L. H. S., Gleason, D. C. and Schiebler, G. L. (1968). 'The roentgenology of tricuspid atresia.' *Semin. Roentgenol.* **3**, 399.

Ellis, R. W. B. and Van Creveld, S. (1940). 'A syndrome characterized by ectodermal dysplasia, polydactyly, chondrodystrophy and congenital morbus cordis: report of three cases.' *Archs Dis. Childh.* **15**, 65.

Emanuel, R. (1970). 'Genetics and congenital heart disease.' *Br. Heart J.* **32**, 281.

— (1971). 'The Holt–Oram syndrome.' Personal communication.

Emanuel, R. W. and Lloyd, W. E. (1964). 'Right atrial myxoma mistaken for constrictive pericarditis.' *Br. Heart J.* **24**, 796.

— and Pattinson, J. N. (1956). 'Absence of the left pulmonary artery in Fallot's tetralogy.' *Br. Heart J.* **18**, 289.

Evans, K. T., Cockshott, W. P. and Hendrickse, P. de V. (1965). 'Pulmonary changes in malignant trophoblastic disease.' *Br. J. Radiol.* **38**, 161.

Evans, W. (1946). 'The heart in sternal depression.' *Br. Heart J.* **8**, 162.

— (1949). 'The heart in endocrine disease.' *Proc. R. Soc. Med.* **42**, 331.

Fallot, A. (1888). 'Contribution a l'anatomie pathologique de la maladie bleue (cyanose cardiaque).' *Marseille méd.* **25**, 77.

Finby, N. and Archibald, R. M. (1963). 'Skeletal abnormalities associated with gonadal dysgenesis.' *Am. J. Roentg.* **89**, 1222.

Fishman, A. P. (1968). *Proceedings of a Symposium on Scoliosis. Action for the Crippled Child Monograph.* Ed. by P. A. Zorab. Edinburgh and London: Livingstone.

Flavell, G. (1943). 'Webbing of the neck with Turner's syndrome in the male.' *Br. J. Surg.* **31**, 150.

Fleischner, F. G. (1962). 'Pulmonary embolism.' *Clin. Radiol.* **13**, 169.

Foliath, F., Burkart, F. and Schweizer, W. (1971). 'Drug-induced pulmonary hypertension.' *Br. med. J.* **1**, 265.

Fontana, R. S. and Edwards, J. E. (1962). *Congenital Cardiac Disease.* Philadelphia: Saunders.

Forsberg, S. A. (1971). 'Relations between pressure in pulmonary artery, left atrium and left ventricle with special reference to events at end diastole.' *Br. Heart J.* **33**, 494.

Friedman, W. F. and Braunwald, E. (1966). 'Alterations in regional pulmonary blood flow in mitral valve disease studied by radioisotope scanning: a simple non-traumatic technique for estimation of left atrial pressure.' *Circulation* **34**, 363.

Fuenmayor, G. (1959). 'Las calcificaciones murales de auricula izquierda, presentacion de un nuevo caso.' *Revta Soc. venezolana Cardiol.* **1**, 247.

Gabriele, O. F., Scatliff, J. M. and Hill, C. (1970). 'Pulmonary valve calcification.' *Am. Heart J.* **80**, 299.

Gabrielson, T. O. and Ladyman, G. H. (1963). 'Early closure of the sternal sutures and congenital heart disease.' *Am. J. Roentg.* **89**, 975.

Gahagan, T. and Green, E. W. (1965). 'Repair of complicated defect in cardiac septum after non-penetrating trauma.' *J. Am. med. Ass.* **194**, 301.

Gahl, K., Sutton, R., Rees, S. and McDonald, L. (1973). 'Correlations of left ventricular cineangiography in coronary heart disease.' In the press.

Gale, G. E., Heimann, K. W. and Barlow, J. B. (1969). 'Double chambered right ventricle—a report of five cases.' *Br. Heart J.* **31**, 291.

Gall, J. C., Stern, A. M., Cohen, M. M., Adams, M. S. and Davidson, R. T. (1966). 'Holt–Oram syndrome: clinical and genetic study of a large family.' *Am. J. hum. Genet.* **18**, 187.

Garcia, R. E., Friedman, W. F. and Kaback, M. M. (1964). 'Idiopathic hypercalcaemia and supravalvular aortic stenosis. Documentation of a new syndrome.' *New Engl. J. Med.* **271**, 117.

Garcia-Palmieri, M. R. (1964). 'Cor pulmonale due to schistosomiasis mansoni.' *Am. Heart J.* **68**, 714.

Gasul, B. M., Arcilla, R. A., Fell, E. H., Lynfield, J., Bicoff, J. P. and Luan, L. L. (1960). 'Congenital coronary arteriovenous fistula.' *Pediatrics* **25**, 531.

Gerbode, F., Hultgren, H., Melrose, D. and Osborn, J. (1958). 'Syndrome of left ventricular–right atrial shunt: successful repair of defect in five cases, with observation of bradycardia on closure.' *Ann. Surg.* **148**, 433.

Gerritsen, T., Vaughan, J. G. and Warsman, H. A. (1962). 'The identification of homocystine in the urine.' *Biochem. biophys. Res. Commun.* **9**, 493.

Giknis, F. L. (1963). 'Single atrium and the Ellis–Van Creveld syndrome.' *J. Pediat.* **62**, 558.

Gleason, D. C. and Steiner, R. E. (1966). 'The lateral roentgenogram in pulmonary edema.' *Am. J. Roentg.* **98**, 279.

Glenn, W. W. L. and Patino, J. F. (1954). 'Circulatory by-pass of the right heart. 1. Preliminary observations on direct delivery of vena caval blood into the pulmonary arterial circulation: azygos vein–pulmonary artery shunt.' *Yale J. biol. Med.* **27**, 147.

Gomes, M. M. and Bernatz, P. E. (1970). 'Arteriovenous fistulas: a review and ten year experience at the Mayo Clinic.' *Proc. Staff Meet. Mayo Clin.* **45**, 81.

Goodwin, J. F. (1967). 'Disorders of the outflow tract of the left ventricle.' *Br. med. J.* **2**, 461.

— (1970). 'Congestive and hypertrophic cardiomyopathies: a decade of study.' *Lancet* **1**, 731.

— and Oakley, C. M. (1972). 'The cardiomyopathies.' *Br. Heart J.* **34**, 545.

Gorlin, R., Klein, M. D. and Sullivan, J. M. (1967). 'Prospective correlative study of ventricular aneurysm. Mechanistic concept and clinical recognition.' *Am. J. Med.* **42**, 512.

Gould, S. E. (1968). *Pathology of the Heart and Blood Vessels,* 3rd edn. Springfield, Ill.: Thomas.

REFERENCES

Grainger, R. G. (1970). 'Transposition of the great arteries and of the pulmonary veins, including an account of cardiac embryology and chamber identification.' *Clin. Radiol.* **21**, 335.

Greenwold, W. E., Dushane, J. W., Burchell, H. B., Bruwer, A. and Edwards, J. E. (1956). 'Congenital pulmonary atresia with intact ventricular septum: two anatomic types.' *Circulation* **14**, 945.

Hallermann, F. J., Davis, G. D., Ritter, D. G. and Kincaid, O. W. (1966). 'Roentogenographic features of common ventricle.' *Radiology* **87**, 409.

Hamby, R. I. and Gulotta, S. J. (1967). 'Pulmonary valvular insufficiency: etiology, recognition and management.' *Am. Heart J.* **74**, 110.

Hampton, A. O. and Castleman, B. (1940). 'Correlation of postmortem chest teleroentgenograms with autopsy findings, with special reference to pulmonary embolism and infarction.' *Am. J. Roentg.* **43**, 305.

Harley, H. R. S. (1961). 'The radiological changes in pulmonary venous hypertension, with special reference to the root shadows and lobular pattern.' *Br. Heart J.* **23**, 75.

Harris, A., Davies, M., Redwood, D., Leatham, A. and Siddons, A. H. M. (1969). 'Aetiology of chronic heart block: a clinico-pathological correlation in 65 cases.' *Br. Heart J.* **31**, 206.

— Gialafos, J. and Jefferson, K. (1972). 'Transvenous pacing in presence of anomalous venous return to the heart.' *Br. Heart J.* **34**, 1189.

— Jefferson, K. and Chatterjee, K. (1969). 'Coronary arteriovenous fistula with aneurysm of coronary sinus: case report.' *Br. Heart J.* **31**, 400.

Harris, L. C. and Osborne, W. P. (1966). 'Congenital absence or hypoplasia of the radius with ventricular septal defect: ventriculo-radial dysplasia.' *J. Paediat.* **68**, 265.

Harris, P., Heath, D. and Apostopoulos, A. (1965). 'Extensibility of the pulmonary trunk in heart disease.' *Br. Heart J.* **27**, 660.

Harrison, C. V. and Lennox, B. (1948). 'Heart block in osteitis deformans.' *Br. Heart J.* **10**, 167.

Hart, F. D. (1969). 'Rheumatoid arthritis: extra-articular manifestations.' *Br. med. J.* **3**, 131.

Hastreiter, A. R., d'Cruz, I. A. and Cantez, T. (1966). 'Right sided aorta. Part I: Occurrence of right aortic arch in various types of congenital heart disease.' *Br. Heart J.* **28**, 722.

Heath, D. and Mackinnon, J. (1964). 'Pulmonary hypertension due to myxoma of the right atrium, with special reference to the behavior of emboli of myxoma in the lung.' *Am. Heart J.* **68**, 227.

Heitzman, E. R., Ziter, F. M., Markarian, B., McClennan, B. L. and Sherry, H. S. (1967). 'Kerley's interlobular septal lines: roentgen pathologic correlation.' *Am. J. Roentg.* **100**, 578.

Hipona, F. A. (1965). 'Pulmonary valvular stenosis with a right-sided aorta and an intact ventricular septum.' *Br. J. Radiol.* **38**, 958.

Holmes, L. B. (1965). 'Congenital heart disease and upper limb deformities.' *New Engl. J. Med.* **272**, 236.

Holt, M. and Oram, S. (1960). 'Familial heart disease with skeletal malformations.' *Br. Heart J.* **22**, 236.

Howarth, S. (1953). 'Cardiac output in osteitis deformans.' *Clin. Sci.* **12**, 271.

Hudson, R. E. B. (1965). In *Cardiovascular Pathology*, p. 1968. London: Edward Arnold.

— (1970). In *Cardiovascular Pathology*, Vol. 3. London: Edward Arnold.

Hughes, R. A. C., Karpur, P., Sutton, G. C. and Honey, M. (1970). 'A case of fatal peri-partum cardiomyopathy.' *Br. Heart J.* **32**, 372.

Hunter, C. (1917). 'A rare disease in two brothers.' *Proc. R. Soc. Med.* **10**, 104.

Hurler, G. (1919). 'Ueber einen Typ multiplar abartungen, vorwiegend am Skelettsystem.' *Z. Kinderheilk.* **24**, 220.

James, J. I. P., Lloyd-Roberts, G. C. and Pilcher, M. F. (1959). 'Infantile structural scoliosis.' *J. Bone Jt Surg.* **41(B)**, 719.

Jefferson, K. E. (1965). 'The pulmonary vessels in the normal pulmonary angiogram.' *Proc. R. Soc. Med.* **58**, 677.

— Rees, S. and Somerville, J. (1972). 'Systemic arterial supply to the lungs in pulmonary atresia and its relation to pulmonary artery development.' *Br. Heart J.* **34**, 418.

Kafkas, P. and Miller, G. A. H. (1971). 'Unusual left ventricular aneurysm in a patient with anomalous origin of left coronary artery from pulmonary artery.' *Br. Heart J.* **33**, 409.

Karlish, A. J., Marshall, R., Reid, L. and Sherlock S. (1967). 'Cyanosis with hepatic cirrhosis—a case with arteriovenous shunting.' *Thorax* **22**, 555.

Keats, T. E. and Enge, I. P. (1965). 'Cardiac mensuration by the cardiac volume method.' *Radiology* **85**, 850.

Keene, R. J., Steiner, R. E., Olsen, E. J. G. and Oakley, C. (1971). 'Aortic root aneurysm—radiographic and pathologic features.' *Clin. Radiol.* **22**, 330.

Keith, J. D., Rowe, R. D. and Vlad, P. (1967). *Heart Disease in Infancy and Childhood*, 2nd edn. New York: Macmillan. London: Collier–Macmillan.

Kelly, D. T. (1965). 'Isolated congenital pulmonary incompetence.' *Br. Heart J.* **27**, 777.

Kent, J. V. (1953). 'The development of rib notching after surgical intervention in congenital heart disease.' *Br. J. Radiol.* **26**, 346.

Kerley, P. (1933). 'Radiology in heart disease.' *Br. med. J.* **2**, 594.

— (1972). In *A Textbook of X-ray Diagnosis*, Vol. 2, 4th edn. Ed. by S. C. Shanks and P. Kerley. London: H. K. Lewis.

Kerr, I. H., Simon, G. and Sutton, G. C. (1971). 'The value of the plain radiograph in acute massive pulmonary embolism.' *Br. J. Radiol.* **44**, 751.

Kirk, R. S. and Russell, J. G. B. (1966). 'Spiral calcification in the ventricular myocardium.' *Br. Heart J.* **28**, 342.

— — (1969). 'Subvalvular calcification of mitral valve.' *Br. Heart J.* **31**, 684.

Kitchen, A. and Turner, R. (1964). 'Diagnosis and treatment of tricuspid stenosis.' *Br. Heart J.* **26**, 354.

— — (1967). 'Calcification of the mitral valve.' *Br. Heart J.* **29**, 137.

Kjellberg, S. R., Mannheimer, E., Rudhe, U. and Jonsson, B. (1958). *Diagnosis of Congenital Heart Disease*, 2nd edn. New York: Year Book Publishers.

Langer, L. O. and Carey, L. S. (1966). 'The roentgenographic features of the KS mucopolysaccharidosis of Morquio (Morquio–Brailsford disease).' *Am. J. Roentg.* **97**, 1.

Leaver, D. G., Sharma, R. N. and Glennie, J. S. (1970). 'Self inflicted ventricular septal defect.' *Br. Heart J.* **32**, 561.

REFERENCES

Levy, M. J., Lillehei, C. W., Elliott, L. P., Carey, L. S., Adams, P. and Edwards, J. E. (1963). 'Accessory valvular tissue causing subpulmonary stenosis in corrected transposition of great vessels.' *Circulation* **27**, 494.

Lewis, K. B., Baum, D. and Motulsky, A. G. (1965). 'The upper limb cardiovascular syndrome. An autosomal dominant genetic effect on embryogenesis.' *J. Am. med. Ass.* **193**, 1080.

Logan, W. F., Jones, E. W. and Walker, E. (1965). 'Familial supravalvar aortic stenosis.' *Br. Heart J.* **27**, 547.

Lyons, H. A., Zuhdi, M. N. and Kelly, J. J. (1955). 'Pectus excavatum (funnel chest), a cause of impaired distensibility as exhibited by right ventricular pressure pattern.' *Am. Heart J.* **50**, 921.

Macartney, F. J. and Miller, G. A. H. (1970). 'Congenital absence of the pulmonary valve.' *Br. Heart J.* **32**, 483.

McCredie, R. M. and Richards, J. G. (1966). 'Combined mitral and pulmonary valve stenosis.' *Br. Heart J.* **28**, 139.

McDonald, A., Harris, A., Jefferson, K., Marshall, J. and McDonald, L. (1971). 'Association of prolapse of posterior cusp of mitral valve and atrial septal defect.' *Br. Heart J.* **33**, 383.

McDonald, A. H., Gerlis, L. M. and Somerville, J. (1969). 'Familial arteriopathy with associated pulmonary and systemic arterial stenoses.' *Br. Heart J.* **31**, 375.

McKusick, V. A. (1966). *Heritable Disorders of Connective Tissue*, 3rd edn. St. Louis: Mosby.

McLoughlin, T. G., Krovet, Z. and Schiebler, G. L. (1964). 'Heart disease in the Lawrence–Moon–Biedl–Bardet syndrome.' *J. Pediat.* **65**, 388.

Magidson, O. and Kay, J. H. (1963). 'Ruptured aortic sinus aneurysms.' *Am. Heart J.* **65**, 597.

Mannheimer, E. (Ed.) (1949). *Morbus Caeruleus: An Analysis of 114 Cases of Congenital Heart Disease with Cyanosis.* Bibliotheca Cardiologica, Fasc. 4. Basel: Karger.

Marfan, A. B. (1896). 'Un cas de deformation congenitale des quatres membres plus prononcée aux extrémités charactérisée par l'allongement des os avec un certain degré d'amincessement.' *Bull. Mém. Soc. med. Hôp. Paris* **13**, 220.

Martelle, R. R. and Moss, A. J. (1962). 'Fifty-three cases of coarctation of the aorta.' *Am. J. Dis. Child.* **103**, 556.

Meadows, W. R. and Sharp, J. T. (1965). 'Persistent left superior vena cava draining into the left atrium without arterial oxygen unsaturation.' *Am. J. Cardiol.* **16**, 273.

Mercer, J. L. (1969). 'Movement of the aortic annulus.' *Br. J. Radiol.* **42**, 623.

Meyer, M. H., Stephenson, H. E. Jnr. and Keats, T. E. (1967). 'Coronary artery resection for giant aneurysmal enlargement and arteriovenous fistula. A five-year follow up.' *Am. Heart J.* **74**, 603.

Miller, G. A. H., Paneth, M. and Gibson, R. V. (1968). 'Right atrial myxoma with right-to-left interatrial shunt and polycythaemia.' *Br. med. J.* **3**, 537.

Moller, J. H., Nakib, A., Anderson, R. C. and Edwards, J. E. (1967). 'Congenital cardiac disease associated with polysplenia. A developmental complex of bilateral left-sidedness.' *Circulation* **36**, 789.

Monge, C. (1948). *Acclimatization in the Andes: Historical Confirmations of 'Climatic Aggression' in the Development of Andean Man.* Translated by Donald F. Brown. Baltimore: Johns Hopkins Press.

Morales, G., Hernandes, O., Fuenmayor, R., Capriles, M. A., Flores, G., Collet, H. and Gonzalez, R. (1962). 'Enfermedad de Chagas: cardiopatia chagasica.' *Archos Hosp. Vargas* **4**, 137.

Morin, Y. L., Foley, A. R., Martineau, G. and Roussel, J. (1967). 'Quebec beer drinker's cardiomyopathy: forty-eight cases.' *Can. med. Ass. J.* **97**, 881.

Morquio, L. (1929). 'Sur une forme de dystrophie osseuse familiale.' *Bull. Soc. Pédiat. Paris* **27**, 145.

Morrels, C. L., Fletcher, B. D., Weilbaecher, R. G. and Dorst, J. P. (1968). 'The roentgenographic features of homocystinuria.' *Radiology* **90**, 1150.

Morrow, A. G. and Behrendt, D. M. (1968). 'Congenital aneurysm (diverticulum) of the right atrium.' *Circulation* **38**, 124.

Mounsey, P. (1959). 'Annular constrictive pericarditis—with an account of a patient with functional pulmonary, mitral and aortic stenosis.' *Br. Heart J.* **21**, 325.

Muller, W. H. Jnr. (1962). In *Gibbon's Surgery of the Chest*. Philadelphia: Saunders.

Munoz-Armas, S., Gorrin, J. R. D., Anselmi, G., Hernandez, P. B. and Anselmi, A. (1968). 'Single atrium.' *Am. J. Cardiol.* **21**, 639.

Murphy, K. J. (1965). 'Pulmonary haemosiderosis (apparently idiopathic) associated with myocarditis, with bilateral penetrating corneal ulceration, and with diabetes mellitus.' *Thorax* **20**, 341.

Murray, R. O. M. and Jacobson, H. G. (1971). *The Radiology of Skeletal Disorders*. Edinburgh and London: Churchill Livingstone.

Nadas, A. S. (1963). *Paediatric Cardiology*, 2nd edn. Philadelphia: Saunders.

Nelson, J. D. (1958). 'The Marfan syndrome with special reference to congenital enlargement of the spinal canal.' *Br. J. Radiol.* **31**, 561.

Neu, L. T., Reider, R. D. and Mack, R. E. (1960). 'Cardiac involvement in Reiter's disease: report of a case with review of the literature.' *Ann. intern. Med.* **53**, 215.

Neufeld, H. N., Lester, R. G., Adams, P., Anderson, R. C., Lillehei, C. W. and Edwards, J. E. (1961). 'Congenital communication of a coronary artery with a cardiac chamber or the pulmonary trunk ("coronary artery fistula").' *Circulation* **24**, 171.

— — — — — — (1962a). 'Aorticopulmonary septal defect.' *Am. J. Cardiol.* **9**, 12.

— Lucas, R. V., Lester, R. G., Adams, P., Anderson, R. C. and Edwards, J. E. (1962b). 'Origin of both great vessels from the right ventricle without pulmonary stenosis.' *Br. Heart J.* **24**, 393.

Nice, C. M., Daves, M. L. and Wood, G. H. (1964). 'Changes in bone associated with cyanotic congenital heart disease.' *Am. Heart J.* **68**, 25.

Noonan, J. A. and Ehmke, D. A. (1963). 'Associated noncardiac malformations in children with congenital heart disease.' *J. Pediat.* **63**, 468.

Obeyesekeve, I. and de Soysa, N. (1970). 'Primary pulmonary hypertension, eosinophilia, and filariasis in Ceylon.' *Br. Heart J.* **32**, 524.

Okin, J. J., Vogel, J. H. K., Pryor, R. and Blount, S. G. (1969). 'Isolated right ventricular hypoplasia.' *Am. J. Cardiol.* **24**, 135.

Oliver, G. C. Jnr. and Missen, G. A. (1966). 'A heavily calcified right atrial myxoma.' *Guy's Hosp. Rep.* **115**, 37.

Ottesen, O. E., Asuquo, U. A. and Rowe, R. D. (1966). 'Peripheral vascular anomalies associated with the supravalvular aortic stenosis syndrome.' *Radiology* **86**, 430.

REFERENCES

Owen, R. A. (1962). 'Total anomalous pulmonary venous drainage with persistent left superior vena cava.' *Clin. Radiol.* **13**, 257.

Paget, J. (1877). 'On a form of chronic inflammation of bones (osteitis deformans).' *Trans. med. surg. Soc. Lond.* **60**, 37.

Parish, J. G. (1960). 'Hereditable disorders of connective tissue.' *Proc. R. Soc. Med.* **53**, 515.

Pearson, K. and Lee, A. (1902). 'On the laws of inheritance in man. Part 1: The inheritance of physical characters.' *Biometrika* **2**, 357.

Perloff, J. K., Ronan, J. A. and de Leon, A. C. (1965). 'Ventricular septal defect with two chambered right ventricle.' *Am. J. Cardiol.* **16**, 894.

Philip, T., Summerling, M. D., Fleming, J. and Grainger, R. G. (1972). 'Aberrant left pulmonary artery.' *Clin. Radiol.* **23**, 153.

Polani, P. E. (1968). 'Chromosome abnormalities and congenital heart disease.' *Guy's Hosp. Rep.* **117**, 323.

Porstmann, R. A., El-Sallab, R. A. and David, H. (1967). 'Pseudo-aplasia of the right pulmonary artery associated with right-sided aortic arch.' *Br. Heart J.* **29**, 527.

Potts, W. J., Smith, S. and Gibson, S. (1946). 'Anastomosis of the aorta to a pulmonary artery in certain types of congenital heart disease.' *J. Am. med. Ass.* **132**, 627.

Poznanski, A. K., Gall, G. C. and Stern, A. M. (1970). 'Skeletal manifestations of the Holt–Oram syndrome.' *Radiology* **94**, 45.

Pridie, R. V., Behnam, R. and Wild, J. (1972). 'Ultrasound in cardiac diagnosis.' *Clin. Radiol.* **23**, 160.

Puigbo, J. J. (1968). 'Chagas heart disease.' *Cardiologia* **52**, 91.

Raftery, E. B., Ahmed, S. and Braimbridge, M. V. (1966). 'Primary sarcoma of the left atrium.' *Br. Heart J.* **28**, 287.

Raghib, G., Ruttenberg, H. D. and Anderson, R. C. (1965). 'Termination of left superior vena cava in left atrium, atrial septal defect, and absence of coronary sinus; a developmental complex.' *Circulation* **31**, 906.

Raphael, M. J., Steiner, R. E., Goodwin, J. F. and Oakley, C. M. (1972). 'Cineangiography of left ventricular aneurysms.' *Clin. Radiol.* **23**, 129.

Reeder, M. M. and Simão, C. (1969). 'Chagas' myocardiopathy.' *Semin. Roentgenol.* **4**, 374.

Rees, R. S. O. and Jefferson, K. E. (1967). 'The Eisenmenger syndrome.' *Clin. Radiol.* **18**, 366.

— (1968). 'The chest radiograph in pulmonary hypertension with central shunt.' *Br. J. Radiol.* **41**, 172.

— and Somerville, J. (1969). 'Aortography in Fallot's tetralogy and variants.' *Br. Heart J.* **31**, 146.

Rodnan, G. P., Benedek, T. G., Shaver, J. A. and Fennell, R. H. (1964). 'Reiter's syndrome and aortic insufficiency.' *J. Am. med. Ass.* **189**, 889.

Rosenbaum, H. D., Lieber, A., Hansen, D. J. and Bernard, J. D. (1966). 'Roentgen findings in ventricular septal defect.' *Semin. Roentgenol.* **1**, 47.

Ross, J. K. and Gerbode, F. (1960). 'The Marfan syndrome associated with an unusual interventricular septal defect.' *J. thorac. Surg.* **39**, 746.

Roy, S. B., Gileria, J. S., Khanna, P. K., Manchanda, S. C., Pande, J. N. and Subba, P. S. (1969). 'Haemodynamic studies in high altitude pulmonary oedema.' *Br. Heart J.* **31**, 52.

Rudolf, A. J., Yow, M. D., Phillips, C. A., Desmond, M. M., Blattner, R. J. and Melnick, J. L. (1965). 'Transplacental rubella infection in newly born infants.' *J. Am. med. Ass.* **191**, 843.

Runco, V., Nevin, H. S., Vahabzadek, H. and Booth, R. W. (1968). 'Basal diastolic murmurs in rheumatic heart disease: intracardiac phonocardiography and cineangiography.' *Am. Heart J.* **75**, 153.

Salle, V. (1912). 'Über einen Fall von angeborener abnormer Grösse der Extremitäten mit einem an Akromegalie erinnernden Symptomenkomplex.' *Jb. Kinderheilk. phys. Erzieh.* **75**, 540.

Salzmann, C., Sutton, G. C., Chatterjee, K., Kerr, I. H. and Miller, G. A. H. (1972). 'Assessment of homograft replacement of mitral valve by chest radiographs.' *Br. Heart J.* **34**, 121.

Schimke, R. N., McKusick, V. A. and Huang, T. (1965). 'Homocystinuria. Studies of 20 families with 38 affected members.' *J. Am. med. Ass.*, **193**, 711.

Schlesinger, F. G. and Meester, G. T. (1967). 'Supravalvar stenosis of the pulmonary artery.' *Br. Heart J.* **29**, 829.

Seymour, J., Emanuel, R. and Pattinson, N. (1968). 'Acquired pulmonary stenosis.' *Br. Heart J.* **30**, 776.

Shaher, R. M., Moes, C. A. F. and Khonry, G. (1967). 'Radiologic and angiocardiographic findings in complete transposition of the great vessels with left ventricular outflow obstruction.' *Radiology* **88**, 1092.

Shawdon, H. H. and Dinsmore, R. E. (1967). 'Pericardial calcification: radiological features and clinical significance in twenty-six patients.' *Clin. Radiol.* **18**, 205.

Shell, W. E., Walton, J. A. and Clifford, M. E. (1969). 'The familial occurrence of the syndrome of mid-late systolic click and late systolic murmur.' *Circulation* **39**, 327.

Shone, J. D., Sellers, R. D., Anderson, R. C., Adams, P. Jnr., Lillehei, C. W. and Edwards, J. E. (1963). 'Developmental complex of "parachute mitral valve", supravalvular ring of left atrium, subaortic stenosis and coarctation of aorta.' *Am. J. Cardiol.* **11**, 714.

Siggers, D. C. and Polani, P. E. (1972). 'Congenital heart disease in male and female subjects with somatic features of Turner's syndrome and normal sex chromosomes (Ullrich's and related syndromes).' *Br. Heart J.* **34**, 41.

Simon, G. (1969). In *Scoliosis*, p. 39. Ed. by P. A. Zorab. London: William Heinemann Medical Books.

— (1972). 'The value of radiology in critical mitral stenosis.' *Clin. Radiol.* **23**, 145.

Sinclair, R. J. G. (1958). 'The Marfan syndrome.' *Bull. rheum. Dis.* **8**, 158.

— Kitchen, A. H. and Turner, R. W. D. (1960). 'The Marfan syndrome.' *Q. Jl Med.* **29**, 19.

Singh, H., Parkash, A., Saini, M. and Wahi, P. L. (1972). 'Bone changes in cyanotic congenital heart disease.' *Br. Heart J.* **34**, 412.

Sokoloff, L. (1964). 'Cardiac involvement in rheumatoid arthritis and allied disorders: current concepts.' *Mod. Concepts cardiovasc. Dis.* **33**, 847.

Somerville, J. (1959). 'Aortopulmonary septal defect.' *Guy's Hosp. Rep.* **108**, 177.

— (1961). 'Gout in cyanotic congenital heart disease.' *Br. Heart J.* **23**, 31.

— (1966). 'Masked cor triatriatum.' *Br. Heart J.* **28**, 55.

— (1971). 'Atrioventricular defects.' *Mod. Concepts cardiovasc. Dis.* **40**, 33.

— (1972). 'Incidence of left superior vena cava.' Personal communication.

REFERENCES

Somerville, J. and Bonham-Carter, R. E. (1972). 'The heart in lentiginosis.' *Br. Heart J.* **34**, 58.

— and Ross, D. (1971). 'Congenital aortic stenosis—an unusual form. Consideration of surgical management.' *Br. Heart J.* **33**, 552.

Sornberger, C. F. and Smedel, M. I. (1952). 'Mechanism and incidence of cardiovascular changes in Paget's disease: critical review of literature with case studies.' *Circulation* **6**, 711.

Stewart, J. R., Kincaid, O. W. and Titus, J. L. (1966). 'Right aortic arch: plain film diagnosis and significance.' *Am. J. Roentg.* **97**, 377.

Sullivan, J. F., George, R., Bluvas, R. and Egan, J. D. (1969). 'Myocardiopathy of beer drinkers: subsequent course.' *Ann. intern. Med.* **70**, 277.

Sutton, G., Harris, A. and Leatham, A. (1968). 'Second heart sound in pulmonary hypertension.' *Br. Heart J.* **30**, 743.

Taussig, H. B. (1962). 'A study of the German outbreak of phocomelia.' *J. Am. med. Ass.* **180**, 80.

— and Bing, R. J. (1949). 'Complete transposition of the aorta and a levoposition of the pulmonary artery.' *Am. Heart J.* **37**, 551.

Teichmann, V., Jesek, V. and Hurles, F. (1970). 'Relevance of width of right descending branch of pulmonary artery as a radiological sign of pulmonary hypertension.' *Thorax* **25**, 91.

Testelli, M. R. and Pilz, C. G. (1964). 'Massive calcification of the myocardium. A report of two cases, one associated with nephrocalcinosis.' *Am. J. Cardiol.* **14**, 407.

Towers, M. K. and Zorab, P. A. (1969). In *Scoliosis*, p. 54. Ed. by P. A. Zorab. London: William Heinemann Medical Books.

Tubbs, O. S. and Yacoub, M. H. (1968). 'Congenital pericardial defects.' *Thorax* **23**, 598.

Turner, H. M. (1938). 'A syndrome of infantilism, congenital webbed neck and cubitus valgus.' *Endocrinology* **23**, 566.

Uhl, H. S. (1952). 'Previously undescribed congenital malformation of heart: almost total absence of myocardium of right ventricle.' *Bull. Johns Hopkins Hosp.* **91**, 197.

Ullrich, O. (1930). 'Über typische Kombinationsbelder multipler Abertungen.' *Z. Kinderheilk.* **49**, 271.

Van Noorden, S., Olsen, E. G. J. and Pearse, A. G. E. (1971). 'Hypertrophic obstructive cardiomyopathy: a histological, histochemical and ultrastructural study of biopsy material.' *Cardiovasc. Res.* **5**, 118.

Van Praagh, R. (1967). In *Heart Disease in Infancy and Childhood*, Chapter 28. Ed. by J. D. Keith, R. D. Rowe and P. Vlad. New York: Macmillan. London: Collier–Macmillan.

— (1968). 'What is the Taussig–Bing malformation?' *Circulation* **38**, 445.

— Ongley, P. A. and Swan, H. J. C. (1964). 'Anatomic types of single or common ventricle in man. Morphologic and geometric aspects in 60 necropsied cases.' *Am. J. Cardiol.* **13**, 367.

— and Van Praagh, S. (1965). 'The anatomy of common aorticopulmonary trunk (truncus arteriosus communis) and its embryological implications: a study of 57 cases.' *Am. J. Cardiol.* **16**, 406.

— Vlad, P. and Keith, J. D. (1967). In *Heart Disease in Infancy and Childhood*, Chapter 25. Ed. by J. D. Keith, R. D. Rowe and P. Vlad. New York: Macmillan. London: Collier–Macmillan.

Varghese, P. J., Allen, J. R., Rosenquist, G. C. and Rowe, R. D. (1970). 'Natural history of ventricular septal defect with right-sided aortic arch.' *Br. Heart J.* **32**, 537.

Varney, R. F., Kenyon, A. T. and Koch, F. C. (1942). 'An association of short stature, retarded sexual development and high urinary gonadotrophic titers in women.' *J. clin. Endocr. Metab.* **2**, 137.

Venables, A. W. (1965). 'The syndrome of pulmonary stenosis complicating maternal rubella.' *Br. Heart J.* **27**, 49.

Waterston, D. J. (1962). 'Treatment of Fallot's tetralogy in children under 1 year of age.' *Rozhl. Chir.* **41**, 181.

Weldon, W. V. and Scalettar, R. (1961). 'Roentgen changes in Reiter's syndrome.' *Am. J. Roentg.* **86**, 344.

West, J. B. (1968). *Frontiers of Pulmonary Radiology*. New York: Grune & Stratton.

Westermark, N. (1938). 'On the roentgen diagnosis of lung embolism.' *Acta radiol.* **19**, 357.

Whitney, B. and Croxon, R. (1972). 'Dysphagia caused by cardiac enlargement.' *Clin. Radiol.* **23**, 147.

Wilkins, L. and Fleischmann, W. (1944). 'Ovarian agenesis: pathology, associated clinical symptoms and the bearing on the theories of sex differentiation.' *J. clin. Endocr. Metab.* **4**, 357.

Williams, B., Ling, J. T., Leight, L. and McGaff, C. J. (1963). 'Patent ductus arteriosus and osteoarthropathy.' *Archs intern. Med.* **111**, 346.

Williams, J. C. P., Barratt-Boyes, B. G. and Lowe, J. B. (1961). 'Supravalvular aortic stenosis.' *Circulation* **24**, 1311.

Wilson, W. J. and Amplatz, K. (1967). 'Unequal vascularity in tetralogy of Fallot.' *Am. J. Roentg.* **100**, 318.

Wood, P. (1958). 'The Eisenmenger syndrome.' *Br. med. J.* **2**, 701 and 755.

— (1968). *Diseases of the Heart and Circulation*. London: Eyre & Spottiswoode.

— McDonald, L. and Emanuel, R. (1958). 'The clinical picture correlated with physiological observations in the diagnosis of congenital heart disease.' *Paediat. Clins N. Am.* **5**, 981.

World Health Organisation (1961). Report of Expert Committee on Chronic Cor Pulmonale. *Tech. Rep. Ser. Wld Hlth Org.* No. 213.

Zutter, W. and Somerville, J. (1971). 'Continuous murmur in pulmonary atresia with reference to aortography.' *Br. Heart J.* **33**, 905.

Index